SuperFoods
HealthStyle

www.booksattransworld.co.uk

SuperFoods
HealthStyle

Proven Strategies for Lifelong Health

Steven G. Pratt M.D. and Kathy Matthews

BANTAM BOOKS

LONDON • TORONTO • SYDNEY • AUCKLAND • JOHANNESBURG

SUPERFOODS HEALTHSTYLE
A BANTAM BOOK: 0553817159
9780553817157

First publication in Great Britain
Originally published in the United States by HarperCollins Publishers Inc.
Published by arrangement with William Morris, an imprint of
HarperCollins Publishers Inc. New York. All rights reserved.

PRINTING HISTORY
Bantam edition published 2006

1 3 5 7 9 10 8 6 4 2

This book is written as a source of information about the effect of foods, vitamins and
lifestyle choices on the body. It is based on the research and observations of the authors.
The information contained in this book should by no means be considered a substitute
for the advice of the reader's personal physician or other medical professional, who
should always be consulted before beginning any diet or other health programme.
The information in this book has been carefully researched, and all efforts have
been made to ensure accuracy as of the date published. Readers, particularly those
with existing health problems and those who take prescription medications, are
cautioned to consult with a health professional about specific recommendations for
supplements and the appropriate dosages. The authors and the publisher expressly
disclaim responsibility for any adverse effects arising from the use or application of
the information contained in this book.

Set in 11.5/13.5pt Sabon by
Falcon Oast Graphic Art Ltd.

Bantam Books are published by Transworld Publishers,
61–63 Uxbridge Road, London W5 5SA,
a division of The Random House Group Ltd,
in Australia by Random House Australia (Pty) Ltd,
20 Alfred Street, Milsons Point, Sydney, NSW 2061, Australia,
in New Zealand by Random House New Zealand Ltd,
18 Poland Road, Glenfield, Auckland 10, New Zealand
and in South Africa by Random House (Pty) Ltd, Isle of Houghton,
Corner of Boundary Road & Carse O'Gowrie, Houghton 2198, South Africa.

Printed in Great Britain by
Clays Ltd, St Ives plc

Papers used by Transworld Publishers are natural, recyclable
products made from wood grown in sustainable forests. The
manufacturing processes conform to the environmental
regulations of the country of origin.

In memory of Al Lowman
1948–2005
agent, friend, mentor

The doctor of the future will give no medicine, but will interest his patient in the care of the human frame, in diet and in the cause and prevention of disease.

– Thomas Edison

The medicine wheel – the traditional Lakota symbol for medicine, health, and balance – is essentially a circle with a cross in the middle. To the east is the spiritual realm, to the north is the mental realm, to the west the physical, and to the south the emotional. To be healthy you must be in balance in all four directions, essentially living in the centre of the circle.

– Donald Warne, M.D., M.P.H.

Contents

Topic Index

Acknowledgements

Once again, Team Pratt (my wife, Patty, and my kids, Mike, Tyler, Torey and Brian, and Mike's wife, Diane) have played an essential and much appreciated role in completing this book. Torey has been my research associate for *SuperFoods HealthStyle*, and could not have done a better job in tracking down the hundreds of studies I reviewed while completing this manuscript. Thanks again to the wonderful employees in my medical office, especially Carol Henry and Maurya Hernandez, for helping me successfully manage my busy clinical practice while working on this book. A special thank-you to my patients, who have cheered me on, provided many insights into what works for them (and what does not), and patiently seen their scheduled appointments change when 'book duty calls'. I appreciate the information about kiwis and avocados provided by my tireless patient Mr Don Rodee.

Thank you, Dr Joe Vinson, for your careful analysis of the polyphenol content of selected foods listed in *HealthStyle* – everyone will love the good news about dark chocolate! I owe a special word of appreciation to Dr Stewart Richer and Dr Victor Sierpina, both good friends and outstanding health care professionals, for their insights, suggestions, and vast knowledge of disease prevention. Thank you to Scripps Health and the Scripps Center for Integrative Medicine, its director Dr Mimi Guarneri, along with Dr Bobert Bonakdar, Rauni King, Karen Struthers, Donna Gilligan and Lori Winterstein, for leading the charge into what I believe will be the model for medical 'healthstyle wellness' care in the twenty-first century. The same can be said for the Calgary Health Region, and two of its employees, Lori Pullian and Joanne Stalinski.

I am blessed to be working with three great SuperFoods

partners and friends – Dr Hugh Greenway, Ray Sphire and David Stern. Debra Szekely, founder of the Golden Door and Rancho La Puerta, continues to inspire me in my own quest to bring optimum health to the world through books such as *HealthStyle*.

I would like to thank Dave Hamburg, the chief operating officer for Vital Choices Seafood. You and your company really 'stepped up to the plate' when it came to providing and developing scientific information relating to the wild Alaskan fish, the backbone of your business. Thanks to Laura Fleming for educating me on the life cycle of wild salmon.

Everyone at William Morrow has been superb. I'd like to give a special thank-you to Michael Morrison and to the world's best editor, Harriet Bell.

No one can write a book like Kathy Matthews. Kathy, I am so thankful to be working with you. Your combination of professionalism, friendship, dedication, wit, sense of humour, and reliability is impossible to match.

I know my close friend, confidant, and agent 'Maestro' Al Lowman is enjoying every word of this book from heaven. It was Al who championed HealthStyle, as he felt strongly, as I do, that this was indeed a twenty-first-century concept.

– Steven G. Pratt, M.D.

SuperFoods HealthStyle has been another wonderful adventure for me and I've enjoyed the help and support of family, friends and colleagues in completing the manuscript.

My husband, Fred, and sons, Greg and Ted, have been endlessly patient with my preoccupation and reduced homemaking for the duration of this project. (Someday, I promise, we will celebrate birthdays and holidays like normal people.)

Once again, Steve Pratt has proven himself to be the most knowledgeable and dedicated professional imaginable. There is nothing about food and healthy living that he doesn't know. The SuperFood partners, Ray Sphire, David

Stern and Hugh Greenway, have been endlessly creative and imaginative as they spread the word on SuperFoods throughout the world. Mark Cleveland has been an imaginative and eager contributor to the SuperFoods concept with his recipes and tips.

The team at William Morrow has been truly wonderful to work with. Harriet Bell is an extraordinary editor – supportive, energetic, and enthusiastic. Michael Morrison, Debbie Stier, Juliette Shapland and many others at Morrow have been tireless in their support of the *SuperFoods HealthStyle* project.

I am in debt to friends who made suggestions, encouraged me and supported this project. They include Dale Blodget, Diane Essig, Lorna Wyckoff, Maggie Peterson, Lori Kenyon, Jon Annunziata and the Island girls – Jean Drumm, Julie Karpeh and Nancy Nolan.

– Kathy Matthews

Introducing Chef Mark Cleveland

Eating well is an important part of HealthStyle, and we all need guidance and inspiration when it comes to putting healthy, delicious food on the table. We are fortunate to have Chef Mark Cleveland help us turn SuperFoods into super meals.

Mark learned to cook as a child from his wise Italian grandma, mastered the concepts of healthy California vegetarian cuisine while in college, and expanded his repertoire of ingredients, techniques, and flavours while living and working in Japan. Once back in California, Mark founded BIAN Personal Chef, a service that specialized in naturally nutritious meals with an international flair. Mark is now busy with his new Avanti Café in Costa Mesa, California. Mark's extensive experience teaching cooking techniques is obvious in the care he's taken in developing HealthStyle recipes.

Conversion Charts

LIQUID MEASURES

US MEASURES	FLUID OUNCES	IMPERIAL MEASURES	MILLILITRES
1 teaspooon	⅙	1 teaspoon	5
2 teaspoons	¼	1 dessertspoon	10
1 tablespoon	½	1 tablespoon	15
2 tablespoons	1	2 tablespoons	30
¼ cup	2	4 tablespoons	56
⅓ cup	2⅔		80
½ cup	4		110
⅔ cup	5	¼ pint/1 gill	140
¾ cup	6		170
1 cup/½ pint	8		225
1¼ cups	10	½ pint	280
1½ cups	12		420
2 cups/1 pint	16	generous ¾ pint	450
2½ cups	20	1 pint	560
3 cups/1½ pints	24		675
3½ cups	27		750
3¾ cups	30	1½ pints	840
4 cups/2 pints	32		900
4½ cups	36		1000/1 litre
5 cups	40	2 pints/1 quart	1120
6 cups/3 pints	48	scant 2½ pints	1350
7 cups	56	2¾ pints	1600
8 cups	64	3¼ pints	1800
9 cups	72	3½ pints	2000/2 litres
10 cups/5 pints	80	4 pints	2250

SOLID MEASURES

US AND IMPERIAL	METRIC EQUIVALENT
1 oz	25 grams
1½ oz	40
2 oz	50
3 oz	60
3½ oz	100
4 oz/¼lb	110
5 oz	150
6 oz	175
7 oz	200
8 oz/½lb	225
9 oz	250
10 oz	275
12 oz/¼lb	350
16 oz/1lb	450
1¼lb	575
1½lb	675
1¾lb	800
2 lb	900
2¼lb	1000/1 kilo
3lb	1kg 350g
4lb	1kg 800g
4½lb	2 kilos
5lb	2kg 250g
6lb	2kg 750g

OVEN TEMPERATURE EQUIVALENTS

FAHRENHEIT	CELSIUS	GAS MARK	HEAT OF OVEN
225°	110°	¼	Very cool
250°	120°	½	Very cool
275°	140°	1	Cool
300°	150°	2	Cool
325°	160°	3	Moderate
350°	180°	4	Moderate
375°	190°	5	Moderately hot
400°	200°	6	Moderately hot
425°	220°	7	Hot
450°	230°	8	Hot
475°	240°	9	Very Hot

Welcome to HealthStyle

HealthStyle is a fresh new way of living. It embraces every aspect of life that promotes health and optimism. HealthStyle is not a diet or an exercise programme or a few isolated principles that promise you'll feel better in a few days or weeks. You're reading this because you already know that's not possible.

You want to live fully, healthfully. HealthStyle recognizes that achieving optimal health in the twenty-first century is a synergy of information, motivation, good habits and inspiration. Many people are aware that the current accepted course of much of traditional medicine – end-stage care of chronic, often fatal, ailments with drugs or surgery – may not be the solution for a long, healthy, fulfilling life. Disease and disability take years and years to develop. Once we experience symptoms, our lives are often changed for ever, usually for the worse. What if you could stop that microscopic cancer cell that showed up in your kidney when you were twenty-five years old and prevent it from thriving? What if by eating a diet high in phytonutrients and fibre, exercising to regulate your metabolism, sleeping enough to maintain a strong immune system – what if all of these and other aspects of your HealthStyle resulted in that tiny cell being flushed harmlessly from your system? What if instead of getting a diagnosis of kidney cancer at age fifty-five after a few years of mild nagging back pain, instead you sailed right on to sixty and seventy and eighty, still playing tennis, still gardening, still enjoying the spring sun on your face?

This is what HealthStyle does for you. The information in this book, if you adopt it, is your ammunition against disease, frailty, and the host of indignities that come with poor health. HealthStyle will help you dodge those potential bullets. With luck, you'll never know how close they came. You'll simply feel good. Energetic. Optimistic. Some sections of this book are expressly designed to help you dodge some of the biggest bullets around. Can the section 'How to Avoid Alzheimer's' or 'How to Avoid Hypertension' guarantee freedom from these increasingly common chronic ailments? Of course not, but you'll increase your odds. And while the end result is not guaranteed, the process is: if you follow the suggestions in this book, you will feel better both physically and emotionally because you'll be doing the best you can to live well on this earth.

If you're reading this book you probably already make some effort to achieve health. Perhaps you have a pretty good diet. Maybe you exercise regularly. Or maybe you hope that your good diet will make you 'immune' from an exercise requirement. Maybe you eat pretty well and exercise but get only about six hours of sleep a night and feel pretty good. But what you don't know is that you're really suffering from a chronic sleep debt that's not only impairing your performance, it could also be promoting hypertension and diabetes as well as impairing your immune system and even promoting obesity.

Health is a web. Each strand is doing a job; no part can be ignored.

Perhaps the big news of HealthStyle is the role that *certain simple habits* play in keeping us at our best. Sleep, attention to our spiritual side, social contacts – all of these affect health in profound and usually unrecognized ways. I find the research studies on these practices particularly exhilarating because they seem to confirm instinct. Doesn't it make sense that achieving what I call 'personal peace' will actually promote health and perhaps even longevity?

My HealthStyle pyramid reflects every aspect of healthy living that I think needs attention. A quick glance at it will help you to get a great overview of how to live a long and healthful life.

THE NUTS AND BOLTS OF HEALTHSTYLE

My first book, the bestselling *SuperFoods*, presented a lively nutrition bible to a public eager for sound, medically based information on foods that promote health and prevent disease. The basic, powerful concept of *SuperFoods* is that certain foods have significant health-promoting abilities. Most people find that when they learn about these abilities it changes their relationship to food: they want to include more SuperFoods in their diets and the inevitable result is a nutrient-dense, lower-calorie, health-promoting diet. The response to this simple idea has been overwhelming. Many people who have struggled with food issues for years have written to tell me that they're eating better and feeling better than ever. I believe this is the simple power of information reinforced by results. When people learn why eating more fibre, more spinach, more blueberries and more wild salmon will make them feel better, they try to do so. And they feel better! So they keep doing it. And they feel even better.

HealthStyle takes the 'best foods' concept one step further and creates a blueprint for optimal health based on the latest peer-reviewed research on the importance of

SuperFoods
H E A L T H S T Y L E   P Y R A M I D

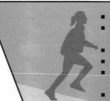

- Aerobic exercise most days (30–90 minutes)
- For those not currently exercising, begin with walking a minimum of 1 hour per week
- Resistance exercises (weight training) 2–3 times per week
- Stress-management practice (15 minutes most days)
- Hydration: Drink 8 or more 8-ounce glasses of water daily (may include tea and/or 100% fruit/vegetable juice)
- Sleep (7–8 hours for most people)

FRUITS: 3–5 servings daily; include berries (fresh or frozen) most days

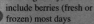

VEGETABLES: Unlimited (minimum 5–7); include dark, leafy greens most days

FOOD FOR THOUGHT:
- Daydream
- Enjoy friendships and laughter
- Spirituality
- Spend some time outdoors each day

SUPPLEMENTS:
- Multivitamin and mineral supplement daily for most people
- Consider fish oil supplement (250–1,000 mg daily)

WHOLE GRAINS: 5–7 servings per day (see SuperFoods List); include whole grain noodles/pasta, tortillas, breads, and cereals

PROTEIN:
Animal Protein: 1–2 servings daily of skinless poultry breast, fish* (see SuperFoods List); may include 3 oz lean red meat every 10 days (*2–4 servings per week)
Vegetarian Protein: 1–3 servings daily of legumes, lentils, soy (i.e., tempeh, tofu), egg whites, eggs (1 per day maximum)

FOR HEALTHY BONES: 1–3 servings daily of non- or low-fat dairy, tofu, soy, fortified soy milk, fortified OJ, fish with bones (i.e., sardines, tinned salmon), shellfish, dark leafy greens

SEASONINGS: Cook frequently with dried or fresh parsley, rosemary, oregano, turmeric, garlic, ginger, citrus zest, chives, red onion and white onion

SAMPLE SERVINGS:
Fruits = 1 medium piece, 1 cup, 1/2 cup juice, 2 tablespoons raisins, 3 prunes
Vegetables = 1/2 cup cooked, 1 cup raw
Grains = 1/2 cup cooked grains/pasta; 1 slice bread
Meat and Fish = 3 oz lean meat, poultry, or fish
Vegetarian Protein = 1 egg, 2 egg whites, 3 oz tofu or tempeh, 1/2 cup cooked beans or lentils
Dairy = 1/2 cup non- or low-fat cottage cheese, 8 oz non- or low-fat yogurt or milk
Fats: 1 oz (24) raw almonds, 14 walnut halves, 1 tablespoon oil, 3/8 avocado

ALCOHOL: If you choose to consume alcohol, we recommend: 1–3 drinks per week for women; 2–8 drinks per week for men

HEALTHY FATS: 1–2 servings daily of nuts, seeds, avocado, extra virgin olive oil, canola oil, soybean oil, peanut oil, flaxseed oil

Up to 100 calories daily dark chocolate, butter, buckwheat honey, sweets, or refined breads and grains exercise, sleep and stress control in your life. 'Peer-reviewed' is important. It means that every bit of information in this book has been published in respected journals. It's not just my theory or a suggestion that seems reasonable. It's actual, proven data. My own feeling is that research data is often mishandled by the media. There's too much focus on single studies that can have conflicting and sometimes alarming results. Many more headlines are written on the one study that confounds previous ones or even common sense. Sometimes animal studies yield results that may not be transferable to humans yet still make headlines and confuse consumers. Except where noted, I rely on studies conducted on humans. I'm convinced that most readers of this book will fall into that category.

Information is one thing; implementation is another, so *SuperFoods HealthStyle* presents information in a seasonal format that is useful to readers searching for practical ways to achieve a healthier lifestyle. How do you 'get out and exercise' when it's sleeting? How do you motivate yourself to choose healthy foods when the holidays roll around and your office is a sea of biscuits and fruitcake? How do you eat a diet rich in fruits and vegetables in January when there seems to be little fresh produce available? We are seasonal creatures. We have physical and spiritual rhythms that change with the weather. Though we sometimes ignore it, we are intimately connected to nature. HealthStyle capitalizes on the seasons by making health recommendations that coincide with the times of year and taking advantage of our natural inclinations.

Nutrition is the cornerstone of HealthStyle. Healthy, whole foods are the foundation of health. And, of course, foods along with the weather change with the season. Our desires ebb and flow. The hearty casseroles that lure us in January hold no appeal in July when we yearn for some grilled fish or perhaps just a salad. The foods in

HealthStyle, the SuperFood recommendations and recipes, are in tune with the seasons. You'll find the freshest and most delicious foods when you eat according to the season.

Each HealthStyle season features some of the original fourteen SuperFoods with updates on their health-promoting abilities as well as new tips and recipes to help you enjoy them more frequently. In addition, I've introduced a few additional SuperFoods as well as SuperSpices. These are foods and spices that have earned their place in the SuperFood pantheon thanks to recent research on their powerful effects on health.

So, again, welcome to HealthStyle. I hope that this book inspires you to live your best year ever. With many, many more to come.

Winter: Season of Resolution

Though the poet may claim that April is the cruellest month, HealthStylers would no doubt pick December. And January, February, and maybe some of March. Winter can be hard on our health. We tend to be less physically active because inclement or cold weather keeps us indoors. We are tempted with holiday foods that we wouldn't dream of eating at other times of the year. The days are shorter: Less daylight makes outdoor exercise a challenge while it promotes more TV watching and thus more snacking. Reduced sunlight affects our moods, making some of us less optimistic and less committed to health goals. Some of us even suffer from SAD (seasonal affective disorder), which makes reduced sunlight an actual health risk.

Don't despair! Winter does have its special beneficial rhythms. We seek warmth in winter – of every kind. Winter draws us inward. We can seize opportunities to be more reflective. Long evenings encourage more family and social time – time to reconnect and cherish the important relationships in our lives. Exciting new evidence demonstrates that these important social contacts keep us healthy as well as happy. The winter holidays are a time of spiritual renewal and give us an opportunity to connect with an often neglected aspect of health – spirituality, or, as we discuss in HealthStyle, Personal Peace. Winter is a perfect time to take stock, make resolutions and look to a healthier new year.

We're about to show you that you can come through winter in healthy style with new and reinforced good health habits. Winter is the time to focus on some new and delicious SuperFoods that will make achieving optimum nutritional health a pleasure. We've got some warming recipes that feature the winter SuperFoods along with some SuperSpices that have impressive health benefits. Just a sprinkle of cinnamon on your breakfast could help control your blood sugar levels and have other positive effects on your health. Here's the really good news: Chocolate is a SuperFood. The beneficial polyphenols in chocolate make it a powerful health promoter. What could be a better winter treat – for your health and your spirit – than a mug of steaming cocoa twirled with a cinnamon stick? Who would have thought that this indulgence could have such positive effects?

Yes, winter can be a challenge for many of us, but it offers special opportunities, and if you adopt the recommendations of HealthStyle, you'll be able to savour the best of the season, improve your overall health profile, and be ready to greet spring in the best shape you've ever been in. You have three months: Make them count towards your better HealthStyle and your better future.

PERMANENT CHANGE

The goal of HealthStyle is literally to help you change your life. You've already taken the first step: You're reading this book. You might be mildly curious – perhaps you'd like to lose a few pounds or eat more healthfully – or you might be absolutely determined to improve your health because a condition or illness has made you realize that your HealthStyle is a life-and-death decision. It doesn't matter how you came to read this book; it should be comforting and encouraging to know that just by doing so, you're going in the right direction. Your goal is change. However, change isn't always so easy. Many of us have tried and failed before. This time will be different because, with the help of HealthStyle, you'll have different skills and constant motivation.

As the winter and the start of the new year are times of recommitment and resolution, it's useful to take a look at the process of personal change. If you are aware of all of the elements of effective change, you'll be more successful in your year of HealthStyle.

In a book published more than a dozen years ago, *Changing for Good*, three psychologists studied thousands of people who were able to alter their lives positively and permanently. The authors learned that change isn't dependent on luck or willpower as many of us believe. It is a *process* that can be successful if certain guidelines are met. As a doctor who actively works to promote health with his patients, I've always known that positive change isn't just a matter of willpower. I've seen too many patients who were determined and committed but who failed to achieve change in the long run for many reasons. Making positive, permanent change is a skill. You can learn how to do it. It's a gradual process of learning to know yourself, learning to set goals, maintaining motivation, and learning what tools you need to reach your goals. I find it useful in winter, when we're starting a new year, to take a close look at the process of change. It will help us as we go forward trying to improve our overall health and well-being.

Life is change. Tomorrow will be different from today. You will be a different person – on molecular, physical and emotional levels – a year from today. Will you be better or worse off? The choice is yours. HealthStyle will put the tools in your hands to improve; you need only decide, each day, to use them.

Some of the life-changing skills I'll describe may seem obvious to you. But each one needs attention if you want to give yourself the best chance for success. Take a minute now and think about each skill and how you can implement it in the season and year ahead.

- One of the important skills of permanent change is the ability to **evaluate yourself** realistically. Take a hard look at the year ahead. What are your goals? How do you want your life to improve? What do you think will be better about your life if you adopt the HealthStyle lifestyle? Do you primarily want to look better by losing some weight? Do you want to extend your active, vital lifespan? Do you want to live to enjoy your grandchildren? Do you want to feel the inner peace that comes with living a healthy and directed life? You probably have enough basic information about health improvement to know the weak links in your own HealthStyle. Maybe it's your diet. Maybe you've never exercised. Maybe the stress in your life is so out of control that you're losing sleep and feeling anxious all the time. Or perhaps you have a very specific issue – high cholesterol, a family history of heart disease, being overweight, a recent diagnosis of type II diabetes. Whatever your health issue, look it square in the face. One year from now, one year of HealthStyle, and you are going to be a different person.
- Change doesn't happen by wishing it so. **You must make the decision to change.** It's not enough to think about how your life *could be better*. You have to determine

that *you will make it better*. Too often we daydream about change. We often think about how nice it would be if we were healthier, if we ate better, if we exercised. We have a moment of resolve when stepping on the scale or sitting in the doctor's office. But we never actually *decide to take action*. You'll be surprised at how empowering it is actually to make a decision to veer from your routine. Winter is the perfect time for a personal revolution. Make a promise to yourself that by this time next year, you're going to be better. Commit to it by writing it down right here, right now: -

_____

You're going to feel better and maybe even look better. You've got nothing to lose and everything to gain.

■ Of course, you have to do more than read this book, you have to **take active steps** to incorporate suggested changes in your life. HealthStyle doesn't insist that you follow a single blueprint for success. You'll learn how to make decisions based on your lifestyle and tastes and on what changes will work for you. You'll be shown how to substitute good health habits for poor ones. This isn't as hard as it might seem, because there are literally hundreds of ideas in this book that will help you. As you go through the year of HealthStyle, you'll pick and choose the tips that work for you. Sometimes you'll have to push yourself a bit to make these changes work. But if you've made the decision to change and you refer back to your written commitment, you will surely keep on track and your HealthStyle year will be a success.

■ You must **keep motivated**. HealthStyle acknowledges: Its core is motivation. Anyone who makes a commitment to change knows that it's important to search for motivation everywhere. You'll find it in the headlines. Former President Bill Clinton's heart surgery was motivating for many people who had been cavalier about their heart health. Many people were shocked that someone who seemed so vigorous, who had lost weight and seemed to be exercising – someone who certainly got good medical care – suddenly found that he needed major heart surgery to avoid a possibly fatal heart attack. Calls to cardiologists spiked in the weeks following Clinton's surgery.

Simple facts are extremely motivating. People tell me all the time that my first book, *SuperFoods*, convinced them to change their diets because the data they read in the book spoke for itself. If there's powerful research evidence that, for example, blueberries have a positive effect on brain function, why wouldn't you eat them? The HealthStyle data on food, exercise, sleep, personal peace and a host of health issues will convince and motivate you as well.

One interesting and exciting aspect of positive change is that motivation grows and strengthens as a result of the positive actions you're taking. Improvement is self-reinforcing. All my patients tell me this and I've found it to be so in my own life. When you eat well, you feel better and want to continue eating well. When you exercise, you have more energy and want to continue exercising and eating well. If there's any magic bullet to health improvement, that's it: *Act better to feel better to get better.*

■ **You need support from friends and family.** You need to make decisions about how to ask for help and who will help you. Perhaps you should tell your children that certain foods the family is eating will ultimately cause health problems, but sometimes it's hard to resist these foods, so you need their help. Maybe they can help prepare salads at dinnertime. Maybe they can help prepare some healthier recipes. If they feel like collaborators rather than victims of change, they're far more likely to be enthusiastic supporters. Don't forget co-workers.

Ask their support in avoiding sugary treats on coffee breaks or at office parties. Suggest a quick, healthy lunch followed by a walk with an office mate instead of a fatty, high-calorie midday extravaganza. So many more people are health conscious these days, but may be shy about speaking up. If you suggest providing fruit instead of doughnuts at the next meeting, others will surely embrace your suggestion. When we put out healthy snacks at my office – grapes, carrots, peppers, nuts – they disappear as quickly as any junk food would.

- **You need rewards.** Many people think of rewards in this context as a major gift to oneself, like a new coat or theatre tickets or even a trip. This is fine if it works for you and your budget, but I prefer to think of rewards in smaller, everyday terms. Rewards are stepping-stones to a goal. They help you cross a river of temptation and conflicting demands. For example, buy that fancy green tea or a soothing CD if you reach your week's exercise goals. Treat yourself to some new exercise clothing or a reflexology session once you go a month without junk food. Call a friend you haven't spoken with in ages as a reward for skipping dessert at a buffet. You know yourself best and you know what your short-term HealthStyle goals are. Connect those goals with rewards. Think up creative rewards as you go along, and when something threatens to derail your efforts, search for the stepping-stone that will keep you on the right path. Write down these reward ideas. One of my patients told me that every Sunday evening she writes a note to herself about her week's reward if she sticks to her goals. One week it was splurging on a basket of exotic fruit. Another week she treated herself and a friend to a house tour in a nearby city.

Cold-Weather Cholesterol

Did you know that blood contains less water in winter, slightly concentrating cholesterol? This means your total cholesterol reading could be a bit higher in winter than in summer. A new study published in 2004 has found that cholesterol levels naturally fluctuate throughout the year. Researchers at the University of Massachusetts Medical Center in Worcester tracked 517 healthy people for a year and found that their cholesterol levels tended to rise in the winter and fall in the summer. The biggest changes occurred in those with elevated cholesterol and in women. Their levels fluctuated by as much as 18 points. The seasonal variation put 22 percent more patients over the official high-cholesterol mark of 240 mg/dl in winter than in summer. Cold-season readings could lead to a misdiagnosis of high cholesterol for up to three million Americans, the researchers estimate. Best bet: Get several checks, make sure that at least one is in the spring or autumn, when levels are at a midpoint.

EXERCISE

Eating alone will not keep a man well; he must also take exercise. For food and exercise, while possessing opposite qualities, yet work together to produce health.

– Hippocrates, fifth century

It's a new year, time to look at the most important elements in your HealthStyle. We're tackling the most challenging habit first – exercise – because it's perhaps the single critical change you can make in daily life – along with eating SuperFoods – that will improve your health, your spirits and your future.

You must exercise. It's that simple. You cannot fully realize the benefits of HealthStyle if exercise is not a part of your life. If you're thinking right now that this is where you tune out because you've never been able to exercise, let me tell you something that should be encouraging: I have a whole new approach to exercise that works even for confirmed couch potatoes. First I want you to understand how important exercise is to your future health. Once you understand how exercise amplifies all the good things you're doing for your health and how powerful a tool simple movement is in preventing disease, I'm sure you'll resolve to get active.

Here's a way to think about exercise that will motivate you: You are dangling by a line – a lifeline – over the abyss. That line is keeping you alive, keeping you a full participant in life, keeping you hanging on. You want this line to be as strong and reliable as possible. It's made up of four strands woven together. On your 'healthline' the four strands are nutrition, exercise, adequate sleep and personal peace. Together, they make up a powerful, reliable health insurance. The synergy of their separate powers can keep you alert, flexible, energetic and optimistic for a long, long time – maybe, with a little luck, to near age 100. Neglect one of these strands and you're in jeopardy. Every fast-food binge, every sedentary month, every frantic year of uncontrolled stress, sleepless nights and spiritual voids fray a few strands in the healthline. Of course, you may be lucky – you may never break a sweat in your life or you may eat fast food daily for half a century and never suffer any consequences. This scenario is highly unlikely but not impossible. Do you want to take the chance of hanging by a frayed rope? Do you want to trust to luck that the other strands will hold?

If you are reading this book you're probably looking to improve your health and if so, exercise must become part of your daily routine. Yes, I'm repeating myself, but exercise is that important. Now here's the good news: It's time to simplify our approach to exercise. Too many of my patients have been turned off by recommendations that are confusing or don't suit their lifestyles. I have a solution: the HealthStyle ERA Exercise Programme, which will be described in detail later once I've demonstrated how important exercise is. It's a simple programme and I've yet to meet someone who can't do it.

Perhaps you already exercise regularly. If so, that's great: Keep it up. Most people find that once they begin an exercise programme, they see results and stick with it. So bear with me while I convince those who don't exercise, or who've tried and failed, to make physical activity part of their daily lives.

A Nation and a World at Rest

First, a little background . . . We were born to move. That's literally true. We are here today because many generations ago our ancestors were running around procuring food. The equation was simple: Move or die. In fact, it's been estimated that Paleolithic man burned approximately 1,000 calories a day and consumed about 3,000 calories a day. Today, in affluent Western nations, we consume approximately 2,100 calories a day and *burn only about 300 calories in daily activity*. A little quick maths will tell you that we burn less than a third as much as our ancestors did in daily calories. As recently as a century ago, 30 percent of all the energy used in the workplace came from human muscle power. Today, the workplace is operating on brain power: Only a tiny percentage of us use our muscles for anything more demanding than moving a computer mouse. It's not only that we don't expend energy at work, we hardly spend energy at all. With our power mowers, TV remotes and vacuum cleaners that push themselves, and our reliance on cars to get anywhere, we have come to a near total standstill as far as energy expenditure is concerned.

Statistics highlight the facts: Nearly 30 percent of American adults are entirely sedentary and another 46 percent don't get enough exercise. That means only about a quarter of Americans get sufficient exercise.

Sedentary individuals may lose 23 to 35 percent of muscle mass over the course of their adult lives. This loss causes a loss of strength and balance, and an overall physical decline.

Do you think that while you might not be Olympic athlete material you certainly get lots of daily activity? Think again. When researchers from the CDC (Centers for Disease Control and Prevention) evaluated more than 1,500 people who claimed to be walkers, they found that only 5 percent of the surveyed group actually walked enough to realize any benefits.

Where does this leave us? With a genetic makeup that thrives on lots of daily activity and a relatively low caloric intake, we are living in a world that encourages the exact opposite. In other words, we now are watching a lethal mix of a genetic makeup suffering from the toxic circumstances of **increased** daily calorie intake and **decreased** daily activity. It's no wonder that chronic diseases are rampant in our culture.

Obviously we cannot change our genetic heritage. But we can change our behaviour: Lower calories; increase exercise!

One in three Americans over age fifty is *completely* sedentary.

Benefits of Exercise

The benefits of exercise are truly extraordinary. Indeed, if some clever salesman could sell exercise as, say, 'The E Technique', and convince people of all the benefits they'd gain from using this technique, he would be a billionaire! Here's how exercise can help you live better today and as the years go by:

- Exercise can make your heart stronger.
- Exercise burns calories and helps you maintain a healthy weight. Exercise is essential for keeping off lost weight.
- Exercise decreases inflammatory markers (e.g., C-reactive protein).
- Exercise helps to control your blood sugar and thus helps to manage or prevent diabetes.
- Exercise can improve circulation, which has myriad beneficial health effects.
- Exercise can decrease blood pressure.
- Exercise increases your cognitive ability, including your ability to concentrate and remain alert.
- Exercise before or after a meal diminishes the postprandial rise in potentially harmful triglycerides (a type of fat).
- Exercise decreases your risk for metabolic syndrome.
- Exercise can decrease the levels of 'bad' low density lipoprotein (LDL) cholesterol, and increase the levels of 'good' high density (HDL) cholesterol.
- Exercise boosts the immune system.
- Exercise can reduce back pain.
- Exercise lowers your risk for upper respiratory infections.
- Exercise helps relieve arthritis.
- Exercise lowers your overall risk of dying prematurely.
- Exercise can make you stronger and more flexible.
- Exercise, particularly weight-bearing exercise, can make your bones stronger.

- Exercise increases your level of endorphins – brain chemicals that increase your sense of well-being. Thus exercise can improve mood and could even fight depression.
- Exercise reduces the frailty of old age.

In one study conducted in northern California, approximately 20 percent of the subjects reported that they had had *no vigorous activity for the past twenty years*! In this study, 13 percent of the colon cancer cases could be attributed to physical inactivity.

- Exercise is an essential activity to prevent cataracts and age-related macular degeneration.

There's no question that the positive benefits of physical activity are extraordinary. Here is a list of the diseases and conditions that exercise can help prevent and/or improve:

- Coronary artery disease
- Heart disease
- Stroke
- Colon cancer
- Endometrial cancer
- Breast cancer
- Prostate cancer
- Osteoporosis
- Obesity
- Type II diabetes
- Depression
- Dementia
- Cataracts and macular degeneration
- Chronic lung disease
- Arthritis
- Disability

This is an impressive list. Keep in mind that many of the physiological benefits will occur *immediately*. While preventing dementia or osteoporosis or coronary artery disease would probably rank as a top long-term goal, you don't have to wait till old age for the benefits of exercise to kick in. Exercise will give you an immediate boost in mood, mental acuity and overall energy levels. This isn't surprising when you appreciate the dramatic effect that physical activity has on the human body. Yes, you're sweating a bit, probably breathing heavily, and perhaps you feel your muscles aching. However, here's what's happening on a cellular level when you're active: You're increasing the activity of free-radical scavenging enzymes, improving immune function, increasing circulating T- and B-lymphocytes, reducing body fat, increasing gastrointestinal motility, altering hormone levels, improving insulin resistance, reducing triglyceride levels and providing beneficial effects on the inflammatory response. Appreciating the intensely synergistic effects of physical activity makes it easier to see why its health benefits are so extraordinary.

> **Exercise Keeps You Young**
> Guess what? Much of the overall physical and mental decline we experience between the ages of thirty and seventy has *more to do with a sedentary lifestyle* than with the ageing process. Exercise slows the deterioration of a host of bodily systems. It helps reverse impairments in sleep, sexual and cognitive functions as well as loss of muscle mass and bone strength.

Exercise and the Brain

Most of us know that exercise affects our bodies. That's pretty obvious. We become stronger, sometimes slimmer and more flexible. I've found that many people are amazed to learn that exercise has a dramatic effect on the brain. Even those of us who think we can live with some extra body fat or less flexibility or even a higher disease risk will be motivated to exercise when we realize that doing so helps preserve our brains! I'm going to go into detail on this aspect of exercise because it affects everyone (with particular benefits for women, for men, for older people and for parents) and because it's a powerful incentive to get moving.

It's dismaying to learn that the human brain begins to lose tissue early in the third decade of life. *The average lifetime losses are estimated at roughly 15 percent of the cerebral cortex and 25 percent of the cerebral white matter.* This loss of tissue is closely related to declines in cognitive performance during the same period.

Exercise to the rescue. In a meta-analysis of eighteen controlled studies conducted over the past forty years it was found that aerobic exercise improves cognitive ability in people over fifty-five. Interestingly, the people who showed the most dramatic improvement were previously sedentary. Moreover, relatively brief programmes (one to three months long) provided as much benefit as moderate programmes (four to six months long), though, as you might guess, the longer time a subject exercised, the greater the overall improvements.

There are now other studies that show similar results. *Better cardiovascular fitness will produce a brain that is more plastic and adaptive to change.*

A study published in 2003 demonstrates that physical exercise actually stimulates physiological changes in the brain. In this study, researchers scanned the brains of fifty-five people aged fifty-five to seventy-nine and tested their aerobic fitness. Then, using MRIs, researchers found that physically fit subjects had less age-related brain-tissue shrinkage than subjects who were less fit.

One study of normal people fifty-five years old and older

showed that the areas of the brain most gravely affected by ageing also showed the greatest benefits from aerobic fitness.

We now have confirmation that the role of cardiovascular fitness as a protector and enhancer of cognitive function in older adults has a solid biological basis. In a nutshell, the simplest and most inexpensive way to delay the effects of senescence on human brain tissue is to get up out of your chair and start moving.

Personally, I find the brain-boosting benefits of exercise powerfully motivating. Many of my patients, especially older people, agree. It's frightening to think that you could face a future with diminished mental ability. Most of us could imagine a happy life despite many disabilities, but cognitive decline is not one of them.

One study found that physical inactivity was an even greater risk to health than tobacco smoking. In this study, conducted on a Chinese population, one-fifth of deaths of those over age thirty-five in Hong Kong in 1998 were due to physical inactivity.

Especially for Women

Women have special challenges when it comes to physical activity, but also particular benefits to gain when they are active. Women begin with a disadvantage in the fitness wars: Their reserves of muscle mass are considerably lower than those of men. They are generally weaker than men, with more body fat and less muscle tissue. As they age, their loss of musculoskeletal capacity affects them sooner and more pervasively than men. They begin to feel the impact of reduced fitness at least ten years before men.

Sadly, the statistics tell us that women are even less active than men: Over 70 percent of adult women do not engage in any regular activity. And women stand to gain a great deal from better fitness – maybe even more than men. One study of 5,721 women found that fitness was twice as strong a factor in preventing death than in men. In another study, previously sedentary women who became active halved their mortality rates from all causes.

Most unfortunately, women who are sedentary often suffer from the results of decline *before they're even aware it's happening.* Half the women in the United States die of cardiovascular disease, and nearly two-thirds of women who die suddenly from cardiovascular disease had no previous symptoms. Also, elderly women can begin to suffer frailty, loss of mobility, balance, and so forth, which might never have occurred had they been physically active. Studies have shown that women in their sixties and seventies, compared with those in their twenties, have lost 30 to 39 percent of their former strength. Again, women often find they're beginning to suffer the damaging results of a sedentary lifestyle before they even realize the extent of their decline.

Exercise has been *proven* to reduce a woman's risk for coronary artery disease, stroke, type II diabetes, breast and colon cancer, as well as osteoporosis.

There is very good news for women, however, on what they stand to gain from regular physical activity. For one thing, adding exercise to your life can lower your risk of cardiovascular disease – the number-one killer of US women. Additionally, there's evidence that improved fitness, regardless of any changes in weight, blood pressure or lipid levels, improves your overall health picture. This is extremely good news for women because it puts the focus back on basics: Work on overall fitness with exercise and diet and you'll make giant strides in improving your overall health status. Once you get moving, pay attention to your optimum weight, blood pressure and cholesterol levels.

I've already mentioned that exercise can reduce a woman's risk for cardiovascular disease. An important meta-analysis concluded that physically active women had half the heart disease of those who were sedentary. Even more exciting for some women: *Vigorous* activity is not necessary for lowering your risk of cardiovascular disease. Women who walk one hour a week had half the coronary artery disease as those who were sedentary. As little as one hour a week of walking yields a lower risk for heart disease, and the walking need not be fast-paced to prove beneficial. The time spent walking was more important than the walking pace. Here's the little bonus I share with my women patients who are totally sedentary: One recent study of more than eighty thousand women showed that the greatest decrease in disease risk is a result of boosting activity from less than one hour a week to between roughly one and two hours a week. This is not at all difficult to achieve! In this study, walking conveyed approximately the same benefit as more vigorous activities among the middle-aged and older women.

Check out the fitness planner for women at MealsMatter.org. You can find it at http://www.mealsmatter.org/EatingFor Health/Tools/wfp.aspx.

In addition to a reduction in cardiovascular risk, women derive other important benefits from exercise. Women, particularly early postmenopausal women, must work to fight the bone loss that occurs as they transition to a post-menopausal state. Exercise – especially weight training – plays an important role in fighting bone loss and resulting osteoporosis.

There's also evidence that regular workouts help reduce the hot flushes and night sweats associated with menopause. A Swedish study followed 142 menopausal women who did not use hormones. Regular exercisers in this group reported half the number of moderate and severe hot flushes compared with those who did no regular exercise. Eight years after this initial study, additional research showed that only 5 percent of very active women experienced several hot flushes compared with 14 to 16 percent of women who were sedentary. In this study, weight, smoking or hormone therapy could not explain the difference.

Young women who exercise just a few hours a week in their teenage years can lower their likelihood of developing breast cancer by 30 to 35 percent. The operating theory is that exercise, even in relatively small doses, promotes a kind of biological shield against cancer.

Especially for Men

Many men have an all-or-nothing approach to exercise. The 'no pain/no gain' concept really appeals to them (even though it's now generally recognized as *ineffective*). They're either weekend warriors, sweating it out for two hours on the squash court every Saturday, or total couch potatoes, enjoying their golf and tennis on the big screen. For those of you who go crazy on the weekends and are stiff, sore and immobile for the rest of the week, it's time to educate, moderate and recalibrate your exercise habits with the new HealthStyle ERA Exercise Programme (see page 55). For those of you who haven't moved since your last PE class in school, hear that sound in the distance? It's the whistle of your new HealthStyle PE instructor getting you back in action.

The health benefits of physical activity are just too powerful to ignore. If you skipped earlier sections in this chapter outlining the specific benefits of exercise, go back and read them now. You need to believe that the effort of physical activity is worth it.

Men have some advantages over women when it comes to health. Yes, women do live longer but the gap is closing. In general, men are larger and tend to have more lean muscle mass. This means that their bodies burn calories more readily than women's bodies. Indeed, preserving and increasing that lean muscle mass is one of the goals of exercise.

While men have the potential for dramatic health gains when they adopt an exercise programme, they are often stymied by simple bad habits and the belief that they'll never get back to the 'fighting form' they enjoyed in their teens and twenties. I often see a certain look in a patient's eyes when I recommend exercise. It says, 'Don't waste your breath, Doc. I'll listen, if you insist, but there's no way I'm giving up the remote control. I'm not an athlete and I'm not joining a gym.' Here's my favourite response to that look. One study tells the heartening story of middle-aged men who had had a thirty-year layoff from exercise. The study showed that in six months, the effects of those sedentary thirty years were actually *reversed* with a programme of exercise training. These guys had really declined in thirty years, too. Their weight had increased by 25 percent, their body fat had doubled, and their aerobic capacity had decreased by 11 percent. Despite all that, in six months they were able to achieve the same degree of cardiovascular fitness they'd enjoyed as *twenty-year-olds*. The moral of the story is that when it comes to fitness, it's never too late. I've found that many male patients are inspired by this story.

It's a very sad fact of life that most people who are not engaged in athletic or workout activity lose a very large proportion of their physical strength and physical work capacity *before they even notice that something is wrong.* Tragically, some people cross the threshold of disability and find themselves unable to participate actively in life, an end result that could have been very different with an easily achievable amount of physical activity earlier on.

Remember that big gains in fitness can be achieved without fanatical and intense activity. One study at the University of Colorado found that after a three-month exercise period that consisted primarily of walking, a study of groups of sedentary men with an average age of fifty-three had improved their endothelial function – a key contributor to vascular health – to a state comparable to that of men who had exercised for years.

It's well known that exercise has impressive beneficial effects on the heart and the circulation. It's not surprising that anything that improves the circulation could improve erectile function, and indeed it's true. One Harvard study that included some 31,000 men between the ages of fifty-five and ninety found that men who exercise only thirty minutes a day are 40 percent less likely to develop erectile dysfunction than sedentary men. Given that about 20 percent of men in their sixties and 30 percent of men in their seventies have erectile problems, a little exercise could go a long way to improving the lives of many men and their partners.

Arthritis and Exercise

If you have arthritis, you may be reluctant to begin an exercise programme. More than half of people over age sixty-five have some degree of this painful disabling condition. It's estimated that by the year 2020, sixty million, or 18 percent of the population, will have to deal with the day-to-day impact of arthritis. While it's often difficult for arthritis sufferers to think about exercise, the fact is that research has shown that exercise can give symptomatic relief. Arthritis sufferers should keep the following in mind: Exercise must be pursued on a regular basis because once discontinued, muscle strength and symptom relief are quickly lost.

- Exercise programmes should have an aerobic component that brings you to 50 or 60 percent of your maximum heart rate for twenty to thirty minutes, three to four times a week (see page 68).
- Resistance training – lifting weights – should be a part of your programme. Beginners should start with four to six repetitions to avoid muscle fatigue, and two to three sessions a week is sufficient.
- Tai chi (see page 51) is also an excellent exercise for arthritis patients because it achieves strength, stretching and aerobics all in one.

Especially for Older Adults

Old age isn't what it used to be. Today we see senior citizens on the tennis court, in marathons and on the bike trail as well as on cruise ships and shovelboard courts. We're lucky to live in a time when a vigorous old age seems not only desirable but possible. It's inspiring to see older people who are as active and engaged in life as any twenty-something. And given that the over-eighty-five segment of the population is the largest growing of all, we can hope to see more and more of them and maybe eventually join them ourselves. If you're over sixty-five and sedentary, *exercise may be the single most important habit you can adopt to improve your overall health and well-being.* The evidence is overwhelming. One study revealed a 23 to 55 percent lower mortality rate in highly active men and women over age sixty-five.

If you think that there's not much point in exercising if you're older because you're not really interested in being physically active, you're ignoring the fact that as we age, the benefits we get from exercise – and our own goals – change. Younger people usually worry more about fitness, appearance and weight. Older people get those benefits from exercise and more: As balance, mental health and maintaining sexual activity become higher priorities, exercise becomes the best tool for achieving them.

Exciting news for older people is that they stand to gain the most from exercise. For example, a number of studies have demonstrated that older women and men show similar or greater strength gains compared with young individuals as a result of resistance training. In one study, older men responded to a twelve-week progressive resistance-training programme by more than doubling knee extensor strength and more than tripling knee flexor strength. This refers to keeping the major strength and function muscles of your legs strong. In another study with elderly men working on their quadriceps with resistance training, the average increase in strength after eight weeks of resistance training was a very impressive 174 percent.

Exercise for the Sick and the Well
Exercise is for everyone, always. Remember, while traditional medicine rarely addresses this issue, exercise has been shown to alter the expression and consequences of a disease that is already present. What this means is even if you already have an ailment or chronic disease, or mobility restriction such as confinement to a wheelchair, exercise can probably help you. Get guidance from a medical professional, but don't miss out on the benefits of physical activity.

One of the great threats of old age is a condition known as sarcopenia. Sarcopenia refers to the loss of muscle mass and decline in muscle quality observed with increasing age. Sarcopenia is also linked to functional decline, osteoporosis, impaired thermoregulation (the ability to control body temperature) and glucose intolerance. Sadly, the effects of sarcopenia can compound: As their physical capacity declines, many older people avoid physically stressful work and thus become increasingly sedentary and increasingly vulnerable to overall decline.

The best way to fight the ravages of sarcopenia is to exercise. Ample evidence demonstrates that decreasing physical activity levels are related to the development of disability in older adults.

An essential key to improvement in fitness in elderly people is resistance training. Only the loading of muscle and resistance training – weight-lifting exercises – have been shown to avert loss of muscle mass and strength in older folks. Studies have shown that even very fit older people – those who run or play tennis for example – do not have the muscle mass and strength of older people who engage in weight training. Weight training can build muscle and strength. In one study, a weight-training programme of three to six months was able to increase muscle strength by an average of 40 to 150 percent. The National Institute on Aging in the US says that even frail, inactive people in their nineties can more than double their strength in a short period with simple exercises.

There's another advantage to resistance training. Elderly people who have been sedentary may have impaired balance and weakened muscles: Aerobic activity could risk a fall. But once a regular programme of simple resistance exercises has begun, both weakness and impaired balance will improve. Resistance training also maintains joint health and function because a joint, particularly knees, elbows and shoulders, is only as strong as the muscles around it. The National Institute on Aging offers exercise videos for seniors. One shows how to use household items like chairs and towels to tone and strengthen muscles. It costs only $7 and comes with a book of instructional information and charts to track your progress. Call 800-222-2225.

Good news for older people: Even if you have periods of inactivity, you'll still benefit from the effort you put into strength training. In one study, people aged sixty-five to eighty-one trained over a two-year period. They exercised twice a week for one hour, performing two to three sets of both upper and lower body exercises at up to 80 percent of the heaviest weights they could once lift. They were still able to lift up to 24 percent above their baseline three years after discontinuing strength training. Control subjects who performed no strength training over the five years saw declines in strength across the board.

HealthStyle Exercise ERA for Older People

If you're a senior – age sixty-five and older – shift the order of the HealthStyle ERA Exercise Programme (see page 55). Begin with R for Resistance Training. Go slowly and keep at it. Depending on your age and physical condition, you can incorporate the first part of the programme – Exercise Opportunities – when you feel able.

Here are some tips for older folks – those age sixty-five and older – who are ready to add exercise to their lives:

■ If you have a family history of heart disease or are under care for a medical condition, check with your health care professional before you begin to exercise. You might want to get a complete physical and perhaps take a stress test if your health care provider advises.

- Wear comfortable clothing and footwear that is appropriate for the activity.
- Seniors generally need to take more care with warm-ups and cool-downs: Don't neglect these exercises. Your muscles need to prepare for activity to avoid injury. If walking is your activity of choice, walk slowly for five or ten minutes before you up your pace, or slowly jog in place for five minutes before your workout to gradually increase your heart rate and core temperature. The idea is to get your muscles and tendons prepared for activity. Cool down after exercising with five minutes of slower-paced movement and some stretching. This prevents an abrupt drop in blood pressure and helps alleviate potential muscle stiffness.
- If you walk, choose a place that is safe, well-lit, and free of traffic, and make sure the walking surface is smooth and regular. Shopping malls can be great places to walk.
- Take it easy. Start slowly and increase your activity intensity slowly. The most common cause of injury and exercise dropouts is going too fast. In general, don't increase your training load – the length or frequency of workouts, the intensity, or the distance – by more than 10 percent a week.
- If you're exercising for more than a half hour and/ or you're exercising in warm, humid conditions, be sure to drink 4 to 8 ounces of water every fifteen minutes. Your body can lose more than a pint of water in an hour. Seniors often find that their sense of thirst is not a reliable guide, and adequate hydration is important.
- A good primer on weight-bearing exercises is *Growing Stronger: Strength Training for Older Adults*. Look for the interactive Growing Stronger Programme as well as the book itself at www.nutrition.tufts.edu/growing

stronger/. You can download the book for free or purchase a copy at the site. Two other useful resources include the American College of Sports Medicine at www .ACSM.org or 800-486-5643 and the National Strength and Conditioning Association at www. ACEFITNESS.org or 800-825-3636.

Tai chi is an excellent form of exercise for middle-aged people and seniors. Consisting of a series of gentle postures combined in slow, continuous movements, tai chi emphasizes deep, diaphragmatic breathing and relaxation. It's a low-intensity exercise that claims to develop balance and coordination, and helps maintain strength and emotional health. Tai chi promotes good health, memory, concentration, balance and flexibility, and is also said to improve psychological conditions such as anxiety, depression and the negative health developments normally associated with ageing and a sedentary lifestyle. Tai chi has also been shown to improve balance and reduce falls in elderly people. It definitely conveys the benefits of an aerobic activity in a very appealing format. In one interesting study, people who practised tai chi for twelve weeks even enjoyed an impressive drop in blood pressure. One of the big pluses of tai chi is that it has a high adherence rate – few people drop out once they experience the pleasure and health benefits of this graceful exercise programme. Check to see if there's a tai chi class at your local Y or adult education centre; health club; college or university; city recreation department; or local martial-arts school.

It's especially encouraging for older people to know that even if they have periods of inactivity, they'll still benefit from any effort they put into strength training. (See 'Resistance Training', page 63, for more information on this.)

Back pain keeping you from exercising? Cross that excuse off your list. Many people, including doctors, are fearful that exercise will cause excessive wear on spinal structures and thus encourage back pain. In fact, research has shown that exercise has no effect on the development of back pain and that trunk muscles in lower-back-pain patients are frequently weaker than in healthy individuals. Indeed, exercise can reverse back impairments and result in a more functional, pain-free back. If you suffer from back pain, ask your health care professional about stretching and strengthening exercises. Researchers at Harvard Medical School report the average reduction in back pain with this type of strengthening treatment is 35 percent. They note improvements in 80 percent of patients. Start slowly and keep at it; as muscles strengthen, your pain will likely decrease.

Especially for Parents

Mum and Dad, you are probably aware of the sad truth: Our kids are couch potatoes. Many of them have become still lifes. What most parents are unaware of is the fact that their kids are facing future health problems of major proportions if their sedentary lifestyles are not abandoned. As parents, we must make every effort to ensure that our children incorporate plenty of physical activity in their daily lives. The best way to do this is to set a good example. Be active yourself and encourage your kids to be active with you. Turn off the TV and go for a bike ride or a walk or a hike.

In 1999, 14 percent of American adolescents aged twelve to nineteen were overweight. This is three times the number of overweight adolescents we saw two decades ago. The Centers for Disease Control and Prevention, the Atlanta-based arm of the federal government charged with the nation's public health, has published research showing that 60 percent of overweight five- to ten-year-old children already have at least one risk factor for chronic disease: elevated fats in the bloodstream, elevated blood pressure or high insulin levels. Type II diabetes, formerly known as adult-onset diabetes, is now affecting children and adolescents. This is an absolute disaster, as the complications of this serious disease include cardiovascular disease, organ damage, vision problems and amputations. As people develop diabetes at younger and younger ages, the complications will ultimately take a toll on younger and younger people.

The tough truth for parents today is that electronic media are more popular than time spent playing outdoors. There is some positive news: There are **video games** that promote movement. The EyeToy series by Sony has a motion-tracking camera and players move their bodies to make screen characters do the same. Similarly, players of the Spider-Man 2 Web Action Video Gaming System must move their bodies to move characters on-screen. Dance Dance Revolution is a floor pad with lighted arrows to show where to step to music. I know some adults who exercise to this.

Of course, an obvious problem with inactive children is obesity. An obese child may not be concerned about future health issues, but will certainly be concerned with the social issues that arise from being overweight. Social discrimination can cause low self-esteem and depression at a particularly critical time in a child's life.

Encouraging exercise, along with healthy eating habits, is a crucial step that all parents should take to preserve their children's future health. Here are some simple steps you can take to become a family on the move:

- Keep in mind that kids should be physically active about sixty minutes each day.
- Encourage your kids to participate in sports for fun. Eliminate the pressure; emphasize the joy.
- Be active yourself. Be a role model.
- Plan active family outings. Hiking, bike riding and ball playing are great ways to spend time together.
- Limit TV and video/computer-game time. These two nonactivities are the biggest drains on kids' time and the biggest encouragements to a sedentary lifestyle. Forty-three percent of teens watch more than two hours of TV daily. Encourage alternative activities.
- Provide a safe environment for your children and their friends to play actively. Provide healthy snacks and drinks, sports equipment and encouragement.
- Don't drive them everywhere. Whenever possible, safe and practical, encourage your kids to walk or ride their bikes to friends' houses and/or school.

Promote safe places to exercise in your community, such as bike paths, running paths, walking trails. Find out if school facilities can be used by the community for activities like adult basketball, football, volleyball, and other exercise activities.

Use Your Head

I hope you're convinced that you need to exercise. Before you move a muscle, however, I want you to use your brain. It's your best asset when it comes to exercise, because success in changing your habits is all about motivation. You've probably heard that roughly 50 percent of people who begin an exercise programme drop out in the first six months. This usually is not because their bodies stopped working (due to injury, for example), but rather because their motivation dried up. Don't let that happen to you. In one study, the single most important factor that kept people on track with their exercise was that they made it a priority. Interestingly, the people in this study did not focus on their physical appearance nearly as much as on their desire to be fit. I have found this to be true with my patients. The people who are most interested in achieving their best HealthStyle seem to be the ones who manage to stick with their resolutions; those who are focused largely on their appearance often get discouraged when and if they don't see immediate results and they quit.

Exercise improves Fido, too! A very interesting recent study showed that older dogs were able to learn new tricks – with the help of improved diet and exercise. The forty-eight beagles in the study were divided into four groups that got either standard care; a diet supplemented with food-derived antioxidants and supplements; standard care plus exercise; or a special supplemented diet plus the extra play and exercise routine. The older dogs clearly benefited most from the supplemental diet and exercise programme. All twelve of the older beagles who got the SuperDog diet and the SuperDog exercise routine could solve a difficult problem compared with eight to ten dogs that got only the enriched diet and two of eight dogs who got no special treatment.

Your New HealthStyle Exercise ERA

I wish I could tell you exactly what to do in terms of exercise. If there were one, single, ideal exercise programme, believe me, I'd tell you. But people and lifestyles are too varied. Actually, that's the fun of it. You have to find activities that suit you – ones you actually enjoy. Pleasure is a great motivator. You have to exercise at a time of day that works for you. With a friend? Alone? With your dog? Doesn't matter. All that matters is that you do it. You don't even have to stick to a single programme. Change with the seasons if you like. Who knows, maybe it was seasonal change that first inspired cross training! Don't feel that exercise is a grind. Sometimes it is, but most of the time it shouldn't be. Are you warmed up now? It's time to get down to it . . .

At the beginning of this exercise discussion I told you that I had a new, simple, flexible approach to getting active. Here it is: the HealthStyle Exercise ERA. Extensive recent research has demonstrated that there are three important aspects to an optimal exercise programme, and the HealthStyle ERA incorporates them all:

Exercise Opportunities
Resistance Training
Aerobics

The HealthStyle ERA Programme will make it easy for you to think about exercise because, after all, it begins in your brain. Many of us are confused into immobility. The ERA programme will set you free.

Before You Begin

Consider your overall health. Do you have any particular health problems? Do you have heart disease, severe arthritis or other chronic health conditions? If so, talk to your health care professional before you begin to exercise. Maybe this is the perfect time to schedule a complete physical.

The Three-Pronged Exercise Attack

If you're going to do the best for your body in terms of exercise, you've got to fulfil three goals: Increase your overall everyday movement (Exercise Opportunities), do weight training (Resistance Training) and adopt some level of aerobic activity (Aerobics). If just reading about this makes you want to nap, be reassured: Start with just the first goal, Exercise Opportunities. I've never met anyone who was unable to take this first step. And very few fail to move on to the next one . . .

Think Outside the Block

I've found that the most common single excuse that people use to avoid exercise is lack of time. Do you put off exercising because you don't have a 'block' of time? Why bother to walk around the block if you only have ten minutes, right? Many people believe that exercise has to be done in one relatively long stretch of time. This misunderstanding is keeping too many of us stuck to the sofa. A guiding principle of Exercise Opportunities is that big blocks of time are not essential to achieve physical fitness. While sixty to ninety minutes of physical activity is optimal, thirty minutes a day is sufficient and beneficial. Best of all, thirty minutes of physical activity can be a fifteen-minute walk in the morning, ten minutes of vigorous housework, and five minutes of jogging in place while you watch the news. So don't let limited time stop you from gaining the powerful benefits of regular exercise.

Think you can't get real benefits from this kind of 'scattershot' activity? In one report, the Cooper Institute recruited 235 relatively sedentary men and women for a study called 'Project Active'. Half of the group worked out in a gym three to five times a week. The others were in the 'lifestyle' group: They incorporated physical activities such as walking and stair climbing into their everyday lives. After two years, by almost every measure, men and women in the lifestyle group enjoyed the same benefits as those in the gym group. People in the lifestyle group were even

57

burning the same number of extra calories from activity as the hard-core gym folk and they achieved the same improvements in fitness.

Those who think they have not time for bodily exercise will sooner or later have to find time for illness.
— *Edward Stanley, the Earl of Derby, 1873*

How Much Is Enough?

Sixty minutes of exercise daily? Thirty minutes of high-intensity activity daily? Twenty minutes of weight training and a half hour of aerobics? Most people quite reasonably ask, 'How much exercise?' But frequently their real question is: 'How little exercise can I get away with?' Many patients wonder if they can exercise a little but eat a lot better. Or maybe lose some weight and then stop exercising. Or maybe skip exercise entirely and improve their diet radically. Many people who do their best to exercise are completely discouraged when they learn that what they thought was a good exercise programme doesn't come near to a newly announced 'goal'.

How much is enough? This is the simple question that has kept too many people from enjoying the benefits of physical exercise. The 'experts' don't help because, human nature being what it is, if there's any level of confusion on what one should do, it's too easy just to shrug your shoulders and settle onto the sofa with the remote. There has been some confusion about the recommendations for the optimum amount of physical activity. We've heard recent updates in these recommendations from the new Dietary Guidelines, the American Heart Association, and the American College of Sports Medicine as well as the National Academy of Sciences Institute of Medicine. Many people have found conflicting recommendations to be confusing and discouraging.

Here's the answer: Aim for thirty minutes of at least moderate physical activity on most days. That's a baseline goal. Everyone can achieve that. Once that becomes a regular habit, push the bar a little higher. Sixty to ninety minutes of activity on most days is optimum.

For every pound of muscle you build, your body burns an extra 35 to 50 calories a day.

Exercise Opportunities means seizing every single chance you get to move your body in the course of the day. It's a state of mind. You probably know people who are exercise opportunists. They walk to the shops or take a bike ride on a sunny morning. Many people think of exercise as something that they must add to their day in a big block of time – the gym before work or the exercise class in the evening or the forty minutes on the treadmill at some odd hour of the day. All of these approaches are good – *if you can achieve them*. But there are many, many people who have never been able to work exercise into their day because they don't have time, they can't afford a gym, or they simply don't like to 'exercise'. If this describes you, Exercise Opportunities is the answer. Exercise Opportunities is a mind-set that works physical activity into every bit of your day – much like our ancestors did. You don't consciously 'exercise'; rather, you make a concerted effort to move whenever possible. You'll be surprised how quickly the perpetual motion of Exercise Opportunities can add up to real gains in terms of all the benefits associated with physical activity. It burns calories so you can maintain a healthy weight (or simply lose weight) and it builds muscles.

There is no 'someday' on your calendar. Schedule exercise on a real day! How about today?

There are countless ways to create Exercise Opportunities (EO) in your day. If you consider how modern technology has eliminated virtually all movement from your life, there are numerous ways to work it back in. Consider the tin opener. Do you have an electric tin opener? Think of it as a symbol of physical decline! Every appliance that keeps you from moving your muscles is also keeping you from being healthy. Well, I know that's a bit exaggerated. But if you started using your muscles instead of electricity for more of your daily chores, you might well be healthier and stronger. Once you begin to adopt an EO mind-set, you'll see activity around every corner.

The first and most obvious activity is walking. Walk whenever you can. Walk to work if possible. Walk to the supermarket, to the post office; walk the kids to school. Take a walk with a friend, a spouse, a child or a dog. Take every opportunity to get up and stretch your legs. Many of my patients have told me that this simple bit of advice has changed their lives. Instead of jumping into the car or onto public transportation without a thought, they now consider if they can turn their journey into a walk. Remember that life is not always about speed – the errand that takes you an extra half hour may be the errand that's saving your life!

Thinking about cycling to work? In one study, those who did so experienced a 39 percent lower mortality rate than those who did not – even after adjustment for other factors.

Here are a few Exercise Opportunities suggestions. Some I use myself; others have been suggested by patients who delight in finding new ways to spend energy.

At Home

- Use the stairs. Some businesses are even posting signs near the lifts suggesting that workers use the stairs when possible. I always climb the stairs in my building and, in fact, in addition to jogging up three flights to get to my office regularly, I sometimes run up and down a couple of times just to get my blood flowing.

- Do things standing up! If you're talking on the phone, folding laundry or even writing out a shopping list, stand up. If there's a step nearby, do calf raises: Hold on to a banister to steady yourself, put the ball of your foot on the edge of the step, and press your heel downward, and lift yourself up. Repeat a few times for each leg.

- When you walk, walk faster. Pick up the pace and even a short walk can give you a bit of a workout.

- Do housework yourself, with gusto. Vacuum to music. Dust those high shelves.

- Walk the dog. Often. Take him out two or three times a day. Once he's used to this routine, he'll nudge you to keep to it.

- Turn everyday chores into brief exercise sessions: Waiting for the water to boil? The oven to heat up? Do side stretches and leg lifts. I do push-ups against the kitchen counter or steps.

- Don't just watch TV: Use an exercise bike or do sit-ups or use weights while you watch. Keep a set of hand weights right next to the remote control.

- An hour of evening TV has about fifteen minutes of commercials. If you do some sit-ups or weight-training exercises during these ads, you'll be *halfway* to your basic goal of a half hour of daily exercise.

- Carry bags to the car instead of putting them in a shopping trolley when possible and practical. Try lifting them (as much as you comfortably can) with your arms extended as you walk home or to the car.

- Park the car farther from the shop than you'd like! This is an old one but it works.
- Do your own gardening. Rake fallen leaves. Shovel snow.

If you have ideas for more Exercise Opportunities, share them with us at www.SuperFoods.com. We'd love to hear from you.

At Work

Most of the time you're probably sitting at a desk, but EOs abound if you pay attention.

- Get off the bus or train early and walk the remaining distance.
- Instead of meeting a friend or colleague to have lunch or coffee, meet to take a walk.
- While sitting at your desk, put your arms straight out in front of you and grab your elbows with opposite hands. Stretch slowly to the right, then to the left.
- Do seated leg lifts. Sit at the edge of your seat and do five straight leg lifts and five bent leg lifts with each leg.

Don't let traffic slow you down. See it as an exercise opportunity. Pull in your tummy at a red light and hold it till the light turns green. Stretch your neck by dropping your head from one side to the other.

On the Road

Travel can be a special challenge, but it offers its own opportunities for exercise.

- Stay in a hotel with a fitness centre. They're very easy to find these days. Make sure that the centre is open at convenient hours.

- Travel with a skipping rope and use it in your hotel room. This is especially useful if your hotel doesn't have a fitness centre.
- Walk, walk, walk as you explore new places. You'll see much more than you would in a car or on a bus.

Resistance Training

Resistance training, or weight training, is your best friend when it comes to fitness and longevity. It preserves lean body mass. Remember sarcopenia – that loss of muscle that causes countless health problems as you age? Resistance training is going to help prevent it. If you're in your late thirties or early forties, you're probably already losing muscle mass at a rate of about a quarter pound a year. You need to hang on to that muscle or lean body mass. Lean body mass is metabolically active – it burns more calories than that other body mass, fat – and thus it helps you keep your weight down. Resistance training will also boost your bone density and balance – both particularly important as the years go by.

Head Games
Don't feel like exercising today? Take a minute and think about how you'll feel at 9:30 tonight. Pretty disappointed in yourself, no doubt. Turns out that anticipated regret can be a great motivator. In a recent study, folks who took the time to think about how bad they'd feel if they skipped their workout were more likely to do it. Take time each morning to think about how you'll feel at the end of the day if you don't follow through on your exercise plans.

There's another bonus to resistance training. Do you still fit into those five-year-old jeans? If not, like many people you're experiencing a gradual piling on of pounds that seems part and parcel of the ageing process. There are many popular theories to account for this phenomenon, most of which imply that there's no escape from middle-aged spread. Well, those supertight clothes are not inevitable. Your resting metabolic heart rate (RMR) accounts for about 60 percent of your daily metabolism or calorie burn. Starting at about age thirty-five or forty, muscle mass begins to decline and with this decline comes a decline in RMR. A lower RMR burns fewer calories. The end result is that what you ate at age twenty-five to maintain a healthy weight can, at age forty-five, make you fat. Fortunately, there's a simple solution to this: Lift weights! You're not looking to build giant muscles – all you're interested in is preserving the muscle mass of your youth, maintaining a higher RMR and thus burning more calories. Who knows, you might just be able to zip up those turn-of-the-century jeans!

There's plenty of excellent information out there on weight-training programmes. If you're a beginner, check out a few of the sources I'm listing here. If you're experienced, good for you. You probably already know the benefits of weight training. If you're unsure how to proceed, invest in a couple of sessions with a personal trainer or join a group class to get you started.

An excellent website that introduces a complete programme of resistance training is the Center for Disease Control and Prevention site Growing Stronger: Strength Training for Older Adults. Although it's geared for older people, it's useful for anyone just beginning a strength-training programme. *http://www.cdc.gov/nccdphp/dnpa/physical/growing_stronger/*

At the American College of Sports Medicine you can download a brochure 'Selecting and Effectively Using Free Weights' or get a free copy by sending a self-addressed, stamped, buisness-size envelope to: ACSM National Center, P.O. Box 1440, Indianapolis, IN 46206-1440.

Here's a simple, basic programme for a beginner:

- If you're healthy, you can probably begin weight training today. If you're frail, arthritic, on medications for chronic ailments like osteoporosis or diabetes, check with a health care professional or exercise therapist before you begin.
- Get some weights.
- Find a comfortable place to use them. You'll need a chair, some steps or a sturdy stool.
- Wear loose-fitting, comfortable clothes.
- Get started!

How often do you have to do these weight-training exercises? The American College of Sports Medicine would like to see you weight-train two or three times a week. If you can do three, great; if not, make twice weekly your regular goal. It's only going to take you a half hour to forty-five minutes – enough time to watch your favourite show and pause for a drink of water. Schedule one session for Sunday morning and you can talk back to the political shows while you train. Do it again one evening and you're all set.

How Much Weight?

In order for resistance training to be effective you have to keep increasing the weight as you go along. If you've been lifting two-pound weights for a year, it's not bad but it's not weight training. To determine how much weight to lift, start with a low amount. The ideal training regimen is four sets of eight to ten repetitions. If you find on the fourth set that it is easy to complete the repetitions, then you need to start adding weight. So if you can easily do four sets of eight reps using three-pound free weights, it's time for you to move up to five-pound weights.

Aerobic Exercise

This is the last part of the HealthStyle ERA Programme. If you've managed to work on the other two parts, you know you're ready for aerobic exercise.

What is aerobic exercise? It's activity that involves the repetitive use of large muscles to temporarily increase your heart rate and your respiration rate. Aerobic exercise improves your cardiorespiratory endurance, working your heart and lungs to promote cardiovascular fitness. That's the key to aerobic exercise – cardiovascular fitness. It's the reason you do it and the reason it keeps you young and vigorous and energetic.

Cardiovascular fitness is seen by many as the single best measure of changes that occur in the body with ageing. Your cardiovascular fitness normally declines by 8 to 10 percent per decade for both men and women after age twenty-five. That means if you're fifty years old, you could already be 25 percent less fit than you were at twenty-five. That's the bad news. The good news is that it's not that difficult to regain youthful fitness if you're willing to devote a minimum thirty minutes most days of the week to this end. Indeed, while you may never be as fit as you were at twenty, studies have shown that even people in their eighties have not lost the ability to improve their aerobic fitness level.

Deciding to exercise is a Big Decision. It's easier for many of us to make Small Daily Decisions. Decide to exercise today!

Brisk walking, running, swimming, cycling, aerobic classes, stair climbing, aerobic exercise videos, cross-country skiing, hiking, football, rowing, skipping, singles tennis and basketball are all examples of aerobic exercise. If you already participate in one of these activities – excellent! You're looking to a healthier future. If, on the other hand, you're one of the millions of people who don't get enough exercise, it's time to change your ways.

And, yes, I know you don't have time. Few of us have time to exercise if we don't make it a priority. We all have too much to do. That's why you have to be both clever and determined when it comes to aerobic exercise. You have to find one activity you can count on – something you can do easily and frequently and that you enjoy. For many of my patients, that's walking. Almost everyone can walk – outside in good weather, at a shopping centre in bad weather, with a friend or with music or a book on tape. (For more information on walking, see page 135.)

There are many excellent books on aerobic exercise that contain detailed information and inspiration. You'll find a list of them at the end of this chapter. My goal here is just to get you started. I'm extremely happy when a patient goes from zero to even twenty-five in the fitness race. If HealthStyle has helped you get moving, I'd love to hear from you. Get in touch with me at www.SuperFoods.com.

Thirty minutes a day most days of the week is the ideal beginning goal for exercisers, but many sedentary people think even that sounds like a lot. If that describes you, here's what I suggest: ten minutes. Decide that you're going to do some aerobic activity for ten minutes most days this week. Maybe a brisk walk around the block. Maybe it's ten minutes of bike riding or a short spell on a rowing machine, stationary bike or stair climber. Just do it. Look at your watch and go. If you want to continue for longer, great. If ten minutes is all you're ready for, great. Just do it almost every day this week and for the next couple of weeks.

Before too long you'll find that you're ready for more than ten minutes. But don't rush: It's better to get those ten brisk minutes in each day, building up a good physical and psychological foundation, than to do an hour one day and then give up because you're sore or you can't find that much time the next day. Slow but steady. That's what will get you to an active, healthy old age.

What's Aerobic?

How do you know you're exercising 'aerobically'? Patients sometimes get confused about what level of activity is considered to be 'aerobic'. The best way to measure this is to check your heart rate, which I'll describe shortly. It's not essential to know your heart rate, and if that's going to discourage you or slow you down, forget about it and just focus on this: You're exercising aerobically if you're breathing rapidly but can still carry on a conversation, and you begin to perspire about five to fifteen minutes after beginning the activity, depending on the air temperature.

Here's how to gauge your activity level: Your heart responds to changes in your activity levels. When you work harder, it beats faster. Your target heart rate for aerobic exercise is 60 to 80 percent of your maximum heart rate. Most of the time when you begin working out your heart rate should be at 60 to 70 percent of your maximum, occasionally going up to 75 or 80 percent. Here's the standard formula for estimating your maximum heart rate:

Maximum Heart Rate: 220 minus your age in years
Target Heart Rate: 60 to 80 percent of maximum

Remember, aerobic exercise is going to amplify all the good things you do to keep yourself healthy. It will help keep your weight down, it will make you feel optimistic and in control of your life, it will make you strong and flexible and better able to participate in life, and it will reduce your chances of developing many chronic diseases. If you walk briskly just three hours a week – that's a half hour on six days or even four half-hour sessions and four fifteen-minute sessions – you will:

- Reduce your risk of stroke by 30 percent
- Reduce your risk of type II diabetes by 30 percent
- Reduce your risk of heart disease by 40 percent
- Reduce your risk of osteoporosis
- Reduce your risk of some types of cancer
- Boost your immune system

age	Target Heart Rate (50–75%)	Avg. Maximum Heart Rate (100%)
20 years	100–150 beats per minute	200
25 years	98–146 beats per minute	195
30 years	95–142 beats per minute	190
35 years	93–138 beats per minute	185
40 years	90–135 beats per minute	180
45 years	88–131 beats per minute	175
50 years	85–127 beats per minute	170
55 years	83–123 beats per minute	165
60 years	80–120 beats per minute	160
65 years	78–116 beats per minute	155
70 years	75–113 beats per minute	150

Tips for Long-term Exercise Success

The HealthStyle ERA Exercise Programme is the answer
for busy people who need to get exercise into their lives.
Many of my patients have adopted it. Trying an exercise
programme is easy; sticking with it is the challenge. I've
kept ERA open-ended and flexible for that reason, because
a rigid programme, even if it's quickly adopted, may be
quickly abandoned. ERA is more an Exercise HealthStyle:
You live it day by day. It's like eating: You do it every single
day; some days you do it better than others, but you never
stop.

Here are some tips to help keep you on track on your
new ERA:

- If you've been sedentary for a long time, are overweight or have chronic health problems, see your
  health care professional before you begin any exercise
  programme.
- Make it fun. Whatever exercise you choose to do, make
  it a pleasure. Find an exercise buddy or work out while
  watching your favourite movies or while listening to
  books on tape.
- Wear comfortable clothes. It was recently discovered
  that people burned more calories on 'casual' days at
  work. This is probably because they feel more comfortable in their clothes and are more eager to move about.
  Wear walking shoes when you can and you might well
  walk more.

A New Winter SuperFood
Dark Chocolate

A source of:

■ Polyphenols

FOR THOSE WHO ENJOY IT, TRY TO EAT: about 100 calories of dark chocolate daily, adjusting your calorie intake and exercise appropriately

We've saved the best news for when you need it the most. As you slog through the winter doldrums, here's the health update that could carry you through until spring: Dark chocolate is a SuperFood. For many of us, this is a dream come true. The interesting thing is that many people have told me that once they think of chocolate as a food that's beneficial to health, even though they still love and enjoy it, because it's no longer 'forbidden', they're somehow less tempted to gorge on it.

This news doesn't mean that you should toss out the oatmeal and fill your cupboards with chocolate. Pause for a moment and let the HealthStyle chocolate watchwords sink in:

■ Keep your daily dark chocolate intake to about 100 calories per day.
■ Eat only *dark chocolate.*

First, and most important, is the amount of chocolate: You can't eat as much as you want. It's high in calories and eating too much of it can sabotage your other HealthStyle achievements. If you eat excessive amounts of chocolate, *you can gain weight.* Depending on your weight and activity level, chocolate should be a small treat, a little healthy indulgence that will have to be accounted for in your overall calorie intake/activity equation.

When you do indulge in chocolate and you're looking for a health benefit, choose *dark chocolate*. Milk chocolate or white chocolate (the latter isn't even real chocolate) won't do. While both contain some of the beneficial polyphenols (though in lower amounts than dark chocolate), preliminary data sugests that the presence of milk in the chocolate somehow mitigates the effectiveness of the polyphenols.

Here, in a nutshell, is the good news: Dark chocolate seems to contribute to lowering blood pressure, increasing blood flow and ultimately contributing to a healthy heart.

It's a myth that chocolate is loaded with caffeine. While there is some caffeine in chocolate, it's not much. In a typical chocolate bar, the caffeine content ranges from 1 to 11 mg. An 8-ounce cup of coffee has about 137 mg of caffeine.

What Makes Dark Chocolate a SuperFood?

Yes, there's the taste . . . the creamy melt-in-your-mouth deliciousness. But when it comes to health, it's none of the above. It's the polyphenols.

Polyphenols: The SuperNutrients

One of the most abundant phytonutrients in the human diet, their total daily dietary intake can easily exceed 1 gram per day, which is much higher than that of all other classes of phytonutrients and known dietary antioxidants.

To give it some perspective, this is about ten times higher than the majority of our vitamin C intake and about one hundred times higher than our dietary intake of vitamin E and carotenoids. Polyphenols act as antioxidants, anti-inflammatories, antimutagens, antimicrobials, antivirals and antifungals. They help protect our DNA and inhibit the growth of unwanted blood vessels. They decrease LDL-C oxidation, elevate HDLs, promote blood vessel dilation, decrease blood pressure, have beneficial effects on capillary permeability and fragility, work in synergy with vitamins C and E, lower the risk for cardiovascular disease, and lower the risk for some cancers. They also seem to play a role in turning on 'good' genes and turning off 'bad' ones.

Whoever first thought to smash a yellow, hard-shelled cocoa pod, scoop out the cocoa beans meshed in the pulpy inside, and turn them into one of nature's most delicious and versatile foods? We can only be grateful. The cocoa beans that yield the chocolate we love come primarily from Africa, Asia or Latin America. It takes approximately four hundred cocoa beans to make one pound of chocolate. The beans are processed into a sticky paste called chocolate liquor, which is then used to make chocolate products. The humble chocolate bar is the product of cocoa butter, chocolate liquor and sometimes powdered cocoa, which is combined with sugar, emulsifiers and sometimes milk. Chocolate is about 30 percent fat, 5 percent protein, 61 percent carbohydrate and 3 percent moisture and minerals. The magic in the mix as far as health benefits are concerned is the polyphenols, specifically the flavonols.

Flavonols are plant compounds with potent antioxidant properties. Cocoa beans, along with red wine, tea, cranberries and other fruits, contain large amounts of flavonols. Research is now suggesting that the flavonols in chocolate are responsible for the ability to maintain healthy blood pressure, promote blood flow and promote heart health.

Chocolate doesn't just have some flavonols; it has lots. Here's a chart that gives a sense of comparison:

Flavonol Content of 100 Grams of Various Foods

apple	111 mg
cherry	96 mg
dark chocolate	**510 mg**
red wine	63 mg
black tea, brewed	65 mg

Chocolate and Blood Pressure

In the early 1990s, a physician and researcher at Brigham & Women's Hospital and Harvard Medical School, Dr Norman K. Hollenberg, was interested to observe that the Kuna Indians, the indigenous residents of the San Blas Islands of Panama, rarely develop high blood pressure even as they age. Studies indicated that neither their salt intake nor obesity was a factor in this seeming immunity. Moreover, when the islanders moved to the mainland, their incidence for hypertension soared to typical levels, so their protection from hypertension was probably not due to genetics. Hollenberg noticed one facet of Indian culture that might play a role: The San Blas Island Kuna routinely drank about five cups of locally grown, minimally processed, high-flavonol cocoa each day. He gave the study subjects cocoa with either high or low amounts of flavonols. Those who drank the high-flavonol cocoa had more nitric oxide activity than those drinking the low-flavonol cocoa. The connection between the ability of the nitric oxide to relax the blood vessels and improve circulation and thus prevent hypertension seemed obvious. Hollenberg is continuing his investigation. He recently completed a pilot study that found that subjects who drank a cup of high-flavonol cocoa had a resulting increased flow of blood to the brain that averaged 33 percent.

Another interesting study looked at the blood flow effects of high-flavonol cocoa compared with low-dose aspirin. The study compared how blood platelets reacted to a flavonol-rich cocoa drink versus a blood-thinning dose of 81mg aspirin. It seems that the twenty- to forty-year-olds who participated in this study enjoyed similar blood-thinning results from both the cocoa and the low-dose aspirin. It must be noted that the effects of the flavonol-rich cocoa were more transitory than those of the aspirin.

Sip your way to winter health . . . Need another reason to curl up by the fire with a mug of cocoa? In a recent study, researchers at Cornell University found that a mug of hot cocoa has nearly twice the antioxidants of a glass of red wine and up to three times those found in a cup of green tea. Make your cocoa with 1% low-fat, nonfat milk or soymilk and sweeten it with minimal sugar. Avoid cocoa mixes, as they are high in sugar or artificial sweeteners and some contain trans fats. And Dutch-process cocoa is cocoa powder that has been treated with alkaline compounds to neutralize the natural acids. It's slightly milder than natural cocoa, but it has lower levels of flavonols so, for health purposes, stick with natural cocoa.

Chocolate and Atherosclerosis

Research suggests that atherosclerosis begins and progresses as a gradual inflammatory process. It normally involves years of chronic injury to the lining of the blood vessels. As the lining – or endothelial cells – is damaged, atherosclerotic plaques, or fatty deposits, are formed on the walls of the blood vessels. These plaques both impede the flow of blood and can rupture, leading to a blood clot, which could precipitate a heart attack or stroke.

Chocolate to the rescue. The polyphenols in chocolate act to relax the smooth muscle of the blood vessels. In addition, it seems that these polyphenols also inhibit the clotting of the blood. In a 2001 study, volunteer subjects were given a commercial chocolate bar containing 148 mg of flavonols. The end result was that the volunteers showed reduced levels of inflammation and beneficial delays in blood clotting at two and six hours after ingesting the chocolate.

What About the Fat?

Ordinarily, foods that are high in fat would never make it to SuperFood status. Chocolate is the rare exception for a variety of reasons. While chocolate is approximately 30 percent fat, the fat in it, known as cocoa butter, is approximately 35 percent oleic acid and 35 percent stearic acid. Oleic acid is a monounsaturated fat that has been shown to have a slight cholesterol-lowering effect. Stearic acid is a saturated fat, but it does not raise blood cholesterol levels. At least two studies have shown that chocolate consumption does not raise blood cholesterol in humans. Indeed, in one three-week trial, forty-five healthy volunteers were given 75 grams daily of either white chocolate, dark chocolate or dark chocolate enriched with polyphenols. As you might guess, since white chocolate has no chocolate liquor and isn't real chocolate, it had no effect, but the dark chocolate increased HDL ('good' cholesterol) by 11 percent and the enriched chocolate increased HDL by 14 percent. As higher HDLs are known to decrease the risk of cardiovascular disease, the argument for including chocolate in your diet is strong.

Consumer Alert
The amount of flavonols in chocolate can vary widely depending on how the cocoa beans are harvested and

processed. Chocolate producers are trying to maximize the polyphenol content in their products. Watch for new, healthier types of chocolate to hit the marketplace in the near future. Look for those containing at least 70 percent cocoa solids.

Chocolate: Some Buyer's Tips

When buying chocolate select dark chocolate with a high level of cocoa solids. The higher the amount of cocoa solids, the more polyphenols the chocolate will contain. Manufacturers are getting wise to consumer interest and you'll soon notice more of this type of labelling on chocolate. Look for at least 70 percent cocoa solids.

Using Chocolate

The best way to get chocolate into your life – for your health – is to eat just a square or two daily.

Dried SuperFruits

It's winter and the supply of ripe, fresh fruit in the supermarket may be discouraging, but don't give up. Dried fruit can be a good source of health-promoting nutrients, as their benefits remain and are actually concentrated if you measure them by volume. Indeed, dried fruits have a greater nutrient density, greater fibre content, increased shelf life, and significantly greater polyphenol content compared with fresh fruit (except for vitamin C; there's little of it in dried fruit).

It's getting easier to find variety in dried fruits beyond raisins, dates and prunes in local markets. Blueberries, cranberries, cherries, currants, apricots and figs are now more readily available. One thing to think about when you buy dried fruit is pesticides. Some fruit is heavily sprayed with chemicals to prevent pests and mold. Of course, when the fruit is dried, the chemicals are concentrated. Blueberries and cranberries are not a heavily treated crop, but strawberries and grapes (and thus raisins) are, and so I buy organic dried fruit when possible. Avoid dried fruit that has been sweetened with high-fructose corn syrup.

Top-ranked dried fruits are apricots and figs, which share the highest nutrient score. Dried plums are second, followed by raisins, dates and dried cranberries. So don't miss out on the fibre, vitamins, minerals, phytonutrients, potassium and complex carbs to be found all year round in dried fruits. Add dried fruits to oatmeal in the last five minutes of cooking, to quick breads, cookies and other baked goods. Don't forget that raisins make great lunchbox snacks. A recent study suggests that, contrary to what most of us used to think, the phytonutrients in raisins actually decrease the risk of cavities.

Don't think that any chocolate dessert is now a health food. Fresh fruit is still the best sweet treat there is. I enjoy eating a square or two of chocolate as an evening treat after dinner. Even just one or two small pieces are satisfying.

Winter SuperFood Update
Oranges

A source of:

- Vitamin C
- Fibre
- Folate
- Limonene
- Potassium
- Polyphenols
- Pectin

SIDEKICKS: lemons, white and pink grapefruit, kumquats, tangerines, limes
TRY TO EAT: 1 serving daily

Once upon a time, an orange at Christmas was a welcome gift for young and old alike. A bolt of pure, intense colour and sweet tropical flavour, an orange is always a treasure but particularly in the middle of winter. Every bit of the orange is a delicious, healthy treat that should be savoured, particularly in winter when the sources of the nutrients they offer are most limited.

Most of us know that vitamin C is important to health. In fact, we've all heard so much about vitamin C in years past that we've come to think of it as almost an 'old-fashioned' vitamin; it doesn't seem nearly as interesting as some of the nutrients that have captured media attention in recent years. This is a mistake, since a steady supply of vitamin C is crucial to our current and future health because it wages a constant battle against serious diseases like cancer as well as everyday afflictions like the common cold. Did you know that vitamin C is the primary water-soluble antioxidant in your body? It's in the first line of defence both inside and outside cells, protecting against the ravages of free-radical damage. Humans, along with primates, guinea pigs and a few bird species, cannot manu-facture vitamin C in their bodies and thus need constant replenishment of this crucial vitamin from dietary sources. As just one orange supplies nearly a quarter of my daily dietary vitamin C recommendation – along with a host of other significant nutrients – you can see why this delicious fruit and its sidekicks deserve their status as SuperFoods.

HealthStyle Holiday Gifts
Winter is the season of giving, but sometimes, in all the stress of shopping and preparing for the holidays, our own

needs fall by the wayside. Here are some suggestions for how you can keep healthy and relaxed while handling the demands of the season. Put one or two of these on your own gift list:

- A gym membership. Take along a friend if you like. Make gym dates and keep them. This can be the best gift of all, as it will keep you healthy and destressed all year long.
- A session or two with a personal trainer. A really helpful idea if you're beginning to exercise or getting back on the exercise track.
- A subscription to a healthy cooking magazine.
- An exercise video or DVD.
- An 'exercise basket' with a set of dumbbells, an exercise ball, a tape or DVD, etc.
- A pedometer and a book on walking, or books on tape or music to listen to while you walk.
- A healthy cookbook.

It's alarming how many of us are deficient in this readily available vitamin. While the RDA for vitamin C is 90 mg for adult males and 75 mg for women, up to one-third of Americans, for example, consume less than 60 mg of vitamin C daily. This inadequate intake of C could be having serious negative health implications. And the truth is that the RDA for vitamin C is, to my mind, too low. What's a more beneficial amount of C? The optimal daily intake of vitamin C should be 350 mg or more a day from food.

While oranges are extremely rich sources of vitamin C, they also provide other nutrients that work hard to preserve your health, including over 170 different phytochemicals and more than 60 flavonoids. The phytonutrients in citrus include flavanones, such as hesperidin and naringenin, anthocyanins, hydroxycinnamic acids, and a variety of other polyphenols. One of the flavanones –

hesperidin – seems to be the most important flavanone studied thus far, as animal studies have shown that it lowers high blood pressure and cholesterol. These nutrients working together have anti-inflammatory, anti-tumour, antiviral, antiallergenic, and blood-clot inhibiting properties, as well as the powerful antioxidant abilities they share with vitamin C. Here are just some of the serious conditions that the nutrients in oranges work to prevent:

- Cancer
- Cardiovascular disease
- Stroke
- Rheumatoid arthritis
- Asthma
- Osteoarthritis
- Diabetes
- Macular degeneration
- Cataracts
- Birth defects
- Cognitive decline

Once you appreciate the vital role of oranges and their sidekicks in keeping you healthy, you'll make a point of regularly including them in your diet.

Citrus and Disease

Cancer begins in the body long before any sign or symptom indicates the disease is growing and spreading. One instigator of cancer is DNA that is damaged by free radicals. One of the functions of vitamin C is to protect the DNA from free-radical damage and prevent cancer before it even begins. One study called 'The Health Benefits of Citrus Fruits', which was released by an Australian research group, CSIRO (Commonwealth Scientific and

Industrial Research Organization), reviewed forty-eight studies showing that a diet high in citrus fruits provides impressive protection against some kinds of cancer. The evidence seems to indicate that citrus can be particularly helpful in preventing the development of DNA damage and possibly cancer in areas of the body where cellular turnover is particularly rapid, such as the digestive system. Thus citrus shows evidence of lowering the risk for oesophageal and oropharyngeal/laryngeal (mouth, larynx and pharynx) cancers as well as stomach cancers. Diets that are rich in citrus fruits can lessen the risk of these cancers by as much as 50 percent.

There's also evidence that citrus can act to help reduce your risk of developing lung cancer. We know that consuming foods rich in beta-cryptoxanthin – the orange-red carotenoids that are found in high amounts in oranges (as well as in corn, pumpkin, papaya, tangerines and red peppers) – may significantly lower lung cancer risk. In one study, dietary and lifestyle data was collected from 63,257 adults in China over eight years. During this time, 482 cases of lung cancer were diagnosed. However, those eating the most cryptoxanthin-rich foods showed a 27 percent reduction in lung cancer risk. It was also found that even smokers who ate the most cryptoxanthin-rich foods enjoyed a 37 percent reduced risk of lung cancer when compared with smokers who ate the least amount of these foods.

In one study, drinking about two glasses of orange juice a day (about 500 ml) increased the vitamin C concentrations in the blood by 40 to 64 percent.

The same CSIRO study cited earlier also gave ample evidence that citrus is an important factor in preventing cardiovascular disease, primarily due to the folate in citrus, which works to lower the levels of homocysteine – a significant risk factor for cardiovascular disease. The potassium in citrus works to lower blood pressure and this, too, lowers the risk of cardiovascular disease.

Citrus fruit can also help to mitigate cardiovascular disease because of its ability to prevent the oxidation of cholesterol. Free radicals oxidize cholesterol. Only after being oxidized does cholesterol stick to the artery walls, building up in plaques that may eventually grow large enough to impede or fully block blood flow, or rupture to cause a heart attack or stroke. Since vitamin C can neutralize free radicals, it can help prevent the oxidation of cholesterol. One study found that including a glass of orange juice in your daily diet can help reduce the risk of stroke. In this study of over 114,000 men and women, one serving per day of citrus juice resulted in a 25 percent reduced risk of stroke.

In one interesting animal study, hamsters with diet-induced high cholesterol were fed a diet that included 1 percent polymethoxylated flavones (PMFs) – a class of compounds found in citrus peels – and it was found that their blood levels of LDL ('bad') cholesterol were reduced by 32 to 40 percent. This result led researchers to speculate that the PMFs in citrus could lower cholesterol more effectively than statin drugs, and without side effects. PMFs, including nobiletin, are found exclusively in citrus fruit. The Dancy tangerine reportedly has the highest PMF total – about five times the amount found in other sweet orange varieties. Nobiletin and other PMFs also exhibit anti-inflammatory, antimutagenic and anticancer properties. While more research needs to be done on this, it does argue for the value of consuming well-washed citrus peel in a variety of foods.

Arguably the most important *flavanone* in oranges, *hesperidin* has been shown to lower high blood pressure as well as cholesterol in animal studies, and to have strong anti-inflammatory properties. What is important is that most of this phytonutrient is found in the peel and inner white pith of the orange, rather than in its liquid orange centre, so this beneficial compound is too often removed by the processing of oranges into juice.

The vitamin C and other phytonutrients in oranges also seem to be of benefit in preventing asthma, osteoarthritis and rheumatoid arthritis – all inflammatory conditions. Free-radical damage to cellular structures and other molecules can result in painful inflammation as the body tries to clear out the damaged parts. Vitamin C, which plays a role in preventing the free-radical damage that triggers the inflammatory cascade, is associated with reduced severity of asthma, osteoarthritis and rheumatoid arthritis. In one study, diets high in vitamin C appeared to decrease the risk of an inflammatory joint condition called 'inflammatory polyarthritis'. Inflammatory polyarthritis is a form of rheumatoid arthritis. It usually involves two or more joints. Compared with people whose diets were highest in vitamin C, subjects in a study whose diets were lowest in vitamin C had three times the risk of inflammatory polyarthritis.

Interesting recent research on animals shows promise that citrus fruits could play a helpful role in lowering the risk for the development of diabetes. In this study, two of the polyphenols in citrus – hesperidin and naringenin – significantly lowered blood glucose levels. When compared with the control groups, the animals consuming these polyphenols enjoyed a 20 percent reduction (hesperidin) and a 30 percent reduction (naringenin) after five weeks of supplementation. There was also a favourable increase in insulin and leptin levels, and several other studies have shown that people with type II diabetes have significantly

84

lower leptin levels than nondiabetic patients. Remember that lower leptin levels are associated with an increase in obesity. While further studies in humans are needed, it is always encouraging to be reminded that in the natural whole foods pharmacy of SuperFoods there are phyto-chemicals that show great potential to decrease rates of chronic disease, and to prove useful in treating disease.

Perhaps vitamin C is most well known for helping to prevent the common cold. It turns out that the evidence supports this claim. One cup (8 ounces) of orange juice has been shown in studies to help maintain a healthy immune system, which can reduce susceptibility to illness. Studies also report that vitamin C may help shorten the duration or lessen the severity of a cold.

> Citrus peel and the white membrane beneath it is a major source of dietary pectin. Dietary pectin plays a role in decreasing LDL ('bad') cholesterol, glucose and insulin levels. My mother always insisted that we kids eat the white part of the citrus skin for that reason.

The C Solution

Are you getting enough vitamin C? A single navel orange, at only 64 calories, provides 23 percent of my daily dietary vitamin C recommendation of 350 mg or more. (That same navel orange provides 9 percent of the adult male RDA and 10 percent of the adult female RDA.) Remember that the concentration of vitamin C in orange pulp is double that found in the peel and ten times that found in the juice. This means you should make a point of buying orange juice with pulp. But even if you eat an orange a day and drink high-pulp orange juice, you still may be below optimal intake. In fact, only a limited number of fruits and vegetables are rich in vitamin C. Here are the top common sources of vitamin C. Try to make them a regular part of your daily diet.

Vegetables

1 large yellow pepper	341 mg
1 large red pepper	312 mg
1 large orange pepper	238 mg
1 large green pepper	132 mg
1 cup raw chopped broccoli	79 mg

Fruits

1 guava	165 mg
1 cup fresh strawberries	94 mg
1 cup cubed papaya	87 mg
1 navel orange	80 mg
1 medium kiwi	75 mg
1 cup cubed cantaloupe	68 mg

Juices

1 cup fresh orange juice	128 mg
1 cup orange juice from concentrate	97 mg
1 cup Pomegreat	50% of DV*

* mg amounts not available

If you take a vitamin C supplement, it's best to take it in the form of ascorbic acid with added bioflavonoids. Your body can absorb only so much vitamin C at one time, so take it in doses of, say, 250 mg at a time twice a day rather than 500 mg once a day. If you do take supplements, make sure to keep your daily supplement intake below the Food and Nutrition Board's tolerable upper limit of 2,000 mg a day. In my opinion, 1,000 mg of supplemental vitamin C is more than enough to optimize health benefits from this vitamin.

Oranges in the Kitchen

It's usually easy to find oranges in the supermarket. Normally, the oranges, lemons or grapefruit with the most juice will be smaller ones with a thinner skin. Once you get oranges or any other citrus fruit home, store them either on the counter or in the fridge. They'll keep for about two weeks, but don't store them in plastic bags, which encourages mould growth.

Orange juice in a carton will stay fresh for two to four weeks once opened, though the amounts of vitamin C in any carton will vary depending on processing. To give orange juice a C boost, squeeze some lemon juice into it along with some orange or lemon zest.

All citrus fruits will yield more juice if kept at room temperature and rolled on the countertop before juicing. If you have an abundance of oranges, juice them, freeze the juice in ice cube trays, and store it in the freezer. Don't forget to zest oranges before juicing and save the zest to use in a variety of recipes.

How to get citrus into your daily life:

■ Eat oranges, tangerines or kumquats every day. Keep a few on hand in the kitchen for quick snacks. Slice oranges to accompany grilled meats.

- A spinach salad with red onion slices and mandarin orange segments is delicious and easy to prepare. Look for tinned mandarin oranges packed with as little sugar as possible.
- Grilled grapefruit halves are a delicious winter treat. Drizzle each half with a tablespoon of honey and sprinkle with cinnamon, then grill for a few minutes until golden.
- Add thinly sliced oranges on top of fish before grilling or baking.
- Add orange juice to a fruit smoothie.

French Toast à l'Orange

Serves 4

This is a healthy, low-fat breakfast with a delicious orange flavour. Top with yogurt and honey.

3 egg whites or 2 omega-3 eggs
½ cup soy or nonfat milk
½ cup orange juice
Zest of 1 orange
½ teaspoon cinnamon
4 slices whole-wheat bread, stale

Whisk the eggs until blended, then whisk into the egg mixture all the ingredients except the bread. Soak the bread briefly in the egg mixture. Fry the bread slices in a medium frying pan just until brown. Serve with yogurt topping.

Orange-Poppyseed Dressing

A delightful dressing to use on spinach salad or fruit salad throughout the year.

½ cup extra virgin olive oil
Zest of ½ orange
Juice of 1 orange

Juice of 1 lemon
2 tablespoons honey
1 tablespoon poppyseeds or toasted sesame seeds

Put all the ingredients in a lidded jar and shake until blended. Refrigerate for 2 hours or overnight to let flavours develop.

Keeping Active Indoors

Sure, it's cold and perhaps snowing where you live, but that's no excuse to become a blob. Keep up with your exercise programme no matter the weather. Here are some tips:

- If you're doing housework – vacuuming, dusting, making beds – try to do it to music. Dance music with a good beat will keep you moving and will turn a light activity into a moderate one.
- Double shop. When visiting the shops take a brisk walk around the interior of the indoor shopping centre before you even begin to shop. Unless you're at an enormous mall, this tactic will add ten or fifteen minutes to your visit and, if you walk briskly, you could be one third or even halfway through with your daily activity goal by the time you head home.
- Take a dance class. Many of us are in the habit of going out to dinner as a relaxing activity, but dance classes are fun and can be something to look forward to on a dark winter evening.
- If you sit at a desk all day, you especially need an active break. Set a timer and every hour or so get up and do something. Walk to another office to deliver paperwork or confer with a colleague, get a cup of tea, use the water cooler on another floor, or just go up and down a flight of stairs a few times.
- Borrow an exercise tape or two from the library and use them! Ask the librarian which ones are especially popu-

lar. Ask a friend or spouse or child to do one with you a couple of times a week in the evening.

- Go ahead and watch your favourite TV show. But do it actively. Use a skipping rope during the commercials. (This can be a real challenge: A commercial break can seem quite long if you're skipping!) Lift weights as you watch. Do a few sit-ups and some push-ups. Get the family to join you.

- Ask a friend or family member to commit to a walk/run event for charity. For information on walking events, check out: the Ramblers' Association and the Long Distance Walkers' Association at http://www.ramblers.org.uk and ldwa.org.uk

- Get a large inflated exercise ball with an instructional video. There are endless exercises – sit-ups, push-ups, leg work – you can do with these. There are some good exercises to try with a ball at this site: http://www.getfit.com.au/html/exercises/ball.html.

- Another good option for exercise is the many Curves centres. Check out their website for more information: www.curves.com.

Winter SuperFood Update
Beans

A source of:

- Low-fat protein
- Fibre
- B vitamins
- Iron
- Folate
- Potassium
- Magnesium
- Phytonutrients

SIDEKICKS: All beans are included in this SuperFood category, though we'll discuss the most popular and readily available varieties, such as pinto, kidney, chickpeas, lentils, string beans (or green beans), sugar snap peas, green peas. TRY TO EAT: at least four ½-cup servings per week

Top Exercise Videos

There are so many great workout videos and DVDs available. It's easy to find one that you're going to enjoy when bad weather keeps you inside. To find something you'll stick with, borrow tapes or DVDs from the library and use them a few times before you commit to buy one. Here are a few that most people find effective and fun:

- Leslie Sansone – *Walk Away the Pounds*
- Kathy Smith – *Timesaver – Lift Weights to Lose Weight*
- Jamie Brenkus – *8-Minute Workouts*
- Petra Kolber – *Trainer's Edge Cardio Interval Training* (You need some weights for this one.)
- Kari Anderson – *Angles, Lines & Curves II*

I love spreading the good news about beans. They're one of my favourite SuperFoods for many reasons. Of course, most important are their health benefits. One recent study of older people revealed that those who regularly ate beans had a *significantly lower risk of overall mortality* compared with non-legume eaters. In fact, for every 20 grams of beans consumed daily, they experienced an 8 percent lower risk of mortality. It's not surprising then that bean eaters live longer given the multiple health benefits of the lowly bean.

Here's why everyone should make beans a part of their regular diet. Research has demonstrated that regular consumption of beans can:

- Lower cholesterol
- Combat heart disease

- Reduce cancer risk
- Stabilize blood sugar
- Reduce obesity
- Relieve constipation and decrease diverticular disease risk
- Reduce hypertension risk
- Lower risk of type II diabetes

If the health benefits weren't enough, the practical reasons for eating beans would push them into the top ranks of desirable foods. Beans are versatile and delicious. Stars in many signature dishes from around the world, they adapt beautifully to myriad seasonings and cooking methods. They're great served hot or cold. They're inexpensive and, fresh or tinned, readily available all year round. Beans are a perfect winter SuperFood, hearty, filling, a great addition to soups, casseroles and a host of winter dishes. And you don't have to go out in the snow to shop for them. Just stock up on them when convenient. With a tin of beans in the cupboard, you have the beginning of a healthy, nutritious, delicious and almost instant meal.

An important consideration when exploring the health benefits of beans is that they're an all-star source of vegetable protein. In an era when high-protein diets have become popular, it's important to understand that there are a variety of protein sources, and there is some evidence that eating more meat and dairy products in place of carbohydrates is linked to greater coronary heart disease mortality. In one study of over 29,000 postmenopausal women who were initially free of cancer, coronary heart disease and diabetes, it was found that the women who ate the most vegetable protein instead of either carbs or animal protein were 30 percent less likely to die from heart disease.

Don't forget that fresh beans, like peas, green beans and string beans, which are readily available in both restaurants and markets, are quick to cook and offer the health benefits of dried or tinned beans.

Beans offer a much healthier source of protein. Just one cup of lentils provides 17 grams of protein with only 0.75 gram of fat. Two ounces of extra-lean trimmed sirloin steak has the same amount of protein but six times the fat. We don't know why different sources of protein have different health effects, but it could be that vegetable protein delivers minerals, vitamins, and phytonutrients that promote health, or perhaps vegetable protein has a more positive effect on our hormones.

Beans offer many healthy components with virtually no fat and very few calories. Loaded with fibre – an often-neglected aspect of a healthy diet – they're also a rich source of antioxidants. Indeed, black beans are as rich in the antioxidant compounds anthocyanins as are grapes and cranberries. In a recent study, researchers found that the darker the bean, the higher the level of antioxidant activity. Black beans were the stars, followed by red, brown, yellow and then white beans. Interestingly, the overall level of antioxidants found in black beans was ten times that of oranges.

Beans are also an excellent source of folate, which helps to lower levels of homocysteine. Elevated levels of homocysteine are a risk factor for heart attack, stroke, dementia and vascular disease. Just one cup of cooked black beans provides 64 percent of the DV (daily value) for folate.

Magnesium is another heart helper in good supply in beans. A kind of natural calcium channel blocker, magnesium relaxes the arteries and veins, thus reducing blood pressure and improving blood flow. A cup of black beans provides over 30 percent of your DV for magnesium.

A recent study analysing the antioxidant content of over one hundred different foods found that beans – particularly red, kidney, pinto and black beans – are the highest vegetable sources of these disease-fighting compounds.

Recent studies confirm beans' power to lower heart attack risk. One study that followed almost ten thousand Americans for nineteen years found that people eating the most fibre of the type found in beans – 21 grams per day – had 12 percent less coronary heart disease and 11 percent less cardiovascular disease compared with those eating the least fibre – 5 grams daily. One cup of cooked chickpeas contains a whopping 13 grams of fibre.

The abundant soluble fibre in beans works hard to stabilize blood sugar levels. Beans provide the steady, slow-burning energy that keeps glucose levels well regulated. A stable blood sugar is helpful not only for controlling diabetes but also for weight management. Beans provide bulk with minimal calories. They fill you up, minimizing hunger and maintaining energy levels throughout the day.

One recent study revealed that eating beans – or at least relying on vegetable protein – could reduce the risk for gallbladder surgery. In this study, women who ate the most vegetable protein from sources like beans and nuts were least likely to need gallbladder surgery. While we knew that vegetable protein seemed to inhibit gallstone formation in animals, now there's evidence that it can play a protective role in humans as well.

Beans in the Kitchen

It is so easy to get more beans and other legumes into your diet. You can cook your own, save money, and have the luxury of picking from a wide variety of dried beans. Or you can buy tinned beans and at a moment's notice have a delicious, healthy meal on the table.

If you're a dried-bean fan, you'll have to plan ahead, as most methods of cooking beans require an overnight soaking. You can cut prep time by cooking the beans in a pressure cooker. Whatever method you choose, cooking beans requires very little attention. Cooking them in batches allows you to freeze them and always have some on hand. Beans freeze well in plastic freezer bags. Don't forget to label the bags with the type of beans and the date. When you shop for dried beans, make a point to buy them only from markets with a good turnover. Old beans won't cook up well, and you can waste hours trying to get them tender. If you buy beans from bulk bins, make sure the bins are clean and covered. If you buy dried beans in bags, avoid the ones with powder in the bags, as that can indicate age.

A great introduction to legumes is lentils. Lentils are quick to cook – no soaking required – and very versatile. Add a bit of curry powder to give them an Indian flavour or some chopped garlic, celery and olive oil for a more traditional spin. Most lentils take about twenty minutes to cook in boiling water. Cook up a batch and keep them in a plastic container to eat as a side dish or to add to broth with other seasonings for an almost instant, filling, healthy soup.

Tinned beans are the solution to quick, easy bean meals. The drawback to using tinned beans can be the sodium levels they contain: Some are unacceptably high. Look for low-sodium or no-salt-added beans, which are becoming increasingly available or, alternatively, rinse the beans in cold water, which will remove much of the salt. Keep a variety of tinned beans in the cupboard for a quick meal. It's helpful to mark the tops of the tins with the date purchased so you can use them in order of freshness.

*

Here are some ideas on how to get beans into your life:

- To make an 'instant' black bean soup, add a tin of low-sodium black beans to a jar of salsa and thin it with vegetable or chicken stock. Add oregano, chilli powder, and Tabasco to taste. Mash some of the beans and return them to the pot to thicken the soup.
- Sprinkle chickpeas on a salad for a boost of flavour, texture and protein.
- Mash chickpeas or black beans with finely chopped garlic and chopped red onions or spring onions. Fill a whole-wheat pitta or wrap with the beans, sprouts or some shredded romaine lettuce, and some chopped tomatoes for a packable lunch.
- For a great salad, combine a half cup of black beans, a few spoonfuls of salsa, some diced red onion and diced avocado.
- Roast green beans by placing them in a single layer in a baking tray, drizzle with olive oil, and sprinkle pepper and perhaps some finely diced garlic on top. Roast in a preheated 400°F oven for about twenty minutes, shaking the pan a few times during cooking.

Best Bean Salad

A simple salad to mix up in the morning and serve as lunch or as a side dish to a dinner entrée. Add some chopped parsley or coriander, as desired.

One 15-ounce tin low-sodium black beans, rinsed and drained
One 15-ounce tin low-sodium red kidney beans, rinsed and drained
2 tablespoons red wine vinegar
2 celery stalks, finely diced
1 small red onion, finely diced

1 fresh tomato or ½ cup tinned tomatoes, chopped,
   juice discarded
2 to 3 tablespoons extra virgin olive oil
Salt and pepper to taste

Mix all the ingredients together in a bowl and refrigerate for an hour or two before serving.

Winter HealthStyle Focus
How to Avoid Diabetes

Diabetes, and a national scourge called prediabetes, are both worldwide time bombs that we will soon see detonate. Few families will remain unaffected. We're looking at diabetes in the winter because two important risk factors for the disease – sedentary lifestyle and obesity – seem to be particular winter issues.

If you're over age sixty, you have a one in five chance of already having diabetes. If you're a young person reading this and you think you don't have to worry about diabetes until you're older or maybe not at all, you may well be wrong. In America, for example, one in five people has a condition known as prediabetes, and many are completely unaware of their precarious state in terms of future health.

Too many of us have been lulled into thinking that chronic health conditions like diabetes are easily managed these days with sophisticated drugs. While chronic ailments are managed better than ever before, it's important to recognize the potential severe consequences of living with a condition like diabetes. The complications of this disease can include cardiovascular disease, cognitive decline, stroke, kidney failure, nerve damage, vision loss and even amputation. As the risk of diabetes increases among young people and the possibility of living with the disease for a number of years becomes a reality for many, the long-term physical, emotional and financial devastation of people's lives becomes a huge burden. To live for ten years with diabetes is one thing; to live for fifty years with it is another thing altogether, in terms of both personal cost and actual health care cost. And of course, many people are not so lucky as to live for fifty years with diabetes: It's a significant cause of premature death.

Here's perhaps the most important thing you need to know about diabetes: You can dramatically lower your risk of developing the disease, and you can help control it if you already have it, by making informed choices and adopting HealthStyle as your way of life.

Diabetes is a condition that is characterized by a high level of sugar in the blood (hyperglycaemia). That's probably the most distinguishing fact about diabetes, but what is most important for you to know is that it affects virtually every cell and organ in the body. The old saying goes that a physician who treats diabetes knows the most about how the human body works because this disease affects every part of it.

There are two types of diabetes: type I, or juvenile diabetes or insulin-dependent diabetes, and type II, or adult-onset or non-insulin-dependent diabetes. With insulin-dependent, or type I, diabetes, the pancreas does not make insulin and thus blood sugar levels rise uncontrolled in the body. In type II, or non-insulin-dependent, diabetes, the tissues resist insulin's efforts to control blood sugar, resulting in uncontrolled glucose levels in the body.

For the purposes of HealthStyle, we're going to concentrate on type II, or non-insulin-dependent, diabetes, because that is the type that is becoming an epidemic. In 2000, approximately 151 million adults worldwide had type II diabetes; it's projected that by 2025, that figure will double to 300 million. It's no surprise that the overall rise in obesity parallels the rise in diabetes, as the two are interdependent: Obesity is an important risk factor for diabetes, and lack of exercise is a major risk factor for both conditions. Worldwide, the estimated number of people who are obese is in excess of one billion.

The shocking news about type II diabetes is that it is a rising plague among children. Type II diabetes used to be called adult-onset diabetes, but today we are seeing a stunning rise in prediabetes among our children. Six million American children, or 25 percent, are obese and one in four of these obese children have impaired glucose tolerance. In 1990, 4 percent of American children were diagnosed with diabetes; by 2001 – only eleven years later – the rate skyrocketed to between 8 and 45 percent of children in ethnically diverse populations, of whom fully 85 percent were obese at the time they were diagnosed. (Indeed, the prevalence of child obesity in America has doubled in the past two decades.) This is a sobering figure, since these children could be facing a lifetime impaired by chronic disease.

A study recently revealed that drinking a glass of tomato juice daily could help reduce the blood-platelet clumping and resulting heart attacks and strokes in people with type II diabetes. As 65 percent of people with diabetes die from complications of cardiovascular disease, such as heart attacks and stroke, tomato juice could be a simple step to take to reduce your risk. Look for low-sodium tomato juice.

HealthStyle is your best defence against developing diabetes as well as your best strategy for controlling it if you've already been diagnosed. Of course, genetics play a role in your risk of diabetes, but for most people the single greatest risk factor is obesity combined with a lack of exercise. A 2001 study suggests that up to 75 percent of the risk for type II diabetes is attributable to obesity. The worldwide obesity incidence is the primary precursor of the type II diabetes epidemic. Lifestyle changes really work when it comes to fighting this disease. In one study, 3,234 people at risk of developing diabetes were divided into three groups: Group One received medication (glucophage) to lower blood sugar and were encouraged to eat a healthy diet; Group Two got a placebo and the same lifestyle recommendations as Group One; Group Three received no medications and no placebo, but had 'intensive lifestyle interventions' involving diet and exercise. By the end of the study, Group Three, the lifestyle group, had a 58 percent decrease in the risk of developing diabetes compared with Group Two. Group One had a 31 percent reduced risk. This and many other studies have come to the same conclusion: Lifestyle – HealthStyle – is the best preventive and treatment for diabetes. Yes, making a commitment to eat well and exercise regularly is more difficult than taking a pill, but these behavioural changes work better, they are cheaper in the long run, and the only side effects are positive ones.

Here's a diabetes preventive that you probably already have in the cupboard: A study of women showed that those who consumed 1 ounce of nuts or peanut butter five times a week or more had a 20 percent decreased risk of developing diabetes.

Here's an outline of the steps you can take to help avoid diabetes or control it if you already have it:

- Maintain a healthy weight. You do not need to reach an 'optimum' weight. For many people, a weight loss of ten to fourteen pounds is sufficient.
- Exercise. Countless studies have demonstrated that exercise improves insulin sensitivity. If you're sedentary, our exercise goal of thirty minutes most days is a good start. You don't have to do it all at once. Ten minutes in the morning, ten at lunch, and ten in the

evening are fine. Find time to walk (see page 135). It's the easiest beginning exercise.

- If you're over forty-five years old, get your blood glucose tested and ask your health care professional how often you should repeat this measurement.
- Reduce your fat intake and pay attention to the types of fat in your diet. In general, a high total fat intake and a high intake of saturated animal fats and trans fats, which are found in many processed foods, are associated with a decrease in the ability of insulin to do its job. Polyunsaturated and monounsaturated fats like extra virgin olive oil have much less tendency to have an adverse effect on insulin sensitivity.
- Increase your fibre intake. In one study of 42,759 men followed for six years, cereal fibre was inversely associated with a risk of type II diabetes. Another study found that people who ate more white bread than whole-grain breads tended to have the highest risk of type II diabetes. Follow a SuperFoods diet and try to get 45 grams on a daily basis of fibre for adult men and 32 grams of fibre for adult women. As whole-grain fibre is so good at lowering insulin resistance, aim for at least 10 grams of whole-grain fibre as part of your total daily fibre intake (see 'Fibre', page 195).
- Increase your intake of fruits and vegetables, especially the carotenoid-rich ones like pumpkins, sweet potatoes, spinach, tomatoes, mangoes, apricots and cantaloupes. This will increase your fibre intake as well as your intake of micronutrients that help promote the efficient use of insulin.
- Eat 1 ounce of unsalted nuts daily.
- Get sufficient sleep. Mounting evidence suggests that sleep deprivation can be a causative factor in diabetes. Curtailing sleep to four hours per night for six nights impairs glucose tolerance and lowers insulin secretion in otherwise healthy, well-rested young men. This

prediabetic condition was entirely reversed when these men paid back their sleep debt (see 'Sleep', page 293).

- Don't smoke.
- If you drink wine, beer or spirits, drink moderately. Published studies suggest a beneficial effect of a moderate (two drinks a day for men; one drink for women) alcohol intake. Don't start drinking alcohol to prevent diabetes. My personal recommendation is a maximum of eight drinks per week for men and three drinks per week for women.
- Pay attention to these nutrients:
  - **Magnesium** has been associated with diabetes: One study of women showed a strong inverse relationship between dietary magnesium intake and the incidence of diabetes. Magnesium is found in whole-grain bread and cereal as well as unprocessed foods like fruits, vegetables, beans and nuts. You should consume the recommended 400mg daily intake of magnesium. One ounce of dry roasted almonds has 86 mg, one half cup of cooked spinach has 78 mg, and one cup of plain low-fat yogurt has 43 mg.
  - Studies have also shown there is an inverse relationship between **calcium** intake (specifically) and dairy intake (in general) called the insulin resistance syndrome. Of course, low-fat or nonfat dairy foods are excellent sources of bioavailable calcium.
  - Additional nutrients such as dietary **vitamin E, chromium, zinc, potassium** and **omega-3 fatty acids** have been mentioned as possibly playing a role in the prevention of diabetes.

People at risk of developing type II diabetes are:*

- White people aged over forty and people from black and minority ethnic groups aged over twenty-five years with:

- A first-degree family history of diabetes (mother, father or sibling)
- People who are overweight (BMI of 25–30 kg/m² and above), and who have a sedentary lifestyle
- Women who have had gestational diabetes (diabetes during pregnancy) – Diabetes UK recommends screening at one year after delivery and then three yearly
- Women with polycystic ovary syndrome who are obese
- Those known to have impaired glucose tolerance or impaired fasting glycaemia

*From Diabetes UK

A New Winter SuperSpice

Cinnamon

What could be more welcome and delicious than a warm mug of apple cider sprinkled with cinnamon or a cinnamony baked apple with crushed nuts on a cold winter day? Cinnamon is welcome all year round, but its special warming scent is a particular treat in the winter months.

Cinnamon, that delightful spice eliciting memories of Grandma's kitchen and the comforts of home, is actually more than a delicious addition to foods. One of the oldest spices known and long used in traditional medicine, cinnamon is currently being studied for its beneficial effects on a variety of ailments. Indeed, recent exciting findings on the power of cinnamon to promote health, in particular its benefits for people with type II diabetes, have elevated it to the status of a SuperSpice.

Cinnamon comes from the interior bark of evergreen trees that are native to Asia. The type we most commonly see in the supermarket is cassia cinnamon (*Cinnamomum cassia*). Known as Chinese cinnamon, it has the sweetly spiced flavour we're familiar with. Varieties of Chinese cinnamon come from China and northern Vietnam. There's also Ceylon, or 'true', cinnamon (*Cinnamomum zeylanicum*), which is sweeter with a more complex, citrusy flavour. Both types of cinnamon are available in sticks (or 'quills') or ground.

Cinnamon and Your Health

Today, we're in the process of learning about the power of cinnamon to affect health, and once you appreciate the special qualities of this mighty spice, I'm sure you'll be eager to use it more frequently.

Perhaps the most exciting recent discovery concerning cinnamon is its effect on blood glucose levels as well as on triglyceride and cholesterol levels, all of which could benefit people suffering from type II diabetes. In one study of sixty patients with type II diabetes, it was found that after only forty days of taking about one half teaspoon of cinnamon daily, fasting serum glucose levels were lowered by 18 to 29 percent, triglycerides by 23 to 30 percent, low-density lipoproteins (LDLs) by 7 to 27 percent, and total cholesterol by 12 to 26 percent. It's not yet clear whether less than one half teaspoon a day would be effective. It's particularly interesting that the effects of the cinnamon lasted for twenty days following the end of the study, leading to speculation that one wouldn't have to eat cinnamon every day to enjoy its benefits. This is great news for HealthStylers and points out once again the benefit of a varied diet of whole foods and spices. The cinnamon – and perhaps other spices and certainly many foods – that you're eating today are affecting your health into the future. Cinnamon by its insulin-enhancing properties is not the only spice to show a positive effect on blood glucose levels. Cloves, bay leaves and turmeric also show beneficial effects.

Try to buy organically grown cinnamon, as it is less likely to have been irradiated. We know that irradiating cinnamon may lead to a decrease in its vitamin C and carotenoid content.

In addition to being a glucose moderator, cinnamon is recognized as an antibacterial. The essential oils in cinnamon are able to stop the growth of bacteria as well as fungi, including the common yeast *Candida*. In one interesting study, a few drops of cinnamon essential oil in about 3 ounces of carrot broth inhibited the growth of bacteria for at least sixty days. By contrast, bacteria flourished in the broth with no cinnamon oil. Cinnamon has also been shown to be effective in fighting the *E. coli* bacterium.

A recent fascinating study found that just smelling cinnamon increased the subjects' cognitive ability and actually functioned as a kind of 'brain boost'. Future testing will reveal whether this power of cinnamon can be harnessed to prevent cognitive decline or sharpen cognitive performance.

Cinnamon in Your Life

What does this exciting news on cinnamon mean to you? While it may not be practical to eat cinnamon on a daily basis, try to incorporate it into dishes when appropriate. If you have been diagnosed with diabetes, make a special effort to increase your cinnamon consumption. Almost everyone is a fan of cinnamon, but we may need a little inspiration to get cinnamon into our diets more frequently. A dash of cinnamon in apple sauce, pumpkin smoothies, and pumpkin pudding or other foods is a delightful treat.

■ Sprinkle cinnamon, a few raisins and walnuts, and a bit of honey, if desired, on a cored apple and bake at 350°F for about 45 minutes until soft for a healthy dessert.

- Make cinnamon toast on toasted whole-wheat bread with some honey and a sprinkle of cinnamon.
- Simmer, don't boil, milk with a teaspoon of vanilla and a cinnamon stick for a few minutes. Drink the warm milk with a bit of added honey or pour over hot oatmeal.
- Combine 1 teaspoon cinnamon with 2 tablespoons honey and 1 cup yogurt. Serve as a dip for sliced fruit or as a dressing for fruit salad. Spoon a dollop on top of hot oatmeal (porridge), whole-grain pancakes, waffles or a crunchy cereal such as Pertwood's Crunchy Organic Cereal.
- Combine equal parts of cinnamon and cocoa. Sprinkle on yogurt and fruit slices.
- Combine 1 tablespoon or more ground cinnamon with 1/2 cup sesame seeds, 1/4 cup golden flaxseeds, and 1/4 cup ground flaxseed meal. Use as a topping on cereal, porridge, yogurt, grapefruit halves or cantaloupe. Whole flaxseeds add crunch and fibre, though you get more of the nutritional value from ground flaxseeds.

Winter SuperFood Update
Oats

A source of:

- Fibre
- Beta glucan
- Low calories
- Protein
- Magnesium
- Potassium
- Zinc
- Copper
- Manganese
- Selenium
- Thiamin

SUPERSIDEKICKS: wheat germ and ground flaxseed (linseed)
SIDEKICKS: brown rice, barley, wheat, buckwheat, rye, millet, bulgur wheat, amaranth, quinoa, triticale, yellow corn, wild rice, spelt, couscous
TRY TO EAT: whole-grain foods that contain a daily minimum of 10 grams of whole-grain fibre

When I first started encouraging people to eat SuperFoods, the one food that a number of people resisted was oats, despite the fact that oats had been endorsed by the FDA in 1997 as a food that could help lower total serum cholesterol levels, and especially LDLs. Oats, particularly oatmeal, had at least for a brief time become a highly touted 'health food'. Why the resistance to oats as well as other whole-grain foods? It was due to the two simple words that for a time transformed the way many people ate: low carbohydrates. When the popular low-carb diets swept into the public consciousness a few years ago, many people eliminated all carbohydrates from their diets. Unfortunately, the low-carb craze oversimplified the issue of carbohydrates in the diet and too many people began to equate carbohydrates with overweight. The disastrous solution for many was a simple equation: eliminate carbs = lose weight.

What this equation ignored was the fact that not all carbs are created equal. While a teaspoon of sugar is a carb, so is a slice of whole-grain bread. While sugar, and refined carbohydrates, should be a very limited part of your diet, whole grains – made from relatively unprocessed grains – are a critical component of a diet that will help you prevent disease and promote health. Anyone who eliminates carbs from their diet does so at the risk of their long- and short-term health.

I'm thrilled to see that we have turned a corner in our appreciation of whole grains. The new food pyramid features whole-grain foods, and even food manufacturers are promoting whole grains. Major cereal producers are boosting the amount of whole grains in their cereals, and there is a new 'whole grain' stamp that appears on food products that are sources of this important component of a healthy diet. This is all excellent news for consumers, who will now have an easier time identifying the true whole-grain products.

Whole Grains and Your Health

Whole grains have been part of the human diet for ten thousand years – ever since man adopted agriculture as a method of providing food. Indeed, for the last three thousand to four thousand years, whole grains were a major portion of the human diet. Whole grains are kernels of intact grains that include:

- The bran: a fibre-rich outer layer that contains B vitamins, minerals, protein and other phytochemicals
- The endosperm: the middle layer, which contains carbohydrates, proteins and a small amount of B vitamins
- The germ: the nutrient-packed inner layer, which contains B vitamins, vitamin E and other phytochemicals

Beginning about 1870, a new type of milling allowed for grains to be 'refined' so that only a part of the grain was used in food products like white flour and white rice. The bran and the germ were stripped away, leaving only a starchy substance that was missing many, if not all, of the whole grains' natural nutrients, antioxidants and phytonutrients. Consumption of whole-grain foods plummeted until few people were consuming anywhere near the amount recommended for health. A study in 2000, for example, found that among Americans twenty years old and older only 8 percent consumed the recommended three servings of whole grains daily. A 2003 study of US children and teenagers found that their consumption of whole grains was less than one serving a day.

Does it really matter if your diet is low in whole grains? If you care about reducing your risk of heart disease, stroke, diabetes, hypertension, certain cancers and various other diseases, yes, it does!

Oats to the Rescue

Oats, one of our most popular whole grains, are a true SuperFood. Low in calories, high in fibre and protein, oats are a rich source of magnesium, potassium, zinc, copper, manganese, selenium, thiamin and pantothenic acid. They're also a valuable source of phytonutrients, such as polyphenols, phyto-oestrogens, lignins, protease inhibitors and vitamin E. It's important to remember that with oats, as with many of the SuperFoods, the synergy of their rich supply of nutrients makes them even more powerful than their individual benefits would imply. Oats are one of my favourite SuperFoods because not only are they health-promoting, they're also inexpensive and widely available.

Here is a rundown of what oatmeal can do for you:

Oats and Heart Disease. There's been a fair amount of press about oats and their ability to reduce cholesterol levels. The soluble fibre called 'beta glucan' that is found in oats seems to be responsible for this beneficial effect. Many studies have shown that individuals with high cholesterol who consume 3 grams of soluble oat fibre a day – roughly the amount in a bowl of oatmeal or porridge – can lower their total cholesterol by 8 to 23 percent. Other studies continue to confirm the benefits of including oats in your diet as a way to reduce heart disease risk. One fourteen-year study at the Harvard School of Public Health of over

27,000 men ages forty to seventy-five found that those with the highest whole-grain intake (about 40 grams per day) cut their heart disease risk by almost 20 percent – but even those eating just 25 grams cut their risk by 15 percent. Another meta-study, which analysed data on 91,058 men and 245,186 women who had participated in ten studies in the US and Europe, found that for each 10 grams of fibre consumed daily, there was a 14 percent reduction in heart disease risk and a 25 percent reduction in the risk of dying from heart disease. The bottom line is that the cereal fibre in whole grains appears to make heart disease much less likely – and less serious if it does occur.

Look for two clues that the foods you're buying contain whole grains:
- Make sure the list of ingredients *begins with the word 'whole'*. Look for 'whole' on all baked goods, including bread, crackers, cereals, pretzels, etc.
- Make sure that the Nutrition Facts on the labels list the fibre content as being at least *3 grams of fibre per serving* for all breads and cereals.

Oats and Diabetes. We're witnessing an epidemic of type II diabetes these days, and so it's encouraging to learn that oats can help to lower the risk for this insidious disease. (See 'How to Avoid Diabetes', page 97.) Epidemiological studies have consistently shown that the risk for type II diabetes is decreased with the consumption of whole grains. Recently, researchers have learned that the same soluble fibre that reduces cholesterol – beta glucan – also seems to benefit people at risk for type II diabetes. We know that people who eat whole grains regularly, especially high-fibre cereals, are less likely to develop insulin-resistant or type II diabetes and metabolic syndrome. In one six-year study of 35,988 older women who were initially free of diabetes, it was found that grains (particularly whole grains), cereal fibre, and dietary magnesium played a strong protective role in the development of diabetes. In another study at Tufts University in the US, researchers found that people who eat three or more servings of whole grains a day, particularly from high-fibre cereals, are less likely to develop insulin resistance and metabolic syndrome, common precursors of both type II diabetes and cardiovascular disease.

Oats and Cancer. There is substantial and growing evidence to indicate that consumption of oats and other whole grains can play a role in reducing the risk of a variety of cancers. We have known for a number of years that there is a link between whole-grain consumption and the reduction of cancer risk. One meta-study of forty observational studies found that men and women who ate whole grains had a reduced risk for twenty types of cancers. More recently, a study at the University of Utah found that high intakes of vegetables, fruits and whole grains reduced the risk for rectal cancer by 28 percent, 27 percent and 31 percent respectively. A high-fibre diet (more than 34 grams of fibre per day) reduced rectal cancer by an impressive 66 percent in this study of over two thousand people.

Oats and Stroke. There is a growing body of research conclusively linking oats and whole-grain consumption to reduced risk of cardiovascular disease and diabetes, but not much attention has been paid to the role that whole grains can play in reducing the risk of ischemic stroke. I'm happy to report that the highly respected Nurses' Health Study offers evidence that whole grains can play a useful role in helping to prevent stroke. In this study of over 75,000 US women aged thirty-eight to sixty-three, it was found that a higher intake of whole-grain foods was associated with a lower risk for ischemic stroke, independent of known cardiovascular disease risk factors.

Oats and Obesity. It stands to reason that eating a diet high in whole grains would help to prevent obesity. One effect of eating whole grains versus refined grains is that the former fill you up. Whole grains are simply bulkier and thus contribute to satiety, or a feeling of fullness. Research supports the idea that a diet that is rich in whole-grain foods promotes optimum body weight. As part of the Nurses' Health Study, researchers at the Harvard School of Public Health followed over 74,000 women from 1984 to 1996, and concluded that women who consumed more whole grains consistently weighed less than women who consumed less whole grains.

Two Top Tips for Boosting Whole-Grain Intake
- Eat whole-grain cereal for breakfast.
- Choose whole-grain breads. Look for whole wheat as the first ingredient and only buy bread with 3 or more grams of fibre per serving.

The SuperSidekicks

Oats are an unusual SuperFood in that they have two SuperSidekicks: flaxseeds and wheat germ. These two foods are unusual because they pack such a nutritional wallop in such small amounts. With the nutritional profile of whole grains, they deserve special consideration and attention as adding these two foods to your diet can make a significant difference in your overall health.

Flaxseeds. Flaxseeds (linseeds) are a SuperSidekick that deserve special attention primarily because they're the best plant source of omega-3 fatty acids. They're a quick, easy way to take advantage of this important nutrient. Flaxseeds are also a powerful source of fibre, protein, magnesium, iron and potassium: an all-round treasure trove of nutrients. Flaxseeds are also the leading source of a class of compounds called lignins, which are phyto-oestrogens, or plant oestrogens. Lignins influence the balance of oestrogens in the body and help protect against breast cancer.

Flaxseeds are available in any health food shop. They're slightly larger than sesame seeds and darker in colour – ranging from dark red to brown – and very shiny. You can buy them whole and grind them yourself, either in a coffee grinder or in a mini–food processor. The seeds must be ground, as the nutrients are difficult to absorb from the whole seeds. Since the oil in flaxseed spoils quickly, it's best to grind them as needed. Some people use a grinder dedicated to flaxseeds, grind them in small amounts, and keep the ground portion in the fridge in a small glass jar. I take another approach by purchasing ground flaxmeal – preground flaxseeds that you can buy in a health food shop – which I keep in the fridge. Sprinkle ground flaxseeds on oatmeal, cereal and yogurt, and use it in smoothies, pancakes, muffins and quick breads. One to two tablespoons of ground flaxseed a day is all you need. This gives you more than the American Institute of Medicine's total daily recommendation for alpha-linolenic acid (ALA, or plant-derived omega-3 fatty acids). Two tablespoons of flaxseed is a safe amount, geared to providing optimal nutrition, and there is no data suggesting that this amount of ALA from flaxseed has any deleterious effect.

The best of all possible SuperFood breakfasts: a bowl of hot oatmeal (or porridge) with raisins or dried cranberries or blueberries, sprinkled with two tablespoons each ground flaxmeal and toasted wheat germ. A great SuperFood summer breakfast is flaxmeal, wheat germ and berries on yogurt.

Wheat Germ

Wheat germ well deserves its status as a SuperSidekick. It's absolutely packed with nutrition. Two tablespoons, at only 52 calories, contains 4 grams of protein, 2 grams of fibre, 41 micrograms of folate, a third of the RDA of vitamin E along with high levels of thiamin, manganese, selenium, vitamin B6 and potassium, as well as reasonable levels of iron and zinc. Wheat germ, like flaxseed, is also one of the few sources of plant-derived omega-3 fatty acids.

Wheat germ contains phytosterols, which play a role in reducing cholesterol absorption. A recent clinical trial reported that slightly less than six tablespoons of wheat germ per day caused a 42.8 percent reduction in cholesterol absorption among the human volunteers in the study.

Like ground flaxseed, wheat germ can be sprinkled on a variety of foods like yogurt and oatmeal. It can also be added to pancake batters and quick breads, sprinkled on baked fish, added to smoothies, and used in many casseroles and other dishes.

Adding two tablespoons a day of wheat germ to your diet can significantly boost your overall nutritional profile and promote your health.

Oats in the Kitchen

Almost everyone is familiar with oatmeal (porridge). It's certainly my favourite winter breakfast. A few of my patients have told me that they make steel-cut Irish oatmeal (which takes about a half hour to cook) in a big batch with cranberries, raisins, cut-up apricots, and other dried fruit, store it in plastic containers, and heat it in portion sizes in the morning for a quick, delicious breakfast. Don't forget about using oatmeal in other recipes such as fruit crisps, turkey meatballs and, of course, oatmeal cookies.

You probably have oats in your kitchen, but you might

want to experiment with other whole grains such as brown rice, pearl barley, quinoa and millet. Here are some tips for getting more whole grains into your diet:

- Make every breakfast an opportunity to eat whole grains. It's the easiest meal of the day in which to include whole grains and it gets your day off to a great nutritional start. Check out the cereals in your cupboard and if they don't contain whole grains, get rid of them and shop for some of the new cereals that tout whole grains as a primary ingredient.
- Use whole-grain breads for your sandwiches. Look for whole-grain tortillas and pitta breads. There are some excellent whole-grain breads on the market that taste great, have no trans fats, and are good sources of whole-grain nutrition and fibre.
- Try the new whole-grain or partially whole-grain pastas that have recently come onto the market. Some are delicious and will give you more fibre and nutrition than traditional refined-grain pastas.
- Substitute brown rice for white rice.
- Purchase whole-grain crackers. They're just as tasty as the less nutritious refined-wheat crackers.

IT'S WINTER: DO YOU KNOW WHERE YOUR VITAMIN D IS?

Days are short, nights are long, and the chances are you're not getting enough vitamin D. A recent US survey found that many adults, particularly those over age fifty, do not reach their recommended daily intake of vitamin D. Many of us are vaguely aware that vitamin D helps preserve bone, but we are now learning that this essential nutrient is also important in protecting us from diseases, including cancer of the prostate, breast and colon as well as non-Hodgkin's lymphoma, rheumatoid arthritis, type I diabetes, macular degeneration, multiple sclerosis, fibromyalgia, gingivitis and muscle aches and pains in elderly people.

Vitamin D is vital in various bodily processes. It maintains normal blood levels of calcium and phosphorus and, by promoting calcium absorption, it helps to form and maintain strong bones. It also works with other nutrients and hormones to promote bone mineralization, which in turn prevents osteoporosis. Vitamin D also seems to play an important role in protecting our immune systems, regulating cell growth and differentiation, and exerting an anti-inflammatory effect.

The Sunshine Vitamin

Vitamin D has a unique feature among essential nutrients: While it's available from food sources, it's also manufactured by the skin and requires ultraviolet light for this process. Women aged nineteen to fifty, as well as men over age fifty-one, eat the least vitamin D-rich food. And, of course, in the winter everyone's exposure to sunlight is limited. Now is a good time of year to check your vitamin D consumption, as your levels of this important nutrient may be lowest.

How Much Vitamin D Do You Need?

America's National Academy of Science set the latest daily vitamin D intake on an age-related scale:

19 to 50 years	200 IU
51 to 70 years	400 IU
71 and above	600 IU

My own recommended HealthStyle goal is 800 to 1,000 IU daily from food and/or supplements.

To put this in perspective, an 8-ounce glass of milk has

about 100 IU of vitamin D. Many of us get most of our vitamin D from fortified foods. In the 1930s, when rickets were a major public health problem in the US, they began to fortify milk with vitamin D. Today, about 98 to 99 percent of the milk supply in the US is fortified. A cup of vitamin D-fortified milk supplies one half of the recommended daily intake for adults between ages nineteen and fifty, one quarter of the RDI for adults between ages fifty-one and seventy, and about 15 percent of the RDI for those over seventy-one.

Here are some excellent fish sources of vitamin D.

Vitamin D per 100 grams (3.53-oz serving)*	
wild sockeye salmon	687 IU
albacore tuna	544 IU
wild silver salmon	439 IU
wild king salmon	236 IU
sardines (tinned in olive oil)	222 IU
sablefish	169 IU
wild halibut	162 IU

* This analysis was conducted for Vital Choices Seafood Inc. by Covance Laboratories, Inc., Madison, Wisconsin.

Ready-to-eat vitamin D-fortified cereals are also an excellent source. Depending on the brand, they supply approximately 40 IU of vitamin D per serving. As you can see, other than fortified milk, fortified cereals and fish, few foods provide a rich supply of this vital nutrient.

Who's at Special Risk?

Some people are at special risk for vitamin D deficiency:

- Older adults. As people age, their skin is less efficient at synthesizing vitamin D and their kidneys are less able to utilize the vitamin. It's been estimated that as many as 30 to 40 percent of older people with hip fractures are deficient in vitamin D.
- People with limited sun exposure. In the winter, this includes many of us. Complete cloud cover halves the energy of UV rays, and shade reduces it by 60 percent. Industrial pollution, which increases shade, also decreases sun exposure. As more of us use sunscreens that prevent skin exposure to UV rays and/or limit our outdoor time to prevent skin cancers, we can become vulnerable to vitamin D deficiencies.
- People with greater melanin in their skin. Melanin is the pigment that gives skin its colour. Darker skin is the result of more pigment. Darker skin is less able to produce vitamin D from sunlight, so dark-skinned people should consume foods containing adequate amounts of vitamin D.
- People with malabsorption disorders. People who suffer from Crohn's disease, pancreatic enzyme deficiency, cystic fibrosis, sprue or liver disease, or who have undergone the surgical removal of part or all of their stomach or intestines can also suffer from vitamin D deficiency.

What's the Solution?

Try to get adequate vitamin D from your diet. Eat fortified low- or nonfat dairy products as well as vitamin D-fortified cereals. Eat the fish listed in the chart on page 117. Spend some unprotected time in the sun. While it's important to use sunscreen most of the time, a sun exposure of 10 to 15 minutes without sunscreen allows sufficient time for vitamin D synthesis and should be followed by the application of a sunscreen with an SPF of at least 15. When you see the sun shining in the winter, take a brisk fifteen-minute walk.

Tomatoes

A source of:

- Lycopene
- Low calories
- Vitamin C
- Alpha- and beta-carotene
- Lutein/zeaxanthin
- Phytuene and phytofluene
- Potassium
- B vitamins (B6, niacin, folate, thiamin and pantothenic acid)
- Chromium
- Biotin
- Fibre

SIDEKICKS: watermelon, pink grapefruit, persimmons, red-fleshed papayas, strawberry guavas
TRY TO EAT: one serving of processed tomatoes or side-kicks listed above per day and multiple servings per week of fresh tomatoes

Tomatoes are an extremely popular SuperFood and it's easy to see why: They're delicious, and in their extremely health-promoting processed form, they're relatively inexpensive and widely available all year round. They're a wonderful SuperFood to rely on in the winter because, in processed form, they're easy to find and make a great addition to winter soups and stews as well as pasta dishes. Despite their chequered past – they were once considered a dangerous food – tomatoes are now enjoyed in cuisines worldwide. Originating in South America, they were first cultivated in Mexico. Today tomatoes are one of the top-selling vegetables around the world.

We owe a lot to the tomato. It keeps us healthy no matter what, even packing a nutritional punch in foods like pizza and ketchup. Research has demonstrated that regular consumption of tomatoes and their sidekicks is associated with:

- Reduced risk of cancer, including prostate, breast, bladder, lung and stomach cancers
- Reduced risk of coronary artery disease
- Reduced risk of sun-related skin damage
- Reduced risk of macular degeneration and cataracts

Tomatoes have received lots of attention over the past few years due to their rich supply of lycopene. Lycopene is a carotenoid, a pigment that is responsible for the rich, red colour of tomatoes. A powerful antioxidant, lycopene seems to be able to protect cells and other structures in the body from oxygen damage. A number of studies have demonstrated that lycopene is a powerful cancer fighter. It's effective in lowering the risk for prostate, breast, digestive tract, cervical, bladder and lung cancers. In addition, lycopene's antioxidant ability seems to make it an important player in the prevention of heart disease.

It's important to remember that it's the synergy of nutrients in a whole food that usually gives it disease-fighting and health-promoting power. In a recent study, it was found that rats that were treated with lycopene in powdered form did not enjoy the protection of those treated with actual tomato powder. The rats that received the food-based lycopene were 26 percent less likely to die of prostate cancer. Those taking the supplement were only slightly less likely to die when compared with those taking nothing.

Tomato Update

Recent research has amplified the good news on tomatoes. In addition to the benefits already widely reported, here are some updates on why it's important to eat tomatoes frequently:

- Recent studies confirm emphatically that a diet rich in tomatoes helps prevent prostate cancer. In a meta-study of twenty-one studies it was found that men who ate the highest amount of raw tomatoes had a 19 percent reduction in prostate cancer risk. Even one 6-ounce daily serving reduced the risk of this disease by 3 percent.

- Exciting new research shows that high lycopene consumption is inversely related to the risk for pancreatic cancer, a frequently deadly, fast-progressing cancer. In this study, data showed that men consuming the most lycopene had a 31 percent reduction in their risk of pancreatic cancer. Among subjects who had never smoked, those whose diets were rich in beta-carotene or total carotenoids reduced their risk by 43 percent and 42 percent respectively.

- Tomato juice has been identified as an effective blood thinner in recent research. People in the study had type II diabetes. They drank 8 ounces of tomato juice or a placebo daily. In three weeks, the platelet aggregation (clumping together of blood cells) in the tomato juice drinkers was significantly reduced. No change was seen in those drinking the placebo. As diabetes can cause blood vessel damage, which encourages platelets to clump and stick to vessel walls and ultimately leads to cardiovascular disease, it's welcome news that a glass of tomato juice a day has potent health benefits.

A daily glass of tomato juice is a good idea not only for those with diabetes but also for anyone susceptible to blood clot formation. People who have recently had a surgical procedure, who travel long distances by plane, who smoke, or who have high cholesterol might all consider drinking a daily glass of tomato juice. Look for low-sodium tomato juice, and if you find that it is too bland, add a dash of hot sauce, a sprinkle of celery salt, a squeeze of lemon juice or a dash of seasoning to improve the taste.

- An impressive body of research confirms the protective nature of tomato-based foods in the prevention of cardiovascular disease. One study published recently followed 39,876 middle-aged and older women who were free of both cancer and cardiovascular disease at the start of the study. After more than seven years of follow-up, those who consumed seven to ten servings each week of lycopene-rich foods were found to have a 29 percent lower risk of cardiovascular disease compared with women who ate fewer than 1.5 servings of tomato foods weekly.

I've always recommended ketchup as an excellent source of lycopene. (It's nice to be able to tell kids, in particular, that there's at least one healthy food at fast-food restaurants!) It turns out that you'll boost your lycopene intake considerably if you buy organic ketchup. In a recent comparison study, it was found that a sample of regular ketchup contained approximately 59 mcg (micrograms) of lycopene per gram while the sample of organic ketchup contained about three times that amount, or about 183 mcg per gram. If you rarely use ketchup, this difference probably won't matter. But if, like many families with children, you use a fair amount of it, it may well be worth getting the extra nutritional benefits of organic ketchup.

While tomato is a major SuperFood, I'd like to call attention to the benefits of its sidekicks watermelon and pink grapefruit. Don't forget that both these delicious fruits are rich in the disease-fighter lycopene. Some experts say that red watermelon is an even richer source of lycopene than tomatoes. It's interesting that nature has provided an all-year-round source of this important nutrient: In the winter, we rely on tomatoes in pasta sauces, soups and stews, while in warmer weather, we enjoy watermelon. Pink grapefruit is delicious all year round. Remember that lycopene needs some dietary fat to be absorbed. This isn't as difficult with tomatoes, as we often eat them with olive oil, but grapefruit and watermelon may take some special effort. When eating grapefruit, follow with a slice of whole-grain toast topped with mashed avocado and a few drops of hot sauce. Enjoy watermelon as a dessert following a meal that has included some healthy fat.

ENJOYING TOMATOES

Although processed tomatoes have greater health benefits than fresh tomatoes, both offer enough pluses to be enjoyed frequently. Remember, tomato skin, like the skin of many other fruits and vegetables, is a powerhouse of nutrients. Given this, it stands to reason that the tomato with the most skin per volume of fruit would be the best, and that's true. Fortunately, the cherry tomato wins the contest, and best of all, these little beauties are available all year round.

Here are some ideas for using tomatoes in your kitchen:

- Roasted cherry tomatoes become sweet as their moisture is removed. Place washed cherry tomatoes in a single layer on a foil-lined baking tray. Drizzle them with extra virgin olive oil and some sliced garlic and bake in a preheated 300°F oven for two hours until they are shrivelled. Transfer to a lidded container and store in the refrigerator until needed. Spread a few on whole-wheat bread with some mashed avocado.

- Spread some tomato-based salsa on top of boneless chicken or turkey parts and bake until done. Sprinkle with a bit of grated mild cheddar at the end of cooking, if desired, and serve with a sprinkle of chopped coriander.

- Tomato paste (purée) is a health food wonder. Since it is particularly rich in lycopene, use it in sauces, soups and stews to boost their nutrient content.

- To make huevos rancheros, sauté chopped onions in a tablespoon of extra virgin olive oil until golden. Add some tinned diced tomatoes and cook until most of the liquid has evaporated. Add some diced jalapeño pepper, if you like. Crack some high-omega-3 eggs into the sauce and cook to your liking. Sprinkle with chopped coriander before serving.

WINTER HEALTHSTYLE RECIPES

Mango Yogurt Cream Sauce

Serves 10

Use this fruity light sauce on desserts such as fruit salad or sponge cake. When mangoes are unavailable, make the sauce with ripe peaches, plums, apricots and/or fresh raspberries or blackberries.

1 medium mango, ripe
1 cup nonfat yogurt
1 tablespoon honey
1 medium lime, zest and juice

Peel the mango and cut the flesh off the stone. Squeeze the stone to release the juice. Place all the ingredients in a food processor or blender, and blend until smooth. Refrigerate until serving time.

Calories: 36
Protein: 1.6 g
Carbohydrates: 8 g
Cholesterol: <1 g
Total fat: 0.1 g
Saturated fat: <1 g
Monounsaturated fat: <1 g

Polyunsaturated fat: <1 g
Omega-6 linoleic acid: <1 g
Omega-3 linoleic acid: <1 g
Sodium: 19 mg
Potassium: 103 mg
Fibre: 0.6 g

Cinnamon Maple Macadamias

Serves 10

These slightly gooey nuts make a great topping for oatmeal or yogurt.

1½ cups macadamia nuts, coarsely chopped
1 teaspoon cinnamon
¼ cup maple syrup

Preheat the oven to 300°F. Toss the macadamias with the cinnamon. Spread on a foil-lined baking tray. Bake until lightly golden and fragrant, about 20 to 25 minutes. Pour the syrup over the nuts and stir to combine. Bake for 5 minutes more, then cool on the baking tray.

Calories: 166
Protein: 1.6 g
Carbohydrates: 8.3 g
Cholesterol: 0.0
Total fat: 15 g
  Saturated fat: 2.4 g
  Monounsaturated fat: 12 g

Polyunsaturated fat: 0.3 g
  Omega-6 linoleic acid: 0.3 g
  Omega-3 linoleic acid: 0.04 g
Sodium: 2 mg
Potassium: 90 mg
Fibre: 1.7 g

Super Fruity Granola

Serves 12

Experiment with these ingredients to create many tasty granola (muesli) variations. If you don't have millet or quinoa, use all oats. Use either rolled oats or a rolled whole-grain blend. Apple juice is suggested here, but try other 100% juice blends like cranberry, mango, peach, pear or pineapple. Dried fruits that work well include raisins, cranberries, cherries, blueberries, banana chips, mangoes, papayas, prunes, peaches and nectarines.

½ cup millet
½ cup quinoa
4 cups rolled oats
1½ teaspoons cinnamon
1½ teaspoons pumpkin pie spice
¼ cup sesame seeds
¼ cup flaxseed meal
½ cup sliced almonds or chopped walnuts
1⅔ cups 100% apple juice
⅓ cup honey or maple syrup
¾ cup chopped dried fruit

Preheat the oven to 300°F. Rinse the millet and quinoa well, and stir with the remaining dry ingredients, except the dried fruit, in a large bowl. Stir in the wet ingredients. Toss well, then spread on a foil-lined baking tray and bake until browned, stirring occasionally, about 30 minutes. Stir in your favourite dried fruits. Store in airtight containers.

Calories: 325
Protein: 9.3 g
Carbohydrates: 55 g
Cholesterol: 0.0

Total fat: 8.7 g
Saturated fat: 1 g
Monounsaturated fat: 3.5 g
Polyunsaturated fat: 3.4 g

Omega-6 linoleic acid: 2.6 g   *Potassium: 403 mg*
Omega-3 linoleic acid: 0.8 g   *Fibre: 7.6 g*
Sodium: 7 mg

Black Bean Soup

Serves 4

Homemade beans can be cooked ahead and frozen, allowing you to put this hearty, delicious soup together in 30
minutes. This soup is also good served chilled the second
day, garnished with some plain yogurt and chopped
cucumber and spring onions. Be sure to pull out the bay
leaves before you ladle the soup into the bowls.

2 tablespoons extra virgin olive oil
3 garlic cloves, sliced
Black pepper
1 teaspoon cumin seeds
1 large onion, chopped
3 celery stalks, sliced
Sea salt (preferably Maldon sea salt)
½ teaspoon dried oregano, optional
1 tablespoon red chilli pepper flakes
2 bay leaves
1 quart (2 pints) low-sodium organic vegetable or
   chicken stock
One 15-ounce can black beans, with their liquid
½ cup pumpkin seeds, toasted

In a large pan, heat the oil over medium-high heat. Add the
garlic and black pepper, and sauté until the garlic is golden.
Add the cumin seeds and toss until the aroma is released.
Add the onion and sauté until it starts to brown. Add the
celery, salt to taste, oregano (if using), and red chilli pepper
flakes, and sauté for a minute longer. Add the bay leaves,

stock and beans, raise the heat to high, cover the pan, and
bring to a boil. Taste and adjust the seasonings, adding a
little more stock if necessary. Serve garnished with pumpkin seeds.

Calories: 411	*Monounsaturated fat: 9.6 g*
Protein: 24 g	*Polyunsaturated fat: 6.6 g*
Carbohydrates: 39 g	*Omega-6 linoleic acid: 5.8 g*
Cholesterol: 0.0	*Omega-3 linoleic acid: 0.3 g*
Total fat: 20.5 g	*Sodium: 742 mg*
Saturated fat: 3.6 g	*Potassium: 1,202 mg*

Bean Salad with Orange Dijon and Balsamic Dressing

Serves 8

This makes a great filling for lettuce or flatbread wraps.
Try Kirby, Persian or Japanese cucumbers which are delicious alternatives to the usual cucumbers.

Dressing
1 large orange, zest and juice
2 tablespoons Dijon mustard
2 tablespoons extra virgin olive oil
3 tablespoons balsamic vinegar
Salt and pepper

Salad
1 medium red onion
1 medium cucumber
15 ounces roasted peppers
1 garlic clove
⅓ cup flat-leaf parsley
15 ounces chickpeas, cooked
15 ounces black beans, cooked

One 15-ounce tin pinto beans
1 pound frozen green peas, thawed

Combine the dressing ingredients in a large bowl and whisk to combine. Dice the onion, cucumber, and roasted peppers, and add to the bowl. Mince the garlic, roughly chop the parsley and add to the salad. Drain and rinse the beans and add along with the thawed peas. Stir to combine. Serve chilled.

Calories: 351
Protein: 18 g
Carbohydrates: 60.2 g
Cholesterol: < 1 g
Total fat: 6 g
Saturated fat: 0.8 g
Monounsaturated fat: 3.4 g

Polyunsaturated fat: 1.3 g
Omega-6 linoleic acid: 0.7 g
Omega-3 linoleic acid: 0.2 g
Sodium: 256 mg
Potassium: 815 mg
Fibre: 17.5 g

Pasta e Fagioli

Serves 8

A thick winter soup of pasta and beans can serve as a hearty lunch or dinner when accompanied by a salad and some rustic whole-wheat bread. I like to use shells, orecchiette, whole-wheat penne or farfalle in this soup. Use fresh herbs when possible. You can substitute marjoram for the oregano. Any combination of white beans (cannellini, small white beans, etc.) will work. And, of course, you can use low-sodium tinned beans if you prefer; one tin is about 15 ounces.

1 pound dried white beans, such as cannellini beans
4 pints low-sodium organic vegetable or chicken
    stock
2 bay leaves

1 large onion, minced
3 garlic cloves, minced
2 tablespoons extra virgin olive oil
One 28-ounce tin chopped tomatoes
4 celery sticks, with leaves, sliced
1 tablespoon dried oregano
¼ cup coarsely chopped basil
1 pound whole-wheat farfalle or penne, cooked
according to package directions
Salt and pepper

Soak the beans in cold water to cover for 6 hours or overnight. Discard the water. Cook the beans in the stock in a large pan with the bay leaves until tender, about 45 minutes, skimming off any foam as it forms. In a small frying pan, sauté the onion and garlic until fragrant and golden. Add to the beans along with the tomatoes and celery with leaves, and simmer for 5 minutes. Skim foam as necessary. Stir in the oregano, basil and salt and pepper to taste. Divide the pasta among the bowls and ladle in the soup.

Calories: 382
Protein: 22.6 g
Carbohydrates: 63 g
Cholesterol: 19 mg
Total fat: 5.3 g
  Saturated fat: 0.9 g
  Monounsaturated fat: 3.2 g

Polyunsaturated fat: 0.8 g
  Omega-6 linoleic acid: 0.3 g
  Omega-3 linoleic acid: 0.1 g
Sodium: 1,159 mg
Potassium: 1,437 mg
Fibre: 16 g

Creamy Tomato-Bean Soup

Serves 6

If tarragon is hard to find, use chervil, basil or parsley.

2 tablespoons extra virgin olive oil
3 garlic cloves, minced
1 large red onion, diced
Salt and pepper
2 pints low-sodium organic vegetable or chicken
   stock
One 28-ounce tin chopped tomatoes
One 15-ounce tin white beans, rinsed and drained
1 tablespoon fresh chopped tarragon

Heat the oil over medium-high heat in a large pan. Add the garlic and stir until fragrant. Add the onion and salt and pepper, and sauté until the onion is tender and translucent. Add the stock, tomatoes and beans. Allow to simmer for about 20 minutes, then stir in the tarragon and remove the soup from the heat. Cool for 15 minutes, then purée, adding a little more stock or water to thin as necessary. Reheat the soup and ladle into bowls.

Calories: 213
Protein: 11 g
Carbohydrates: 29 g
Cholesterol: 0.0
Total fat: 5.1 g
  Saturated fat: 0.8 g
  Monounsaturated fat: 3.8 g

Polyunsaturated fat: 0.5 g
  Omega-6 linoleic acid: 0.06 g
  Omega-3 linoleic acid: 0.05 g
Sodium: 681 mg
Potassium: 573 mg
Fibre: 7.6 g

Cinnamon-Apricot Oatmeal Cookies

Makes 2 dozen

If you can't find barley flour, use whole-wheat flour for a more crumbly cookie. Date syrup can be found in your local deli, or bought online via www.goodnessdirect.co.uk. Measure the oil first, then use the same cup for the sweeteners; they will slide right out of the cup. Grapeseed oil is a healthy neutral-flavoured oil, but extra virgin olive oil works well here.

¼ cup grapeseed oil or extra virgin olive oil
¼ cup pure apple juice
1¼ cups maple syrup or date syrup
¼ cup packed dark brown sugar
1 teaspoon vanilla
2 tablespoons apricot jam
½ teaspoon baking soda
Pinch of salt
1½ cups barley flour or whole-wheat flour
3 cups rolled oats

Preheat the oven to 350°F. Combine the oil, apple juice, syrup, brown sugar, vanilla and jam in a mixing bowl and stir well. Stir in the baking soda and salt, then add the barley flour and oats. Stir to combine. Drop the dough by teaspoonfuls onto parchment-lined baking trays. Bake 15 minutes, or until cookies just start to brown. Allow to cool for 5 minutes, then transfer to a wire rack.

Per cookie:
Calories: 150
Protein: 2.3 g
Carbohydrates: 28.6 g
Cholesterol: 0.0
Total fat: 3.2 g
Saturated fat: 0.4 g

Monounsaturated fat: 1.6 g
Polyunsaturated fat: 1.1 g
Omega-6 linoleic acid: 0.7 g
Omega-3 linoleic acid: 0.2 g
Sodium: 30 mg
Potassium: 128 mg
Fibre: 1.6 g

Spring: Season of Joy

Spring, the very word conjures up images of rebirth, rapidly lengthening days, emerging blossoms and greenery, and the smell of freshness. Spring is a season of joy. The world is once again reborn. It's also a season of focus and energy. It's a time when we undertake new beginnings, a time when we act on the ruminations of winter and seize control of our lives. If we want to reap an autumn harvest, now is the time to plant. It's a time to savour nature and once again feel our connection to the natural changes that are happening around us. Walking is a wonderful way to achieve this, and we'll look at walking as an excellent form of exercise, particularly in spring.

It's time to shrug off the inertia of winter and embrace the energy of a new HealthStyle, a new selection of SuperFoods, and a new opportunity to improve our spirits by taking action.

Spring is on our side: We know that the improving weather boosts our mood. A recent study that involved more than six hundred participants found that people who were randomly assigned to be outdoors during warm and sunny days showed improved mood and memory compared with people who were outside when the weather was not pleasant and compared with participants who spent the time inside. For weather to improve mood, subjects needed to spend at least thirty minutes outside in warm, sunny weather. Here's the key: You must spend time outdoors. You won't enjoy the benefits of the improving weather if you sit at your desk and look out of the window. In fact, in the study mentioned above, researchers found that, contrary to their initial expectations, spending time indoors when the weather outside was pleasant actually decreased mood and narrowed cognitive style. As most of us spend over 90 percent of our time indoors, we've lost out on the natural healthy advantages that wait just outside our front doors.

It shouldn't be surprising that weather and seasons affect human behaviour, given that humans have evolved with seasonal and weather changes since the dawn of man. The point of HealthStyle is to take advantage of nature. Savour it. Use the boost in mood and memory to help you establish new, healthy habits this spring. Begin a walking programme. Fill your fridge with the fresh greens and vegetables of spring. Get active. Encourage your friends and family to become active. Let this spring be the season of your renewal.

Laugh out loud. It's good for your heart. Studies have shown that laughter may reduce the risk of coronary heart disease. In one study, researchers measured three hundred subjects' propensity to laugh in a variety of everyday situations. It was found that, compared with the control group, people who suffer from coronary heart disease were significantly less likely to experience laughter during daily activities, surprise situations, or social interactions, leading researchers to propose that the inclination to laughter may be cardioprotective.

Walking

The weather is improving. The days are a little longer. You're feeling a burst of energy and it's time to take advantage of it all: Start walking! The benefits of exercise are legion. If you're in doubt, read 'Exercise' (page 32). Regular exercise is a must for people who want to reap the most benefits from their new, improved HealthStyle. But perhaps you dread the gym or you're tired of being indoors or maybe you'd just like to try something different. There's one form of exercise that everyone can benefit from and enjoy: walking.

Walking is a form of exercise that I encourage all my patients to participate in. All it takes is comfortable clothing and a good pair of shoes. You could put this book down and head out the door. It's that simple. On the other hand, if you learn a bit about walking and plan ahead, you will have more satisfactory results, both in terms of health promotion and in making walking a staple of your exercise routine.

The HealthStyle goal of a half hour a day of exercise is easy to meet when you walk. Indeed, if you walk with a friend, you may find yourself achieving the optimum goal of one to one and a half hours of exercise daily. Walking is also a good supplement to any other fitness programme. Walking is a good choice for people who are just beginning a fitness programme or for elderly people who are uneasy about more vigorous exercise.

Many people think that walking for exercise doesn't yield much in the way of results. The fact is that walking briskly for 1 mile (brisk walking usually means 3.5 to 4 miles per hour) burns nearly as many calories as running a mile at a moderate pace. Even slow walking (about two miles per hour) confers some benefits. There's no question that walking at a moderate pace for thirty to sixty minutes burns stored fat and can build muscle and thus speed up your metabolism. Walking an hour a day is also associated with cutting the risk of heart disease, breast cancer, colon cancer, diabetes, osteoporosis and stroke. In a Harvard study of over 72,000 female nurses, it was found that walking as little as an hour a week, at any pace, reduces the risk of coronary artery disease. As you might imagine, longer and more vigorous walks – three or more hours a week – yielded a greater risk reduction. The authors of this study concluded, 'Our results suggest that such a regimen (e.g., brisk walking for three or more hours a week) could reduce the risk of coronary events in women by 30 to 40 percent.' The authors also claim that one-third of heart attacks among women in the United States can be ascribed to physical inactivity.

Walking can help prevent disease, and evidence also exists that it may actually promote a lower mortality rate. A study from the Honolulu Heart Program looked at 707 retired men aged sixty-one to eighty-one. Those who walked more than one mile a day had a reduction in deaths during the twelve-year follow-up of about one-third; walking more than two miles a day provided only a small additional benefit. Even after taking into account other activities and other risk factors, the beneficial effects of walking at least one mile a day was evident. The authors of this study concluded, 'Our findings indicate that regular walking is associated with a lower mortality rate. Encouraging elderly people to walk may benefit their health.'

Shape Up America (www.shapeup.org) has useful information on keeping in shape, including tools to help you assess your flexibility, aerobic level, fitness level, etc.

Getting Started

As with any exercise, a little preparation can yield optimum results. Before you begin your walking programme, it's very important to think of it as an actual 'programme'. If you just take a walk now and again, you'll derive some benefit, but the effects will be limited and you're not likely to stick with it. The most important aspect of walking as an exercise is making it a habit and part of your regular routine. If you get used to walking at the same time every day, you don't even have to think about it; you just lace up your shoes and go. Find a time of day that will work for you every day. For many people, it's first thing in the morning, but you may find that just after work or after dinner works best.

Here are some other tips that will help to make your walking routine a success:

Set a Goal. Walk briskly for at least half an hour every day, or one hour four to six times a week. If it's impossible for you to schedule a full half hour at a time, try to work in that much in smaller stretches – say, three brisk ten-minute walks. Almost everyone can manage that amount, although if you break up your walking, it's more difficult to create a programme for yourself and it may be more challenging to reach your goal.

Choose Comfortable, Appropriate Clothes. It's easy these days to find exercise clothing appropriate to any weather conditions. Sports shops carry a wide range of comfortable, attractive clothes that will make your walking workout pleasurable. Supportive, comfortable shoes are critical. If you have a pair of comfortable trainers, they're probably fine, but if you're uncertain whether your shoes are appropriate or if you're walking on variable terrain, it's worth a trip to a good specialist shop to find a pair that will give you support and will be comfortable. Many types of walking shoes are available that have flexible soles and stiff heel counters to prevent side-to-side motion. Warm-weather clothing is easy: shorts and a T-shirt. For cooler weather, you'll want to dress in layers, so investigate fleece for outer layers and fabrics that dry perspiration from the skin as the best choice for a base layer of clothing.

If walking is your primary physical activity, add some simple weight-training exercises a few times a week to your programme (see page 63). Weight training will help you work muscles that don't get used in walking, increase the strength of your musculoskeletal system, and help you to amplify all the health benefits you get from walking.

Make Sure Your Walking Site is Safe and Well Lit. Particularly at night or at dusk, you should make sure your walking site is populated and/or well lit, and that you wear reflective clothing. Walking with a friend is the best choice at night no matter where you walk. Avoid uneven terrain that could cause falls, particularly if you're elderly or if you walk alone.

Walk with a Friend. For some people, walking with a buddy keeps them honest: They won't skip their workout so as not to disappoint their friend. This is a very effective technique not only for sticking with your programme but also for enjoying it more. Chatting with a friend can make the time fly by, and you may find that you're covering even more distance than you'd planned. The buddy can have four legs too. Dogs generally insist on a daily walk and will be delighted with any extra walks they're offered. Many of my patients tell me that their dogs force them outside regularly, and they are grateful for this.

Listen to Books on Tape or Your Favourite Music While You Walk. Either of these two techniques can make your walking time speed by and be twice as pleasurable.

Vary Your Terrain. Walking up and down hills varies the muscles used for your workout. Walking on grass or gravel burns more calories than walking on a track, and walking on sand increases caloric expenditure by almost half. Walking on a track is easiest on your joints and also makes it easy to judge distance.

Pay Attention to Speed and Stride. If brisk walking usually means 3.5 to 4 miles per hour and your goal is a half hour of brisk walking, aim for covering about 2 miles in a half hour. Work out this amount by using a track or, if you don't use a track, drive the distance using your car's milometer to figure out a two-mile distance. Remember that covering more than two miles in that time period or walking more than a half hour may convey more health benefits and will surely burn more calories. Also, if you want to walk faster, instead of taking longer steps, take faster steps. Lengthening your stride can increase the strain on your feet and legs.

Use Walks to Reconnect with Friends and Loved Ones. Walking is a great way to share time with your spouse, kids, parents or significant others at the end of the day or at any convenient time. A walk can be an effective way to enjoy nature, discuss problems and plan the future. One patient told me that her daily walk with her husband helped to keep their fifty-year marriage alive.

Try Walking Sticks or Poles. A walking stick can be helpful for balance, especially for older people or those walking on varied terrain. Enhance your upper-body workout by using lightweight, rubber-tipped poles, available in many sports shops. Walking with poles is like cross-country skiing without the skis. Test the poles for the right size in the shop: You should be able to grip the pole and keep your forearm about level as you walk. Many poles are now adjustable. Nordic Walker, Exerstrider sticks, or Leki poles are three brands that are commonly available. For information on Nordic Walking check out www.nordic walking.co.uk.

Keep a Log. Many people find that keeping a log helps them stick to their goals. Recording the date, distance and time of your walks in a little notebook will help to keep you motivated.

Train for an Event. An excellent way to get motivated is to train for a particular event. Don't think of yourself as a 'marathon man'? You don't have to be. Many events today have categories for people who are walking the course. You'll often find participants who range in age from nine to ninety. You don't have to cover a tremendous distance either; some events, like 5K walks, are well within the range of someone with a few months of preparation, depending on age and physical condition. Check out the Ramblers' Association and the Long Distance Walkers' Association websites for further information (www. ramblers.org.co.uk and ldwa.org.uk).

Take a Walking Holiday. A number of agencies specialize in setting up walking holidays in various areas of the world. These holidays give you an opportunity to slow down, exercise, and see the world while meeting like-minded people or even to arrange your own group to make the trip together. Planning such a trip can give you a training goal as well as a reward.

Ped Power

A pedometer is a motion-sensitive device that resembles a tiny beeper and clips onto your waistband. The recommended goal is ten thousand steps a day. On average, people walk about 5,310 steps in a day, according to a Harris Interactive online poll. That simply isn't enough to maintain optimum health.

Walking ten thousand steps is the approximate equivalent of walking four to five miles. The distance covered depends on the length of your stride.

Many people find that using a pedometer is a great help in reaching exercise goals and particularly walking goals. Pedometers are inexpensive and, while there are variations in accuracy, most people find that just paying attention to how much they move is an eye-opener. I suggest wearing a pedometer for a few days, noting how many steps you're taking. For many people, it's as little as three or four thousand steps a day. Try to add to your baseline total week by week. You may find that adding just fifty steps a day for a few weeks will get you to your ten-thousand-step goal. Many have told me that knowing they needed just a few hundred more steps to reach their daily goal would be enough to get them to take the dog for a walk or to walk to post a letter instead of driving. Wearing a pedometer can be just the encouragement you need to take the stairs instead of the lift, to park a few streets from your destination, and to take a walk at lunch instead of sitting at your desk. Of course, all those steps add up to calories burned, muscles built, and a host of health benefits.

The About Walking website has a wealth of excellent information on everything to do with walking, including charts to measure your progress. Check out http://walking.about.com/.

Calories Burned per Mile by Walking

weight in pounds

speed	100	120	140	160	180	200	220
2.0 mph	65	80	93	105	120	133	145
2.5 mph	62	74	88	100	112	124	138
3.0 mph	60	72	83	95	108	120	132
3.5 mph	59	71	83	93	107	119	130
4.0 mph	59	70	81	94	105	118	129
4.5 mph	69	82	97	110	122	138	151
5.0 mph	77	92	108	123	138	154	169
6.0 mph	86	99	114	130	147	167	190
7.0 mph	96	111	128	146	165	187	212

PORTION CONTROL = WEIGHT CONTROL

Many of us pay special attention to our weight in the spring. We are beginning to wear lighter, more revealing clothes. Summer and the beach and summer activities are ahead, and we all want to look our best when outside enjoying the good weather. Often, when we think about weight and weight control, we think about dieting. Diets can be effective and healthy. I prefer to take a positive approach: Instead of limiting what you can eat, I suggest that you focus on making SuperFoods the largest part of your daily food intake and, instead of limiting food types, limit portion sizes. It's the 'nondiet diet' that can work for a lifetime.

Recently when I was having breakfast in a hotel dining room, I ordered oatmeal (porridge) with a side order of fresh fruit, as I often do. When my order arrived, I almost laughed out loud. The waiter put before me what could best be described as a boatload of oatmeal. The bowl was so large that I could have almost bathed in it. A serving of oatmeal should be about one cup; this bowl contained at least three. Yes, oatmeal is a healthy breakfast. However, eating enough for three people would not make me three times healthier. I'm sure the hotel dining staff felt that they were being lavish in presenting such a grand bowl of food, but in fact these giant-sized portions only make it difficult for those who hate to 'waste' food and/or those who simply eat what's put in front of them as they're being distracted by the table conversation.

It's no secret that many of us eat too much and we pay for our overeating with soaring rates of obesity, diabetes and other weight-related ailments. It's not that we have voracious appetites, but that we've become accustomed to eating huge amounts of food at every meal and have lost our sensitivity to what a portion size should be.

When I started working on this book, I knew that I would have to tackle the topic of weight control. Obesity rates among children as well as adults are on the rise and many people are struggling to lose weight. For many of us, weight control is a significant part of our efforts to achieve optimum health. Diet books are always popular and anything that promises to 'take off pounds' is a sure bet with the public. On the other hand, many people, particularly those who read books like this one, recognize that fad diets and weight-loss supplements won't yield results. I hope that reading this book helps you to understand that extreme modifications or limitations in your diet can have negative long-term effects if your body is being robbed of the nutrients it needs to fight disease and achieve vibrant health.

How can people cope with obesity and/or reduce weight in a healthy but truly effective way? After *SuperFoods* was published, reports from readers came in from around the country and the world. That book was not designed to be a 'diet' book, but many people who followed the recommendations of *SuperFoods* were thrilled to tell me that they were losing weight. This isn't surprising when you consider that the foods recommended in *SuperFoods* – whole, low-fat foods, plenty of fruits and vegetables, lean sources of protein and healthy fats – are bound to crowd out less desirable and more fattening foods. So, shifting to a higher-quality diet will surely show positive results in terms of weight control.

I also know, and readers confirmed this theory, that approaching food with a positive point of view makes an enormous difference. SuperFoods isn't about what you can't eat; it's about what you should eat. This simple fact is tremendously encouraging to people. They don't feel deprived. Their energy is spent on finding tasty, whole foods, not on avoiding 'forbidden' foods.

There was one piece in the weight-loss puzzle missing, however, and it was the one thing that many – even those knowledgeable about nutrition – forgot about. This was the key that would help people finally achieve weight control with an optimum healthy nutrition plan they could live with for ever.

Portion control is the most commonly ignored element of weight control among many people. Even those of us who are eating the right foods are often hampered in our weight-loss efforts due to this single misunderstanding.

It's not surprising that we don't pay attention to portion sizes. For one thing, it seems complicated. How the heck do you judge a 'portion' of salad? Or a portion of baked potato, when potatoes can be anywhere from marble size to baseball size? And food labels can be deceptive. A quick glance at a label might indicate that the food is relatively low in calories. Only closer inspection will reveal that, say, a small bag of cookies that resembles a single portion is designed to feed two and a half people!

Another problem is that most of us suffer from 'portion distortion'. This became apparent when another new food pyramid was unveiled; it recommended five to nine servings of vegetables a day. Many people were shocked. Who could possibly eat nine servings of vegetables daily? Many patients asked me about this and complained that the goal was unrealistic. They no doubt imagined servings like my hotel breakfast bowl and figured they'd have to eat bushels of vegetables a day to comply with the new pyramid recommendations. That's when I knew what the missing link in weight control is for people who are already doing their best to follow a SuperFoods diet. The fact is that many people routinely eat two to three servings of vegetables at one sitting. Getting to nine servings isn't that formidable a challenge. But most people don't really know how big a serving size should be.

Over the years we've grown accustomed to the bigger-is-better notion that affects everything from our cars to our houses to those mounds of mashed potatoes on our dinner plates. We regularly eat in restaurants that serve us the equivalent of two dinners. One recent study found that the portion sizes of many popular restaurants and packaged foods have increased substantially over the past twenty years. Some portions exceed standard recommended sizes by as much as eight times. Many foods and beverages nowadays are two to five times larger than when the items first became commercially available. Chocolate bars, for example, have increased in size more than ten times since they were first introduced. It's got to the point where we'd probably feel cheated if the portions we were served were of normal size.

The Price of Plenty

I'm a big believer in personal choice and self-determination. But the truth is that living the supersized life of steadily increasing portions has made it very difficult for many of us to maintain an optimum weight. Over the years the effect of all those gigantic meals – even the healthy ones – begins to show. Indeed, the average American gains nearly two pounds a year – every year! If you ate just a hundred extra calories a day – for example, the difference between a large and a small potato – you could gain ten pounds a year.

Here's the common scenario: You are served a super-sized soft drink – a mega-42-ounce cup. You drink some of it and are really satisfied after enjoying about 12 ounces – a 150-calorie addition to your daily count. But that giant drink sits there and you absentmindedly sip it until by the time you're ready to toss out the cup you've consumed nearly the entire drink. Now you've sipped away about 410 calories – a whopping dent in your total daily calorie allowance. You didn't really want that much soft drink – or meat or oatmeal or even vegetables – you didn't even really enjoy it, but it was there and so you ate or drank it.

If you've experienced a gradual weight gain over the years, you're not alone. The average American weighs about twenty-four pounds more today than he did in 1960. Why? We move less, thanks partly to all those labour-saving devices, and we eat more foods – fast foods, processed foods – that are high in calories and low in nu-tritional value. However, perhaps the single most important factor is that we're eating larger portions. According to statistics from the Centers for Disease Control and Prevention in the US, the average number of calories Americans eat each day has risen from 1,996 to 2,247 over the last twenty years. That significant increase – 251 cal-ories per day – theoretically works out to an extra twenty-six pounds every year.

A large order of french fries weighs 6 ounces today; in 1960, the only size available weighed in at 2^1/$_2$ ounces.

Many of us don't make the connection between amount of food consumed and weight gain, even though it should be apparent. Indeed, many people think it's more important to cut out fat than to reduce the amounts of food we eat. When the American Institute for Cancer Research asked over one thousand Americans, 'Which do you think is more important in maintaining or losing weight, the amount of food you eat or what kind of food you eat?' a remarkable 78 percent answered, 'The kind of food you eat', and only 18 percent replied that it was 'the amount of food'. This is a serious misunderstanding.

Once upon a time a chair 18 inches wide was standard; today, auditoriums, stadiums and even subway cars are installing new seats that are several inches wider to carry the new, bigger customers.

Here's another very concrete way to look at the problem of portion creep and how misunderstanding portion sizes – and the calories involved – can sabotage weight control. A single large bagel with three tablespoons of cream cheese is close to the caloric equivalent of the following:

3 medium bananas (280 calories)	One large bagel with 3 tablespoons cream cheese
Two slices light bread (80 calories)	
Muffin with 1 tablespoon low-sugar jam (150 calories)	
A cup of oatmeal (100 calories)	
A cup of Cheerios (100 calories)	
Total calories: 710	700

By this measure, the single large bagel is the caloric equivalent of about three and a half breakfasts.

Once upon a time, a bagel weighed 1.5 ounces and was 116 calories. Today's bagels weigh 4.5 ounces and are 350 to 400 calories.

Huge portion sizes are making our lives difficult. It's not that we're stupid; it's just that we don't pay attention. When it comes to eating, most of us are driven by what we see, not by how hungry we feel. Most people eating the giant bagel described above would be full after finishing about a quarter to a third of it; few people would stop there. Large portions encourage you to eat more, and study after study proves it. In one study, adults given a large serving ate 30 percent more calories than when given a small one. Kids are not immune: In another study, children served large portions ate 25 percent more calories. A particularly fascinating study was conducted by Brian Wansink of the University of Illinois. It was called 'At the Movies: How External and Perceived Taste Impact Consumption Volume'. Subjects at a cinema in Chicago were given containers of stale popcorn that tasted pretty terrible. Those who got big buckets ate about 61 percent more than the people who got smaller buckets. When asked to estimate how many calories they'd consumed, both groups guessed they'd eaten about the same amount. What do we learn from this? One lesson is that it's very difficult to judge how much you're eating if the container is oversized. And perhaps the more pertinent lesson is whatever the size of the portion, *and even if it doesn't taste very good,* our impulse is to finish it.

It's time to get control of *how much you're eating* as well as what you're eating.

Get Your Bearings

Do you need to lose weight or maintain the weight you currently enjoy? (So few people need to gain weight that I won't address this challenge here.) Most people have a pretty good idea of where they fall in terms of their optimum weight. If you're uncertain, figure out your BMI (body mass index). Your BMI is a number that relates your height and weight to show approximately how much fat you carry. If your BMI is 25 or more, you're overweight and possibly at risk of adverse health effects. If your BMI is over 30, you're obese and your risk of diabetes and high blood pressure is significant. To calculate your BMI, here's a simple formula:

$$\text{BMI} = \left(\frac{\text{weight in pounds}}{\text{height in inches} \times \text{height in inches}}\right)(\times 703)$$

You can also go to this site, which will calculate your BMI instantly: http://nhlbisupport.com/bmi/bmicalc.htm.

A moderate weight loss of 5 percent of body weight can produce significant health benefits and is a reasonable goal for most people.

Once you know roughly how much weight you need to lose to reach your optimum weight, you have to accept a simple reality that's sometimes difficult to face: You cannot lose weight quickly and expect it to stay off. If you've been gaining a few pounds a year, it may well have taken you ten years to put on the extra weight. If that's the case, you can't reasonably expect to lose it in a few weeks. My recommendation is to not set a timetable. Rather, focus on a more positive goal: eating SuperFoods in proper portions. The weight loss will take care of itself. If you follow the HealthStyle recommendations, you'll be exercising, getting a healthy amount of sleep, and practising stress control. These efforts will help you in your quest to lose weight. HealthStyle is set up in a yearly format because seasonal changes can have both positive and negative effects on our efforts to maintain health. Health takes time; weight loss takes time. Give yourself the HealthStyle gift of a year of effort. I know that if your goal is to lose weight, you will.

You Really Can Do It

Losing weight and maintaining an ideal weight are important goals for most of us. If you are overweight, this single issue can come to dominate your life, affecting countless daily decisions and ultimately becoming the primary lens through which you see yourself. Most overweight people have tried and failed to lose weight. Most of us know that diets don't really work for the vast majority of people – certainly not in the long term. I'm also very concerned about the long-term health effects of many diets. Once you appreciate how an optimum varied diet of whole foods predicts short- and long-term health, it's hard to imagine how you can feel comfortable eating a diet that is extreme in any way.

Here is how you can safely, permanently, healthfully lose weight:

SuperFoods + Exercise + Portion Control

The SuperFood information you need is here in this book. You have the exercise information too (see pages 32–70). If you make time to set and reach goals, you'll look back on the year as a turning point. Give yourself the gift of time – the time you need to be healthy. The final part of the equation – portion control – will take just a bit of focus, but it will be a powerful ally in your efforts.

Portion control really works. In one recent study, controlling portion size was the most effective strategy for losing weight and keeping it off. The study of over three hundred people found that those who included portion control as part of their overall weight-loss strategy – in addition to exercise and healthy food choices – were able to lose more weight and keep it off compared with those who simply exercised and ate healthier foods. Another study found significant differences in weight-loss (and cholesterol and fasting insulin) reduction in women who ate portion-controlled entrées versus those who ate the same proportions of fats, carbs and protein but without portion controls. Both groups met weekly and the non-portion-control group was advised on the recommended number of servings of foods. The study concluded, 'Accurate portion control is an important factor in weight loss success.'

Getting on the PC Bandwagon

You've got to do a little bit of work if you want to make portion control work for you. But the time you put into it in the beginning will pay off sooner than you think. Just remember, you're fighting an entire supersized culture and you won't succeed without a little preparation.

First, you need to learn what a portion size is. Try this: Take out a bowl and pour dry cereal into it. Pour in what you might have for breakfast. Then pour that cereal into a measuring cup. Most people pour out about a cup of cereal. But a portion of cereal is only one half to three-quarters of a cup for most cereals. Pasta is almost always a portion pitfall. Next time you're serving pasta, try the exercise again: Put a portion of pasta in a bowl. Then pour it into a measuring cup. Many restaurants serve about two cups of pasta in a serving. A portion of pasta should be about a half cup!

With packaged foods it's easier to figure out how much you'll be eating because the serving size will be listed on the package. Unfortunately, most of us don't bother to check this information. Right now, pull out some of the packaged foods that you frequently eat and check the serving sizes. Do they correspond to how much you usually eat at a sitting? Following is a list of tips that will help you determine various aspects of portion control, but it's very important that you imprint on your mind what an appropriate portion size actually looks like. Take a few minutes to study this chart:

Food	Serving	Looks Like
Chopped vegetables	½ cup	a rounded handful for an average adult
Raw leafy veggies	1 cup	a fist for average adult
Fresh fruit	1 medium piece	a fist for average adult
	½ cup chopped	a rounded handful for average adult
Dried fruit	¼ cup	1 golf ball or scant handful for average adult
Pasta, rice, cooked cereal	½ cup	a rounded handful for average adult

Ready-to-eat cereal	1 ounce, which varies from ¼ cup to 1¼ cups (check label)	
Meat, poultry, seafood	3 ounces (boneless cooked weight from 4 ounces raw)	deck of cards
Dried beans	½ cup cooked	a rounded handful for average adult
Nuts	⅓ cup	a level handful for average adult
Cheese	1½ ounces (2 ounces if processed cheese)	1 ounce looks like 4 dice

Source: US Department of Agriculture

Check out the pictures and actual sizes of servings on the new food pyramid. Go to the US government pyramid website (http://mypyramid.gov/pyramid/index.html) and in the 'Inside the Pyramid' section; click on the food that interests you. You'll find useful information as well as photos of actual sizes.

Here are some practical tips on how to make portion control work for you:

■ Practise measuring. Fill a measuring cup with the proper size portion of vegetables, rice, etc. Empty it onto a plate so you can see what these serving sizes look like. Take note of how much of the plate is covered; this will help you in the future, even if you only do it once.

- You eat with your eyes as well as your fork, so down-size your dishes. If you're putting a half cup of cereal in a giant bowl, you will feel deprived. Use smaller plates and bowls at home. You can even buy 'portion control' bowls that could be a great diet aid. One set of six pretty nesting bowls that's available online has bowls marked in portion sizes that make serving easy (see www.mesu.us). Of course, you can simply create your own portion-control serving dishes by using measuring cups to determine how much to serve.

- Adjust the balance of food on your plate: A SuperFoods plate is mainly vegetables and healthy whole grains with meat (or fish or a vegetarian substitute) as a side dish. The American Institute for Cancer Research has introduced 'The New American Plate', which offers guidelines about portion size and the balance of foods on your plate. A wealth of material can be found on their website: http://www.aicr.org/publications/brochures/online/nap.htm.

- Don't serve meals 'family style' with platters on the table. It's too easy to continue eating even if you're full when the food is in front of you. Rather, serve food on plates with the appropriate amounts on them. Remember, it takes about twenty minutes to feel satiated. Give yourself some time and you might not be interested in seconds after all.

- Store leftovers in separate, portion-controlled amounts. Consider freezing portions that you won't eat for a while.

- Never eat out of a bag or carton. If you're tempted to eat ice cream from the carton, only buy frozen treats in individual servings.

- If you're eating in a restaurant, consider sharing portions or ask for smaller portions. If the portions are large, make a point of setting some of the food aside and ask the waiter to wrap it for you 'to go'. My wife and I often each order a salad with dressing on the side and then share one entrée. If you simply can't resist dessert, share it with others at the table.

Be restaurant savvy! Some cuisines are notorious for being served in huge portions. Pasta, for example, is often served in amounts that would be sufficient for three or four meals. Chinese restaurants serve abundant portions as well. Some studies have found that Chinese food servings can be up to a pound and a half each, which would be enough to feed four people. Keep this in mind when you order in or eat out. Share portions. Don't be shy about asking for a doggie bag so you can finish the meal at another time. Order steamed vegetables and brown rice, and use both to mix with any other entrées to reduce the calorie, fat and sodium content of an individual portion.

- Consider ordering a 'child's meal' in a restaurant. The portion will be smaller and you'll save money. Some restaurants won't allow this if you're an adult but few will restrict you if you're getting the meal to go.
- Tiny crackers or cookies are deceptive: We often eat more of them than we think we are. Be sure to check their serving sizes and count out the proper amount.
- A pitfall of 'single portion'-sized packaged foods is that sometimes they're not single portions at all. Some small-portion packages are actually meant to be one and a half servings or more. Be sure to check the label before you assume that that tiny package is just one serving.
- Consider repackaging food into serving-size packages at home. You probably wouldn't want to bother doing this with cereal, but it could be helpful with biscuits or

dried fruits, nuts and seeds, popcorn or pretzels. If you measure the appropriate amounts into portion-controlled bags or small plastic containers, you'll be less tempted to overindulge.

■ Fat-free and sugar-free foods still have calories – sometimes as many as their full-fat versions – and those calories count just as much. The same is true for sugar-free foods. Many people think the word 'free' means you can eat all you want. Not so: You still have to check calorie counts and pay attention to portion sizes.

Regular exercise is critical to any weight-loss programme. You must move if you want to lose. Check out the ERA exercise plan (see page 55). You'll find it simple to work into your daily life.

Here is a general idea of what you should be eating:

	Daily Servings
Vegetables	5–7 servings; include dark leafy greens most days
Fruits	3–5
Soy	1 or more
Animal protein	0–2
Vegetarian protein	3–6
Healthy fats	1–2
Whole grains	5–7
High-calcium foods	2–3
Nuts and seeds	5 (weekly)
Fish	2–4 (weekly)

The Satiety Factor

Controlling weight isn't always about eating less, it's about eating smarter. The simple unchanging fact is that weight loss is a result of taking in fewer calories. Adding exercise speeds the process. Calories come in all different sizes. If you're eating SuperFoods and watching portion intake, you don't need to be too worried about calories, but there is a trick that will help speed you on your weight-loss way. Satiety is a term that refers to the feeling of fullness after eating. It's the feeling that, if we listen, tells us we've had enough and it's time to stop. If you can promote feelings of satiety, it will be easier to keep portion sizes appropriate and calorie intake low. There is a simple way to increase satiety: Increase your water intake. Foods that contain a lot of water, in general, are low-calorie-density foods; that is, low in calories and high in volume. Think soups and salads. They fill you up, not out. Barbara Rolls has researched and written extensively on this successful dieting strategy. In her books *Volumetrics* and *The Volumetrics Eating Plan*, she outlines how adding water to foods increases the volume you can consume and the resulting satiety without increasing calories.

Others have confirmed this approach. In one study, researchers found that adding a large, low-calorie salad before the entrée actually reduced overall calorie intake. Study participants were served three cups of salad at 100 calories before their pasta lunch. All study subjects were allowed to eat as much pasta as they liked. Those eating the salad ate 12 percent fewer calories overall compared with those who skipped the salad. Over a year's time, this kind of calorie reduction could lead to about a ten-pound weight loss.

If your diet is primarily made up of SuperFoods, you are already getting a satiety boost. Whole-grain foods, vegetables and fruits are all choices that make you feel full.

It can still help, however, to focus on servings of soups and salads before meals that will help to satisfy you and keep you from overeating.

Note to postmenopausal women who are on diets: A recent study found that postmenopausal women who were dieting absorbed less calcium from food than nondieting women. As women over fifty are supposed to consume 1,200 to 1,500 mg of calcium a day, it appears that women trying to lose weight should shoot for roughly 1,800 mg a day.

A Note on Overweight Kids

It's no secret that too many kids today are overweight. A recent study revealed an interesting, sobering fact: For the first time since the early 1800s, life-expectancy gains could be reversed for our children, who may well live shorter, less healthy lives than their parents. Why? Primarily because of the soaring rates of childhood obesity. Childhood obesity is a large and complex topic. Suffice it to say here that parents should not ignore childhood obesity as 'baby fat'. An overweight child needs adult help and support.

A Kaiser Family Foundation report recently reviewed more than forty studies on the role of media in the nation's dramatic increase in the rates of childhood obesity. The report concluded that the majority of scientific research indicates that children who spend the most time with media are more likely to be overweight. However, contrary to common assumptions, most of the research reviewed for this report didn't find that children's media use displaces physical activities. It seems that children's exposure to billions of dollars' worth of food ads and marketing may be a key mechanism whereby media promotes childhood obesity. The report cites studies showing that the typical child sees approximately forty thousand ads a year on

TV, and the majority of ads targeted to kids are for sweets, cereal, fizzy drinks and fast food. Many of the ads enlist kids' favourite TV and movie characters to sell these foods.

If you have an overweight child, it can be a challenge to tactfully help him (or her) to get back in shape, but it's critically important for the sake of your child's future health to do so. You are your child's best ally in this effort. There are many excellent books available today that will give you guidance on how to cope with the physical and emotional issues of youthful obesity.

Use fizzy drinks as a special treat, and when possible, choose diet drinks. Sugar-sweetened soft drinks contribute 7.1 percent of the total energy intake and represent the largest single food source of calories in the US diet. In general, soft drink consumption tends to be a marker for a poor overall diet and an unhealthy lifestyle. One can a day can lead to a fifteen-pound weight gain in one year if the calories aren't subtracted elsewhere in the diet, but studies support the finding that when people increase their soft-drink consumption, they don't reduce their solid-food consumption to balance things out.

So cut out the fizzy drink for a quick, easy way to improve your diet and lose weight. Substitute with sparkling water and a splash of fruit juice or a squeeze of lemon or lime.

Thirteen Ways to Avoid Childhood Obesity

- Strive for a BMI of less than 25 before becoming pregnant.
- Avoid excessive weight gain during pregnancy.
- Try to breast-feed for twelve months.
- Introduce children to SuperFoods as soon as they begin solid foods.

- Make at least thirty minutes of fun physical activity a daily priority.
- Eliminate foods containing high-fructose corn syrup and/or partially hydrogenated oils.
- Make breakfast mandatory.
- Whenever possible, send your child to school with a homemade lunch and/or snack (e.g., carrots, apples, dried apricots, dried plums, figs, celery with peanut butter, raisins and dates, whole-grain muffins/cookies).
- Have a house rule of no more than one hour daily of TV or computer play time.
- Help your child develop good sleep habits and remember that most teens need eight and a half to nine hours of sleep each night.
- Make family dinners a priority.
- Make fast-food meals an occasional treat, not a habit.
- Encourage three servings daily of low-fat/nonfat dairy foods.

A New Spring SuperFood

Kiwi

A source of:

- Vitamin C
- Folate
- Vitamin E
- Potassium
- Fibre
- Carotenoids (primarily lutein/zeaxanthin)
- Polyphenols
- Chlorophyll
- Glutathione
- Pectin
- Low glycaemic index

SIDEKICKS: pineapple, guava (any variety)
TRY TO EAT: multiple times a week

Cut a kiwi open. Doesn't it look just like spring? It's time to learn more about this superfruit from Down Under.

Kiwis are perhaps the first fruit to be named after a bird – twice. Introduced to New Zealand from China around 1906, the fruit was first known as a Chinese gooseberry (the first bird), probably because, like a green gooseberry, it has pale flesh. As kiwis became more popular, and international demand spread, New Zealanders proudly renamed the fruit after their national bird – the kiwi (the second bird). Now kiwis, or kiwifruit, are popular the world over and deservedly so, as their pale green and delicious flesh, reminiscent of strawberries to some and pineapple to others, offers a potent mix of nutrients that elevate it to the status of a SuperFood.

Kiwi the SuperFruit

While many fruits feature one or two nutrients in their profile, kiwi offers an unusual array of health-promoting substances. Extremely rich in vitamin C, kiwis also offer folate, potassium, fibre, carotenoids, polyphenols, chlorophyll, glutathione and pectin. In addition, kiwis are an unusual source of vitamin E, because most sources of this important vitamin, like nuts and oils, are high in both fat and calories. Kiwi, by contrast, offers its rich nutritional bounty for only about 93 calories for two kiwis. In fact, on a calorie-per-nutrient basis, kiwis have only 3.8 calories per nutrient. Of twenty-seven fruits tested, only cantaloupe (2.6), papaya (2.8), strawberry (2.5) and lemon (2.5) had fewer calories per nutrient.

Kiwis are antioxidant all-stars. Offering a rich bounty of vitamin C – more than the equivalent amount in an orange – kiwis can help neutralize the free radicals that damage cells, ultimately leading to inflammation, which, in turn, can lead to cancer and other chronic diseases. Vitamin C plays such an important role in so many bodily functions, including the immune system, and is associated with preventing so many ailments from asthma and atherosclerosis to osteoarthritis and colon cancer, that it's no wonder that high consumption of the foods containing the vitamin is associated with a reduced risk of death *from all causes*, including cancer, heart disease and stroke.

Kiwi and Your Heart

Kiwis promote heart health by lowering triglyceride levels and reducing platelet hyperactivity, which in turn seems to play a role in the development and stability of athero-sclerotic vascular plaques.

Kiwis can promote heart health by limiting the tendency of blood to form clots. The vitamins C and E in kiwis, combined with the polyphenols and magnesium, potassium, B vitamins and copper, act to protect the cardiovascular system. In one study in Oslo, Norway, people who ate two or three kiwis a day for twenty-eight days reduced their platelet aggregation response – or potential for clot formation – by 18 percent compared with those who ate no kiwis. Moreover, the kiwi eaters enjoyed a triglyceride drop of 15 percent compared with the controls.

Four medium kiwis supply about 1.4 mg of lutein/zeaxanthin. Therefore, this fruit is a nonleafy green source of these two important nutrients, which have been associated with a decreased risk for cataracts, macular degeneration and the development of atherosclerotic plaques.

Kiwis are reported to have a laxative effect, which can be beneficial to all, but especially to older people who are troubled by constipation.

Kiwi in the Kitchen

Kiwis are generally available in most supermarkets all year round. The most common variety is the Hayward, which has green flesh and is covered with brown fuzz. Gold kiwis have a smooth bronze-coloured skin and are pointy at one end. The flesh is mustard coloured and quite flavourful. The gold kiwi is also higher in vitamins C and E, and lutein/zeaxanthin. New hybrids include the baby kiwis, which are green, smooth, about the size of table grapes, and eaten much like them. When you shop for kiwis, choose plump ones that yield slightly to the touch. Avoid those that are shrivelled, mouldy or have soft spots. You can easily ripen kiwis by leaving them at room temperature for a few days, or to speed up the process, put the kiwis in a dry paper bag along with an apple or banana.

Most people don't realize that you can eat the kiwi, skin and all, after rubbing off the fuzz. The skin is actually quite nutritious. If you want to omit the skin, simply slice the fruit in half and scoop out the flesh, or you can slice it into rounds and peel the rounds before serving. If you have an egg slicer, use it to slice kiwis into uniform rounds.

Here are a few ways to get more kiwis into your life:

- Toss diced kiwis into a green salad.
- Purée kiwis into smoothies. They're delicious with bananas and/or blueberries and nonfat yogurt.
- Kiwi chunks make a tasty addition to a turkey or tuna salad.
- Serve kiwis with strawberries and add a dollop of yogurt and a dash of honey.
- Blend kiwis with cantaloupe or other melon, and add yogurt for a creamy, chilled soup. Garnish with blueberries and mint for delightful colour.

- Make a relish of chopped kiwi, red onion, pineapple and orange. Serve with grilled meat or fish.

Remember that you should be trying to get 'Five a Day' of a wide variety of fruits. It's easier to achieve this goal in the spring, when the cascade of ripening fruits beckons from our markets. Here's some information on which fruits will continue to ripen once purchased and which will not:

Never ripen after picking: soft berries, cherries, citrus, grapes, lychees, olives, pineapple, watermelon

Ripen only after picking: avocados

Ripen in colour, texture and juiciness but not in sweetness after picking: apricots, blueberries, figs, melons (except watermelon), nectarines, passionfruit, peaches, persimmons

Get sweeter after picking: apples, kiwis, mangoes, papayas, pears

Ripen in every way after harvest: bananas

Spring HealthStyle Focus
How to Avoid Osteoporosis

We think of our bones as the scaffolding to our bodies. From certain standpoints, this is correct. Our bones are the rigid framework that supports our muscles and soft tissue. But there is a dramatic difference between our bones and a steel scaffold: Our bones are living tissue in a constant state of flux. Bones constantly break down and build up. Indeed, as far as your bones are concerned, you're not the person you were ten years ago; the adult skeleton is replaced about every decade. Bones are also porous. They actually consist of a flexible porous framework of a protein substance known as collagen, plus a lot of calcium phosphate that serves as a mineral filler.

Here are the two most important things to know about

your bones: First, because they're in a constant state of rebuilding, today's diet and exercise are creating tomorrow's bones. Second, we are facing a health care crisis because, as many of us tend to live longer, our bones, abused by poor diet and lack of exercise, aren't up to the task of supporting us into old age. The results: The estimated risk of lifetime fracture exceeds 40 percent for women and 13 percent for men. In fact, approximately ten million Americans are currently diagnosed with osteoporosis and, perhaps more alarming, eighteen million are at risk because of low bone mass.

The Looming Danger

Osteoporosis, or porous bone, is aptly named. If you could see an X ray of osteoporotic bone it would look like Swiss cheese. As you might imagine, when bones become porous they lose strength. The great danger here is fracture. A young person, with strong resilient bones, who experiences a simple broken or fractured bone will heal fairly quickly. An older person who experiences a hip fracture – a common occurrence among seniors with osteoporosis – can find that he has crossed the threshold into disability and worse. For too many older people, a hip fracture can be the cause of nursing home confinement and subsequent immobility and decline. Indeed, in the elderly, hip fractures are associated with mortality in over 20 percent of cases. When you realize that 350,000 hip fractures are reported annually in the US alone, and this number is likely to rise as the number of people over age sixty-five increases, you can see that osteoporosis is a significant health issue.

While genetics plays a role in the development of osteoporosis, there's a lot you can do now to improve your chances of having a strong, flexible skeleton into old age.

- Boost your calcium and vitamin D intake. Calcium is a mineral used in a wide variety of bodily functions. If you're not getting sufficient calcium from your diet, your body will begin to break down the calcium in your bones to use it elsewhere. Vitamin D helps your body both absorb calcium and deposit it in the bones. Many studies have demonstrated that adequate amounts of both calcium and vitamin D will improve bone mineral density. In 1997, for example, researchers found that men and women who were given calcium and vitamin D rather than a placebo enjoyed higher bone density and fewer fractures. Most of us don't get enough calcium in our diets. The typical woman consumes 800 mg of calcium daily from food and supplements, but the recommended level is 1,000 mg daily to 1,200 mg daily for women over fifty years of age. This is of particular concern when you realize that a negative balance of only 50 to 100 mg a day over a period of time is enough to result in osteoporosis. The best sources of calcium are low-fat and nonfat dairy products like yogurt, as well as fortified soymilk and soy foods, cereals, sardines, and tinned wild salmon (with bones), broccoli, spring greens, kale, and calcium-fortified orange juice.
- Adequate vitamin D intake is important to preserve bone strength. Our skin actually makes vitamin D when exposed to ultraviolet rays of the sun. Unfortunately, many of us do not get sufficient vitamin D from either sunlight or dietary sources, so it may be important to consider adding a supplement to your diet. (See 'It's Winter: Do You Know Where Your Vitamin D Is?', page 115.) I recommend 800 to 1,000 IU of supplemental vitamin D3 daily. (All supplemental vitamin D from fish sources is vitamin D3.)
- Resistance exercise plays an important role in preserving

bone strength. Resistance training and weight-bearing exercise like walking stimulate new bone formation. Include this type of exercise in your routine two to three times weekly. (See 'Resistance Training', page 63.) Remember that balance and flexibility to prevent falls are important also, especially as you age. Exercise in general, particularly tai chi, enhances flexibility.

■ Vitamin K is being recognized as an important player in the promotion of bone strength. One recent study in the Netherlands emphasized the importance of vitamin K when subjects who took vitamin K supplements, along with calcium, vitamin D, zinc and magnesium, had significantly less bone loss after three years compared with subjects who took either a placebo or the same supplements minus the vitamin K. The current recommended dose of vitamin K is 90 mcg (micrograms) a day for women and 120 mcg a day for men, but many researchers believe that this amount is too low. Trials are under way to come up with a more beneficial recommendation, but in the meantime if you follow a SuperFoods diet, you'll easily get the vitamin K you need. Vitamin K is particularly abundant in spinach and its sidekicks, especially kale and spring greens.

Many people think that osteoporosis is a woman's disease. While it's true that women can be at high risk because of bone loss during and immediately after menopause, men also are commonly afflicted. US statistics show that one in every eight men over fifty will suffer a hip fracture due to osteoporosis. Men should discuss their risk for osteoporosis with their health care providers and should have bone density tests as indicated.

- Potassium is a real bone booster. Research has shown that people who get a good supply of potassium experience less bone loss than others who do not. Once again, as potassium is readily available in fruits and vegetables, you should have no trouble reaching your HealthStyle potassium goal of 8,000 mg a day if you follow a SuperFoods diet. A single potato has 940 mg of potassium and a banana, 490 mg. (See 'Potassium Power', page 267.)
- Soy can promote healthy bones because its phyto-oestrogens – literally plant oestrogens – seem to boost bone mineral density. I recommend 10 to 15 grams of soy protein a day, which supplies about 50 mg of soy isoflavones. If you have a history of breast cancer in your family, check with your health care practitioner before eating soy.
- Limit alcohol consumption to a maximum of three to seven drinks per week for women and six to fourteen drinks per week for men. Alcohol consumption at these levels may enhance bone mineral density; however, in larger amounts, alcohol decreases the activity of bone-rebuilding cells. The risk for breast cancer in women begins to climb with four drinks per week. My own HealthStyle recommendations on alcohol are one to three drinks per week for women and two to eight drinks per week for men.
- Limit caffeine consumption. Excessive amounts of caffeine can affect bone strength, as it increases the amount of calcium excreted in the urine. Limit your coffee consumption to two cups a day, and don't forget that many brands of fizzy drink contain caffeine as well as phosphates, which tend to pull calcium from the bones. (Noncola soft drinks, by the way, do not contain phosphates.) Consider adding nonfat milk, 1% low-fat milk, or calcium-fortified soymilk to tea and/or coffee, as this helps to counteract any adverse effects of the caffeine.

- Limit your sodium intake. Excessive sodium intake may trigger calcium excretion. Aim for no more than 2,400 mg of sodium per day. Hide the salt shaker, look for low-sodium labels in the supermarket, avoid most processed foods and cured meats, and check the labels on tinned goods for sodium content. Try a salt substitute.
- Watch your intake of vitamin A (in the form of retinol, or so-called preformed vitamin A), as it's a nutrient that in excess will increase your risk for bone fractures. While vitamin A is essential for bone growth, too much of it in the form of retinol can be damaging. Limit retinol intake to a maximum of 3,000 IU daily. There is, by the way, no increased risk of fracture from carotenoid sources of vitamin A.
- Don't smoke. Many people don't realize that smoking, along with so many other health negatives, plays a role in promoting osteoporosis. Although the reasons for this are unclear, there's no doubt that smoking has a negative effect on bone strength, which seems to translate into an increased risk of hip fracture. Indeed, the negative effects of smoking on bone health last up to ten years after quitting.

EAT YOUR GREENS!

One of the great delights of the spring season is the appearance in supermarkets and farmers' markets of the first greens of the season. After months of eating the vegetables of winter – cabbage, swede, carrots (not without their charms, of course . . .) – we finally begin to see the rich greens of the new season, offering a change and a nutritional jump start from the doldrums of winter. Greens are so rich in crucial nutrients that they have indeed earned their reputation as tonics. They abound in carotenoids and vitamin C as well as folate, iron, calcium and fibre. They're truly essential to a healthy diet and a vibrant HealthStyle.

Chard, kale and spinach are more commonly found, but many markets feature unusual and tempting varieties, such as dandelion, pea shoots, watercress, mustard, purple sprouting broccoli, baby bok choy and a host of others. Most can be added to a salad or lightly sautéed with extra virgin olive oil and a minced garlic clove.

Here are some tips:

- Look for fresh-looking, fresh-smelling greens. Avoid any that are yellowed or browned. Avoid any slimy or wilting greens.
- Refrigerate greens and keep them moist but not wet. Roll greens lightly in damp paper towels and store the bundle in a plastic bag (with holes punched in it so humidity doesn't promote spoilage) in the fridge.
- Don't wash greens until just before using.

Some greens are bitter, others are strongly flavoured, and some are a surprising change from the usual bland winter lettuces. Some people, especially children, like their greens with a little added flavour. Here are three quick preparations that will make greens even more appealing:

- Blend 2 tablespoons reduced-sodium soy sauce, 1 tablespoon rice vinegar, 1 tablespoon toasted sesame oil, 1 teaspoon honey (buckwheat honey, if you have it), 2 teaspoons minced fresh ginger, 1 small clove minced garlic, and 1 teaspoon grated orange or lemon rind. Toss these ingredients with cooked greens such as kale, spinach, Swiss chard or even broccoli.
- Blend ¼ cup peanut butter, soy butter or almond butter with 2 tablespoons hot green tea. To this add 1 table-spoon reduced-sodium soy sauce, 1 teaspoon honey

(buckwheat honey, if you have it), 1 tablespoon lime juice, 1 small clove minced garlic, and a dash of crushed red chilli pepper flakes, if desired. Use as a dressing for any cooked greens.

■ Blend ¼ cup balsamic vinegar with 1 tablespoon chopped shallots. Heat in a small saucepan over medium heat until syrupy. Remove from the heat and add 2 tablespoons raisins or dried cranberries and 1 tablespoon extra virgin olive oil. Toss with cooked Swiss chard, kale or spinach.

Spring SuperFood Update
Spinach

A source of:

■ Synergy of multiple nutrients/phytonutrients
■ Low calories
■ Lutein/zeaxanthin
■ Beta-carotene
■ Plant-derived omega-3 fatty acids
■ Glutathione
■ Alpha-lipoic acid
■ Vitamins C and E
■ B vitamins (thiamin, riboflavin, B6, folate)
■ Minerals: calcium, iron, magnesium, manganese and zinc
■ Polyphenols
■ Betaine
■ Coenzyme Q_{10}

SIDEKICKS: kale, spring greens, Swiss chard, rocket, mustard greens, turnip greens, bok choy, romaine lettuce, orange peppers, seaweed
TRY TO EAT: one cup steamed or 2 cups raw most days

You can usually recognize SuperFood fans in the super-market: Their trolleys are loaded with spinach. Nothing makes me happier than seeing how people have jumped on the spinach bandwagon. In the United States, people are now eating five times more fresh spinach than they ate in the 1970s. This is the highest level of spinach consumption since the 1950s, when parents were urging their kids to eat spinach so they'd be as strong as Popeye. There are two reasons for this renaissance of spinach in the diet. For one thing, it's never been easier to prepare spinach for the table. You can buy prewashed baby spinach at most markets. Some spinach can be microwaved right in the bag and put on the table in three minutes. The most important reason for the popularity of spinach is its powerful health benefits.

Spinach, and its green, leafy sidekicks, are among the most nutritious foods on earth. Calorie for calorie, spinach provides more nutrients than any other food. Along with two of my favourites, wild salmon and blueberries, spinach is an all-star SuperFood that packs an incredible nutritional wallop. Low in calories and jam-packed with nutrients, spinach should be a regular part of your daily menu.

Spinach seems to be able to lessen our risk of many of the most common diseases of the twenty-first century. Overwhelming research has demonstrated an inverse relationship between spinach consumption and the following:

- Cardiovascular disease, including stroke and coronary artery disease
- Cancer, including colon, lung, skin, oral, stomach, ovarian, prostate and breast cancers
- Age-related macular degeneration (AMD)
- Cataracts

In addition, preliminary research suggests that spinach may help prevent or delay age-related cognitive decline.

What makes spinach and its sidekicks such powerful health promoters? The list of compounds that have been discovered in spinach is truly impressive. Beyond the iron that Popeye was yearning for, spinach contains carotenoids, antioxidants, vitamin K, coenzyme Q10, B vitamins, minerals, chlorophyll, polyphenols, betaine and, interestingly, plant-derived omega-3 fatty acids. This is a condensed list and it's hard to convey the powerful impact of these nutrients as they work synergistically to promote health.

I am particularly interested in the role of spinach in promoting visual health. My mother spent the last sixteen years of her life suffering from macular degeneration. While her overall health was excellent, the macular degeneration meant that she was unable to drive, watch TV or read – activities that many of us take for granted but are sorely missed when eliminated from our lives.

The macular pigment of the eye helps protect against AMD, and responds very quickly to a rich supply of lutein/zeaxanthin. Within four weeks of increasing your intake of spinach and its sidekicks, you can significantly increase your macular pigment and thus help protect your vision. In effect, the nutrients in spinach function like an internal pair of sunglasses, thereby increasing the SPF (sunprotective factor) of the eye.

Here's what we know about age-related macular degeneration, or AMD. The macula of the eye is responsible for central vision – which we need for close work like writing and sewing as well as distinguishing distant objects and colour. Unfortunately, as many as 20 percent of all sixty-five-year-olds show at least some early evidence of

age-related macular changes. By age ninety, about 60 percent of Caucasians will be affected by AMD, and close to
100 percent of centenarians reportedly have this leading
cause of age-related vision loss. Worse yet, there is no effective treatment for AMD. The good news is that nutrition
can play an important role in preventing AMD. Among the
carotenoids, lutein and zeaxanthin are most strongly associated with a decreased risk of AMD. Spinach and its
sidekick green leafies are important players in preventing
macular degeneration because of their rich supply of the
carotenoids lutein/zeaxanthin and, coupled with dietary
marine-based omega-3 fatty acids (see 'Wild Salmon', page
260), they can offer a powerful reduction of our risk for
AMD. All of the lutein and a significant percentage of the
zeaxanthin found in the macula come from the diet, thus
reinforcing the prescription to eat the best sources of lutein
– spinach and kale – regularly. For those who can't eat
green leafies or fish, DHA eggs, found in virtually every
supermarket, supply very bioavailable amounts of lutein,
zeaxanthin and DHA.

Many people have asked me why I include orange peppers as a spinach sidekick. It's far from green and just as far
from leafy. Orange peppers are a worthy sidekick to green
leafies because of their abundant supply of the carotenoid
zeaxanthin. You can think of them as nature's gift to those
few of us who don't like spinach and other green leafy vegetables. Most people, including children, enjoy eating
strips of orange peppers with a dip or just on their own.
They're also excellent in salads and stir-fries. On those
days when you can't work green leafies into your diet, rely
on orange peppers to give your eyes their zeaxanthin
boost.

While the USDA has yet to analyse orange peppers, I
know from independent research that their supply of these
important nutrients is extremely impressive. Here is a comparison of lutein/zeaxanthin all-stars:

Lutein All-Stars

1 cup cooked kale	23.7 mg
1 cup cooked spinach	20.4 mg
1 cup cooked spring greens	14.6 mg
1 cup cooked turnip greens	12.1 mg
1 cup cooked green peas	4.2 mg
1 cup raw spinach	3.7 mg
1 cup cooked broccoli	2.4 mg

Zeaxanthin All-Stars

1 medium orange pepper	6.4 mg
1 cup tinned sweet yellow corn	0.9 mg
1 raw persimmon	0.8 mg
1 cup degermed cornmeal	0.7 mg

Spinach is a powerful ally in the fight against cancer. A number of studies have shown an inverse relationship between spinach consumption and almost every type of cancer. Researchers believe that it's the rich supply of vitamins, minerals, omega-3 fatty acids, antioxidants and phytonutrients that do the job. For example, spinach and its sidekicks offer rich supplies of glutathione and alpha-lipoic acid – two critical antioxidants. These substances are manufactured in the body, but our ability to produce them subsides as we age. That's when spinach can make an important contribution with its ready-made supply of both glutathione and alpha-lipoic acid. In addition to these antioxidants, spinach supplies the carotenoids lutein/zeaxanthin and beta-carotene that play an important role in our body's anticancer defence systems.

In addition to significant contributions to the promotion of eye health and prevention of cancer, spinach and its sidekicks also promote cardiovascular health. The vitamin C, beta-carotene and other nutrients in spinach work together to prevent oxidized cholesterol from building up in the blood vessel walls. We can't forget about the fabulous folate in spinach. Folate is an important contributor to heart health, as it works, along with B6 and betaine, to lower serum levels of the dangerous amino acid homocysteine. We are learning more every day about the dangers of homocysteine and its association with heart disease, stroke, osteoporosis and age-related cognitive decline. Finally, we must remember that the potassium and magnesium in spinach also make significant contributions to heart health. Both work to lower blood pressure and the risk of cardiovascular disease and stroke.

Salad Sense

Don't rely on fat-free salad dressings if you want a full nutrient boost from salads. Too many people try to cut calories by using nonfat salad dressings. We now know this can inhibit your body's absorption of nutrients from the greens and other vegetables. In a recent study, volunteers ate spinach, romaine lettuce, tomatoes and carrots topped with 2 ounces of Italian dressing containing either 0, 6 or 28 grams of extra virgin olive oil. Blood tests revealed that the people who ate fat-free dressing absorbed a negligible amount of beta-carotene, a carotenoid that's been linked to protection against cancer and heart disease. The highest-fat dressing offered the greatest absorption of beta-carotene as well as alpha-carotene and lycopene. My suggestion is to use homemade dressings (to reduce the sodium level). Try a combination of extra virgin olive oil, balsamic vinegar, ground pepper, salt substitute, and herbs and spices of your choosing. Use the dressing sparingly: Don't drench the greens!

Spinach in the Kitchen

We are really fortunate to be able to buy fresh spinach in so many convenient forms. Perhaps quickest and easiest are the bags of prewashed baby spinach, which can simply be microwaved, bag and all. They take just a minute or two to prepare. Add a squeeze of lemon juice and a drizzle of extra virgin olive oil, and you've got a side dish. Spinach can also be eaten raw in salads. Buy bagged greens carefully, checking for the best-before dates, as some can deteriorate quickly. Check for any dark soggy leaves, since this means the greens are past their prime. Fresh loose spinach is widely available, too, and is always a good choice. Be sure to check for fresh, sweet-smelling leaves. Spinach will only keep for two or three days in the fridge, so plan accordingly. Don't wash loose spinach until ready to serve. Loose spinach can be quite sandy, so wash it carefully in a few changes of cold water.

Here are a few tips on how to get some spinach into your life:

- Hot, steamed spinach is a good side dish, but it's also great cold. I always make extra and eat some for lunch with a drizzle of soy dressing or lemon juice.
- Add spinach and its sidekicks to salads regularly.
- Add spinach to soups and casseroles.
- Dress up steamed or sautéed spinach with a sprinkle of toasted sesame seeds or pine nuts.
- Use spinach in place of lettuce on your sandwiches.

Braised Spinach with Roasted Cherry Tomatoes

This recipe is from a southern SuperFood fan, Lorna Wyckoff, who mentions that, as a transplanted northerner, she's learned to love her greens. Try this with mustard greens, kale, spring greens or Swiss chard.

Preheat the grill. Arrange 8 ounces of organic cherry tomatoes and 2 minced garlic cloves on a foil-lined baking tray. Drizzle with olive oil and salt and pepper. Grill, turning with a spatula every couple of minutes until the tomatoes are browned but not burned.

Heat 1 teaspoon extra virgin olive oil in a large pan over medium heat. Add a diced large shallot and sauté. Add a bag of organic baby spinach leaves, rinsed but not dried, and a pinch of red chilli pepper flakes (optional). When the spinach is just about wilted, add the roasted tomatoes and garlic and cook for another minute.

Krispy Kale

Preheat the oven to 350°F. Trim and cut up a bunch of kale into bite-sized bits. Spread it on an aluminum foil–lined baking tray lightly sprayed with extra virgin olive oil. Bake for 15 to 20 minutes, stirring every 5 minutes or so. Sprinkle lightly with seasoned salt, garlic powder, or any spice you prefer.

Spring SuperFood Update
Soy

A source of:

- Phyto-oestrogens
- Plant-derived omega-3 fatty acids
- Vitamin E
- B vitamins (thiamin, riboflavin, B6)
- Iron
- Potassium
- Folate
- Magnesium
- Selenium
- Saponins
- Phytates

- Phytosterols
- Lunasin
- Excellent nonmeat protein alternative

SIDEKICKS IN FORMS OF SOY: tofu, soymilk, soy yogurt, soy nuts, edamame, tempeh, miso
TRY TO EAT: at least 10 to 15 grams of soy protein daily (30 to 50 mg isoflavones daily; not from isoflavone-fortified products)

Soy, or soya, is perhaps the most misunderstood SuperFood. While its health benefits are undeniable, the controversy surrounding the relationship between soy and breast cancer has obscured the value of this extraordinary food and has made some people nervous about regular soy consumption. I can reassure you that soy is a safe and healthy food when eaten in a whole-food form. Information about the health effects of soy supplements is less clear, so I advise my patients to stick with soy in whole-food form.

There's no question that soy is a health-promoting food. While soybeans have been cultivated in China for more than three thousand years, interest in soy has come relatively recently to the West; today the United States is responsible for more than half of the world's soybean production. We now have a vast body of research that has demonstrated that the value of soy as a healthy food has created a continuing interest in soy and all of its varieties.

The power of soy rests in its benefits as an excellent protein food, its level of essential fatty acids, its supply of vitamins and minerals, its rich supply of fibre, and its health-promoting isoflavones and other phyto-nutrients.

Regular consumption of soy has been associated with:

- Reduced cholesterol and larger and less dangerous LDL cholesterol particles
- Reduced blood pressure
- Reduction of cancer risk, including breast, prostate and colon cancer
- Better management of diabetes
- Reduced proteinuria (protein in the urine) in people with kidney disease
- Lower risk of osteoporosis

In the US in 1999, the FDA allowed soy food manufacturers to make health claims on their packages. They are able to state that soy protein, when included in a diet low in saturated fat and cholesterol, may reduce the risk of coronary heart disease by lowering blood cholesterol levels.

Soy Isoflavones

One of the great confusions about soy has to do with isoflavones. Soybeans are the best-known source of these compounds, which act like antioxidants as well as oestrogens. Two of the isoflavones in soy – genistein and daidzein – reduce the risk of coronary heart disease, mitigate hormone-related cancers and other conditions, and decrease the ability of tumours to grow new blood vessels. Preliminary evidence suggests that genistein decreases the growth of new blood vessels in the retina, which can lead to vision loss from age-related macular degeneration.

The confusion about the health benefits of soy stems from the fact that many people want to take shortcuts and rely on soy products and supplements. Some research suggests that not only is the cancer-preventive ability of soy foods greatly reduced in these supplements and processed soy foods but, indeed, these foods can stimulate the growth of preexisting oestrogen-dependent breast tumours in mice. On the other hand, abundant research evidence exists that demonstrates that soy in the form of whole foods can be beneficial; indeed, soy is a food that has been shown to reduce the risk of breast cancer. Another study has shown that consuming the amount of soy phytoestrogens that would be eaten when soy foods are included in the diet (in women, about 129 mg a day of isoflavones) does not increase the risk of breast or uterine cancer, and appears to be protective. Once again, Mother Nature has produced a product that is more effective and much safer than those produced by man. The complex mixture of bioactive compounds that act synergistically in soy to promote health is found only in whole foods, and I recommend sticking with minimally processed, whole soy foods.

The question does remain whether soy is safe for breast cancer survivors. The most recent expert recommendations from the American Cancer Society provide the following counselling regarding soy during and after cancer treatment: 'Because soy has been associated with oestrogenic effects in some studies, the safety of consuming high amounts of soy from supplements or a soy-rich diet remains unclear: Consumption of up to three servings per day of soy foods [soymilk, tofu, etc] is considered moderate and has not been associated with specific benefit or harm in breast cancer survivors.' I recommend that women who have been diagnosed with breast cancer consult with their health care provider about the safety of consuming soy food products in their individual case.

Isoflavones in Soy Foods

The USDA, in collaboration with Iowa State University, has compiled a listing of the isoflavone content of soy foods. The values are expressed in milligrams per single serving of the food. The foods are listed in descending order of isoflavone content.

	Calories	Fat (g)	Isoflavones
Soybeans, dried, cooked (1 cup)	298	15	95
Soybean sprouts (1/4 cup)	171	9.4	57
Soynuts (1/4 cup)	194	9.3	55
Tempeh (4 ounces)	226	8.7	50
Soy flour, full fat (1/3 cup)	121	5.7	49
Tofu, firm (4 ounces)	164	9.9	28
Soymilk (1 cup)	81	4.7	24
Edamame, cooked (4 ounces)	160	7.3	16

Soy the Health Promoter

There are a host of specific reasons to get soy into your diet, but one excellent reason is that soy is a valuable protein alternative to animal protein. A half cup of tofu provides 18 to 20 grams of protein, which is 40 percent of the daily requirement for most people. That same amount of tofu also provides 258 mg of calcium (more than a quarter of our daily needs) and 13 mg of iron (87 percent of a woman's daily need and 130 percent of a man's). Here's a comparison of the percentage of protein by weight of a few foods: Soy flour is 51 percent protein; whole, dry soybeans are 35 percent protein; fish is only 22 percent protein; hamburger is only 13 percent protein; and whole milk is just 3 percent protein.

Boosting your protein intake isn't in and of itself a goal: The more important aspect of soy as a protein source is that it doesn't contain many of the undesirable components of other protein sources in our diets, in particular, saturated fat but also including hormones, antibiotics, pesticides and other negatives. Finally, even though soy offers the highest-quality protein of any plant food, it's low in calories. Indeed, tofu has the lowest known ratio of calories to protein in any plant food, save mung beans and soybean sprouts.

Soy's benefits go beyond its not being meat. It has long been recognized for having a beneficial effect on blood cholesterol levels. A recent study investigated the effects of soy protein and soy isoflavones on blood pressure and cholesterol levels in sixty-one middle-aged Scottish men who were at high risk of developing coronary heart disease. For five weeks, half of the men consumed diets that contained at least 20 grams of soy protein and 80 mg of soy isoflavones each day. The control group consumed a diet that was without soy but did contain olive oil. The soy consumers were found to have significant reductions in both diastolic and systolic blood pressure. Moreover, their total cholesterol was significantly lower and their HDL ('good') cholesterol was significantly increased. The control group also enjoyed an increase in their HDL cholesterol levels, but their blood pressure was unaffected and their LDL ('bad') cholesterol levels did not drop. The researchers concluded that eating at least 20 grams of soy protein, including 80 mg of soy isoflavones for a minimum of five weeks, would be effective in reducing the risk of cardiovascular disease in high-risk, middle-aged men.

In connection with promoting cardiovascular health, it's significant that soy has been found to lower heart disease risk by increasing the size of LDL cholesterol particles. Small, dense LDL is the most dangerous form of cholesterol. Large LDL, especially when accompanied by adequate supplies of HDL, is considered much less risky. In a study at Tufts University in the US on subjects with high cholesterol, researchers found that those who ate a diet high in soy protein significantly increased the size of their LDL particles compared with periods when they ate diets high in animal protein. The participants were given four different diets, each for a period of six weeks: soy protein with no isoflavones, soy protein enriched with isoflavones, animal protein with no added isoflavones, and animal protein with added isoflavones. The isoflavones had no effect, but soy protein consumption resulted in a decrease in the amount of small, dense LDL and an increase in larger LDL particles compared with animal protein. This is yet another argument for using soy as a regular substitute for animal protein in the diet.

Another way that soy promotes heart health is due to the ability of soy protein to increase blood levels of nitric oxide – a molecule that can boost blood vessel dilation and reduce the free-radical damage of cholesterol and the adhesion of white cells to blood vessel walls. Preventing these events lessens the risk of the development of atherosclerotic plaques. One study on mice found that when fed soy protein diets, the mice had increased levels of nitric oxide metabolites compared with mice that were fed other protein sources.

Soy protein is an excellent food for those who suffer from diabetes, particularly non-insulin-dependent diabetes. The protein and fibre in soy foods can help to stabilize blood sugar levels. There's also evidence that soy protein can help to protect both the hearts and kidneys of diabetic patients from the damage that can be caused by the disease. In a recent study, diabetic patients who were switched to a diet containing 35 percent soy protein and 30 percent vegetable protein showed significant reductions in total cholesterol, triglyceride, and LDL blood cholesterol levels as well as an improvement in kidney function. The researchers concluded that a diet that includes soy protein could reduce the risk of heart disease and also improve kidney function in diabetic patients.

Finally, there is evidence that soy protein, which has a significant fibre content, could play a role in reducing the risk of various cancers, including breast, prostate and colon cancer. Various components of soy have demonstrated anticarcinogenic effects. They include protease inhibitors, phytosterols, saponins, lunacin, phenolic acids, phytic acid and isoflavones. The fibre in soy also plays a role in reducing cancer risk. Fibre seems to be able to bind to some cancer-causing toxins and escort them from the body, thus decreasing the incidence of cancers, particularly colon cancer. It has been noted that in various parts of the world where soy is eaten regularly, the rates of colon cancer, as well as breast and prostate cancer, tend to be lower than the rates in Western cultures where meat proteins are a more dominant part of the diet. A study in mice showed that a combination of soy protein and black tea synergistically inhibited prostate tumour growth. Once again, this demonstrates the beneficial synergy of whole foods in preventing disease.

Soy and Your Thyroid

Many people ask me about soy and thyroid dysfunction. In general, adequate dietary iodine seems to be protective against soy's occasional potential for promoting thyroid hormone abnormalities. In addition, epidemiologic studies show that soy consumption may reduce the risk of thyroid cancer.

There have been questions about whether calcium from soymilk is as bioavailable as the calcium from cow's milk. A recent study reported that calcium absorption from calcium carbonate-fortified soymilk was equivalent to calcium absorption from cow's milk. (Less well absorbed is the calcium in the form of tricalcium phosphate found in some fortified soymilks.) Don't forget to shake the container well before pouring, as the calcium tends to settle on the bottom.

How Much Soy Should You Eat?

It can be difficult to work out how much soy is beneficial to health because many consumers look for amounts of soy isoflavones on soy food labels. Unfortunately, some foods don't list isoflavones. Some others list isoflavone amounts that are inaccurate. And some foods list isoflavone fortification, and I don't recommend relying on added isoflavones. (There isn't enough evidence to confirm the long-term safety of isoflavone-fortified products.) Here's the key to shopping for soy foods: **Check the protein content on the label.** In general, the best way to learn the isoflavone content of a food is to rely on the listed protein content. The protein content of the food is closely linked to the isoflavone content. You can get the benefits of soy with as little as 10 grams of soy protein a day. For example, one-quarter cup of soy nuts has 15 grams of soy protein. While soy nuts are high in calories, most people love to eat a scant one-quarter cup while relaxing at the end of the day. That's all it takes to get the benefit of soy.

Soy in the Kitchen

Some of my patients love soy foods; others do not. Whether you enjoy a tofu stir-fry or have no interest in cooking with soy foods, you can enjoy the benefits of soy in your diet. Many people aren't aware that there are a variety of ways to enjoy soy. Here are a few ideas:

Soymilk. Soymilk is made from soybeans that have been ground, cooked and strained. A wide range of varieties is available in the supermarket, including aseptic packages, which will keep for a long time, or fresh and even fresh, flavoured soymilk. Some people find that the fresh soymilk available in the dairy section tastes the best. Try a few brands until you find one you like, as there's quite a wide variation in flavours. Soymilk can be used as a substitute for cow's milk in baking and in pancakes, muffins and cakes.

A daily intake of 25 grams of soy protein is ideal. Here are some rich sources of soy:

- Four ounces of firm tofu contain approximately 18 to 20 grams of soy protein.
- One soy 'burger' includes approximately 10 to 12 grams of protein.
- An 8-ounce glass (1 cup) of Alpro contains more than 9 grams of protein.
- One soy protein bar delivers 14 grams of protein.
- One-half cup of tempeh provides 16 to 19 grams of protein.
- One-quarter cup of roasted soy nuts contains approximately 15 grams of soy protein.

Soy Flour. Soy flour is made from whole ground soybeans. Use it to supplement other flours and increase the protein content of breads, cakes and cookies. One quarter cup of soy flour has 8 to 12 grams of protein. As it contains no gluten, it can't be used to replace white or wheat flour entirely in baked goods. Use it in quick breads by substituting up to one quarter of the wheat flour with soy flour. When baking yeast breads, replace 2 tablespoons of each cup of wheat flour with soy flour.

Soy Nuts. Soy nuts are soybeans that have been soaked in water and then baked or roasted until they're lightly browned, toasty and crunchy. They're high in protein, isoflavones and soluble fibre. However, they're also high in calories – one quarter cup of soy nuts contains 136 calories and 15 grams of protein – so limit your intake. Read labels carefully when buying soy nuts. Some varieties have lots of added salt, sweeteners and oil.

Edamame. Edamame are green soybeans in their pods. You can find edamame at www.goodnessdirect.co.uk. To prepare edamame, briefly boil the pods in lightly salted water. Kids in particular enjoy popping the soybeans from the pods into their mouths. A cup of shelled edamame contains about 23 grams of protein.

Tofu. Tofu is perhaps the best-known soy food. A white, cheeselike food made from curdled soymilk and shaped into blocks, tofu is available everywhere. You can buy it firm, extra firm, soft or silken. Firm tofu is good for using in stir-fries and soups, or it can be grilled or baked, because it quickly absorbs marinades and flavourings. Even those who don't like tofu in dishes will enjoy silken tofu in smoothies, dips and dressings. Tofu is perishable, so check the best-before date on the package, keep it in a covered container in the fridge, and change the water it soaks in daily.

Tempeh. Popular in South-east Asia, tempeh is made from fermented cooked soybeans, other grains and flavourings. It has a nutty flavour and can be added to chilli or burritos. Or, rinse and cut into patty-sized squares, warm in barbecue sauce, and create a tempeh sandwich.

Miso. Miso, a soy ingredient that is gaining in popularity, adds flavour, depth and incremental amounts of soy isoflavones to foods. It is a staple in Japanese cooking. A fermented soybean paste, miso is made when soybeans and various grains such as rice or barley are cooked and cooled, then inoculated with friendly mould and allowed to culture.

Miso ranges in colour from pale yellow to dark rich chestnut brown and in flavour from sweet to salty. The lighter misos are sweeter, fruity and more subtle, while dark misos are hearty, robust and complex. There are three kinds of miso: shiro miso (white), aka miso (red) and awase miso (blended), plus many varieties within those categories. Experiment with the various types of miso; like vinegars, they are adaptable to different cooking uses.

Miso keeps well in the fridge for several months. Always use a clean spoon to remove some from the storage container. When used raw in dressings or cold preparations, miso adds healthy bacteria to the system, just as yogurt does. If mould forms on the surface, just scrape it off. It is perfectly safe to eat. Miso is high in sodium, so use it sparingly as a salt alternative and avoid using additional salt when preparing a dish using miso.

Mix a scant tablespoon of miso with a cup of warm water for a simple healthful stock. For a vinaigrette or a marinade with a delicately complex flavour, combine 2 tablespoons miso (a mix of two types is nice) with a minced shallot, ½ cup fresh lemon or lime juice with zest, ½ cup extra virgin olive oil and black pepper. Allow the miso to steep in the liquid for five minutes to soften, then whisk until smooth.

Here are some quick and easy ways to get soy into your diet:

- Use soymilk in place of cow's milk in baking and on cereals. These are both good ways to get children to eat some soy, as most won't even notice the difference.
- Sprinkle soybean sprouts on salads and tuck into sandwiches.
- Add soybeans to soups and casseroles.
- Keep some soy flour on hand to mix into pancakes, cakes and other baked goods.
- Add puréed silken tofu to dressings and dips.

Creamy Coriander Dressing

2 cups coriander leaves
1 teaspoon minced fresh garlic
⅛ cup water
One 10.5-ounce package silken tofu
1 tablespoon lemon juice
1 tablespoon reduced-sodium soy sauce

Put the coriander, garlic and water in a food processor and process until blended. Add the tofu, lemon juice and soy sauce and process until smooth. Pour into a bowl, cover, and chill for at least 2 hours before serving.

Creamy Tofu Dressing

Here's a good mayo substitute for sandwiches. It will keep in the fridge for about a week.

One 10.5-ounce package silken tofu
1 tablespoon balsamic vinegar
1 tablespoon honey
1 teaspoon prepared horseradish
1/2 teaspoon finely minced fresh garlic
Dash of dried mustard
Freshly ground black pepper

Combine all the ingredients in a blender or food processor and process until smooth. Adjust the thickness of the dressing to your taste by adding a teaspoon or more of water. Pour into a bowl, cover, and chill for at least 2 hours before using.

A New Spring SuperFood
Honey

A source of:

- 181 different substances including
- Polyphenols
- Salicylates
- Oligosaccharides

SIDEKICKS: none
TRY TO EAT: 1 to 2 teaspoons multiple times a week

No wonder the word 'honey' is a term of endearment. What could be sweeter and more appealing than the rich golden liquid? I've long enjoyed the delights of honey on cereal, toast, yogurt and pancakes, and as a sweetener for green tea, and I'm sure once you know about the nutritional benefits of honey, you'll be eager to use it more frequently.

Honey is much more than just a liquid sweetener. One of the oldest medicines known to man, honey has been used in the treatment of respiratory diseases, skin ulcers, wounds, urinary diseases, gastrointestinal diseases, eczema, psoriasis and dandruff. Today, we know the validity of these timeless treatments, as research has demonstrated that honey can inhibit the growth of bacteria, yeast, fungi and viruses.

The power of honey comes from the wide range of compounds present in the rich amber liquid. Honey contains at least 181 known substances, and its antioxidant activity stems from the phenolics, peptides, organic acids and enzymes. Honey also contains salicylic acid, minerals, alpha-tocopherol, and oligosaccharides. Oligosaccharides increase the number of 'good' bacteria in the colon, reduce levels of toxic metabolites in the intestine, help prevent constipation and help lower cholesterol and blood pressure.

The key point to remember with honey is that its anti-oxidant ability can vary widely depending on the floral source of the honey and its processing. The process begins when bees feast on flowers and collect nectar in their mouths. The bees mix the nectar and enzymes in their saliva to turn it into honey, which is then stored in combs in the hive. The constant movement of the bees' wings promotes moisture evaporation and yield the thick honey we enjoy. The phenolic content of the honey depends on the pollen that the bees have used as raw material. There's a very simple way to determine the health benefits of any honey: its colour. In general, the darker the colour of the honey, the higher the level of antioxidants. There can be a twentyfold difference in honey's antioxidant activity, as one test revealed. For example, Illinois buckwheat honey, the darkest honey tested, had twenty times the antioxidant activity of California sage honey, one of the lightest-coloured honeys tested. Overall, colour predicted more than 60 percent of the variation in honey's antioxidant capacity.

Honey and Your Health

Maintaining optimal blood sugar levels has a positive effect on overall health, and honey seems to contribute to this goal. Indeed, the ancient Olympic competitors relied on foods such as figs and honey to enhance performance by helping to maintain energy levels and restore muscle recovery. In one recent study of thirty-nine male and female athletes, following a workout the participants ate a protein supplement blended with a sweetener. Those who ate the supplement sweetened with honey, as opposed to sugar or maltodextrin, enjoyed the best results. They maintained optimal blood sugar levels for two hours following the workout and enjoyed better muscle recuperation.

There are hundreds of different kinds of honey to choose from, such as clover, buckwheat and orange blossom. Light-coloured honeys are generally mildly flavoured, while dark honeys are more robust.

Perhaps honey's most important health-promoting benefit is its antioxidant ability. We know that daily consumption of honey raises blood levels of protective antioxidants. In one study, participants were given about four tablespoons daily of buckwheat honey while eating their regular diets for twenty-nine days. A direct link was found between the subjects' honey consumption and the levels of protective polyphenolic antioxidants in their blood. In another study, twenty-five healthy men drank plain water or water with buckwheat honey. Those consuming the honey enjoyed a 7 percent increase in their antioxidant capacity. As the US Department of Agriculture estimates that the average US citizen consumes about 68 kilograms of sweetener annually, substituting honey for at least part of this amount would make an impressive contribution to our overall antioxidant status and would no doubt be a significant health promoter.

Never give honey to children younger than a year old. About 10 percent of honey contains dormant *Clostridium botulinum* spores, which can cause botulism in infants.

Honey, long recognized as a healer, has been used for centuries as a topical antiseptic for treating burns, ulcers and wounds. A study in India compared the effectiveness of honey with a conventional wound-healing treatment, silver sulphadiazine, on patients suffering from first-degree burns. Amazingly, in the honey-dressed wounds, early subsidence of acute inflammatory changes, better control of infection and quicker wound healing were observed. Some researchers attribute this effect to the nutrients in honey that promote skin growth and to the antibacterial substances present in honey. While I'm not recommending that you consider using honey topically, its power in this role is further evidence of its wide range of health benefits.

An additional benefit of honey is found in the oligosaccharides it contains. They increase the numbers of good bacteria in the colon, reduce levels of toxic metabolites in the intestine, help prevent constipation and help reduce cholesterol and blood pressure.

Feeling under the weather? Throat sore and scratchy? Try sipping some hot green tea with a spoonful of honey and a dash of red pepper (cayenne). The potent mix of SuperFoods tea and honey along with red pepper can soothe that inflamed throat. Researchers think that the red pepper subdues one of the body's pain chemicals, substance P – a neuropeptide that carries pain signals to the brain – so that you can swallow more comfortably.

Honey in the Kitchen

It's not difficult to find uses for honey in your kitchen. It's an obvious substitute for sugar in tea and other hot and cold drinks. You can also bake with honey, but you will have to adjust your recipe, as the honey may cause foods to brown more quickly. Reducing the oven temperature by about 25°F and using one quarter cup less liquid in your recipe is a good formula. About one half cup of honey equals a cup of sugar.

Don't keep honey in the fridge, since the cold will cause it to crystallize. If the honey does crystallize, put the container in a bowl of warm water and the crystals will dissolve. Avoid heating honey in the microwave because this can alter the taste.

Here are some suggestions for using honey:

- Add a tablespoon to smoothies and shakes.
- A super after-school snack is a sliced apple or pear drizzled with honey and sprinkled with cinnamon.
- Some fruit-on-the-bottom yogurts have quite a lot of sugar. Make your own version by adding a bit of honey and some fresh fruit to nonfat or low-fat plain yogurt.
- Make a honey-mustard salad dressing by mixing a few tablespoons each of honey with Dijon mustard, a drizzle of lemon juice, and about a quarter cup of extra virgin olive oil. Delicious served on peppery greens like rocket.
- A great way to start the morning: Steep 2 green tea bags in 3 ounces hot water for 3 minutes. Squeeze the tea bags into the water and add ½ to 1 teaspoon honey plus 4 to 5 ounces silk vanilla soymilk. Stir and enjoy.
- Toast 1 slice whole-grain bread and spread with natural peanut butter, dark honey and a sprinkle of cinnamon.

Spring HealthStyle Focus
Fibre

HealthStyle is about habits – the everyday behaviours that can boost your health profile and result in vigorous optimum good health. No *single* habit is likely to turn the tide from illness to optimum health, but a *pattern* of good habits can help ensure a vigorous and vital future. My goal is to persuade you to adopt as many HealthStyle habits as you can over the course of a year so that one year from now you'll feel better than ever, and ten or twenty years from now you'll be better yet.

One of the HealthStyle habits I want you to adopt is the fibre habit. Adequate fibre intake is critical for optimum health. Back in the Paleolithic era, the typical Stone-Ager ate about 47 grams of fibre daily. Today, in Western cultures, the average fibre intake is just 17 grams a day. This simply isn't enough. In my opinion, even America's new Food and Nutrition Board of the Institute of Medicine's recently set goal of 38 grams a day for adult men and 25 grams a day for adult women is low. (Their goal for people over age fifty-one is 30 grams a day for men and 21 grams a day for women; lower because of the typical reduced calorie intake at that age.) My own HealthStyle recommendations may be ambitious, but I believe the health payoffs are well worth it.

Here are the HealthStyle Fibre Challenge Goals:

- 45 grams daily for adult men
- 32 grams daily for adult women

For many people, this will be more than double the amount of fibre you're eating today, but it's not a difficult goal to achieve once you learn how to choose high-fibre, healthy foods. Meeting this HealthStyle fibre challenge will have a dramatic synergistic effect on your overall health and it could be the most important single change you can make in your diet.

Other than a nod to bowel health, the role of fibre just doesn't get much respect. In part, this is because we used to believe that as fibre contained no protein, fat, carbohydrates, vitamins or minerals, its role was pretty much to sweep through the digestive system and add bulk. Not much romance there. We thought that fibre was just cellulose and lignan – the woody part of plants – and that its role was to absorb water and keep things moving along. We now know that fibre is not a single substance, but a powerful variety of compounds that have important and broad-ranging effects on various bodily systems.

What is fibre? It is the general name given to all indigestible carbohydrates. All fibre comes from plant foods, including fruits, vegetables, grains and legumes; meat contains no fibre. In the old days, fibre was divided into two categories – soluble and insoluble. While these simple categories have morphed into more sophisticated ones, they still provide a basic understanding of the role of fibre.

Soluble Fibre. This is fibre that dissolves in water. It plays an important role in lowering cholesterol levels and promoting cardiovascular health. It also helps regulate blood sugar levels, thus playing an important role in the management of diabetes. And finally it contributes to maintaining optimum body weight, because high-fibre foods tend to fill you up while being generally low in calories.

Insoluble Fibre. This is fibre that does not dissolve in water. It adds bulk to the stool while it stimulates peristalsis, the intestinal contractions that move food through the digestive system.

Now that we know that both types of fibre are present in many foods, experts prefer to define fibre in relation to its physiological benefits, for example, intestinal transit time (to mitigate constipation and cancer), viscosity (to escort cholesterol from the system) and fermentability (for intestinal health).

If you learn only a few lessons from HealthStyle, one of them should be a new respect for fibre and making an active effort to eat more of it. Fibre is an essential nutrient, vital to our health.

Here's the simple equation: High-fibre foods are also highly nutritious and are associated with health promotion; low-fibre foods are generally less nutritious and are associated with a greater risk of disease.

Another way to look at it is that people who consume

the most fibre-rich foods are the healthiest from the standpoint of a whole host of health markers. In one study, it was found that the amount of fibre that people consume may better predict weight gain, insulin levels and other cardiovascular risk factors than does the amount of total fat consumed.

> My fibre recommendation is based on fibre that is present in whole foods, not in fibre supplements. Fibre supplements may not contain the health-promoting anticancer and cardiovascular-healthy nutrients that are present in whole, high-fibre foods.

What Fibre Can Do for You

A high-fibre diet has a whole host of health benefits, first and simplest being that these foods tend also to be packed with disease-fighting phytonutrients. This would be reason enough to eat them. But there's more: High-fibre foods have been proven to provide very specific health benefits that promote cardiovascular health, digestive health, and improved glucose tolerance, as well as cancer prevention.

Research has shown that a high-fibre diet may lower the risk of coronary heart disease. When soluble fibre mixes with water in the digestive tract, it forms a gel that acts to mop up cholesterol and escort it from the system. In one study, women who consumed the most cereal fibre were approximately 35 percent less likely to develop heart disease compared with those who ate the least fibre. In another study of 42,850 men, the Health Professional Follow-up Study found that during a fourteen-year period there was an 18 percent decrease in the risk of coronary heart disease in men with the highest daily intake of whole grains and, when adjusted additionally for bran intake, those with the highest bran intake had a 30 percent reduced risk of coronary heart disease. A recent body of research has pointed to the association of C-reactive protein with inflammation and resulting heart disease. Another recent study found that high-fibre intake is inversely associated with C-reactive protein (CRP) levels. In this study, those with the highest fibre intake had almost a 40 percent reduced risk of having a high CRP compared with the participants in the lowest quintile of fibre intake.

A high-fibre diet can play an important role in both preventing diabetes and managing it. We know that by slowing digestion, fibre helps reduce the rapid rise in blood sugar that occurs after eating foods that contain carbohydrates. One small study had impressive results for the participants. The study group included thirteen patients with type II diabetes. By the end of the study, those who ate 50 total grams of fibre daily had seen a total cholesterol reduction of 6.7 percent, an LDL cholesterol reduction of 6.3 percent, a triglyceride reduction of 10.2 percent, a very-low-density lipoprotein cholesterol reduction of 12.5 percent, a blood glucose level reduction of 10 percent, and a blood insulin level reduction of 12 percent. These patients achieved these results by consuming unfortified foods, particularly those high in cholesterol-lowering soluble fibre. While it's true that this is more fibre than many people are accustomed to eating, the health benefits were considerable: For example, the decrease in blood glucose levels was similar to that achieved by taking an oral hypoglycaemic drug.

High-fibre foods play a role, in some instances controversial, in fighting cancer. For example, while the relationship between high-fibre foods and colon cancer remains uncertain, at least two observational studies from Europe and the United States have found an inverse relationship between total dietary fibre and the incidence of colon polyps or cancer. It's also been demonstrated that a high dietary fibre intake reduces the risk of rectal, breast, prostate, laryngeal and ovarian cancers. We do know that fibre can play an important role in preventing a recurrence of breast cancer, and now that, thanks to better care, more and more women are living with a history of breast cancer, it's very important to adopt any and all strategies that could prevent recurrences. Epidemiologic evidence over-whelmingly suggests that a diet low in unhealthy fat and rich in fruits and vegetables is associated with a reduced risk for many primary cancers, including breast cancer. This type of diet also reduces the circulating oestrogen levels in breast cancer survivors and could potentially stave off recurrence. In one study of breast cancer survivors, the intervention group had a significant increase in fibre – from 22 to 29 grams a day – and a significantly lower intake of fat. These women found that their levels of oestrogen decreased significantly, and analysis of the data showed that this change was independently associated with the increased fibre intake, but not the decrease in fat intake. As the author of the study said: '. . . dietary strat-egies that reduce oestrogen stimulation . . . may help reduce risk of recurrence and improve the likelihood of survival in women with a history of breast cancer.'

Good news for those of us trying to maintain an opti-mum weight: A high-fibre diet has been conclusively associated with healthy weight maintenance. It's generally thought that fibre may decrease calorie intake and pro-mote weight loss by inducing satiety – the feeling of fullness – as well as reducing blood glucose concentrations following a meal. We know that soluble fibre intake has been shown to be inversely associated with long-term weight gain. In a recent study, the daily consumption of either three apples or three pears (both fruits are high in soluble fibre) was associated with weight loss in overweight women.

And finally, the old news is still good news: A high-fibre diet promotes normal bowel function and helps prevent constipation, haemorrhoids and diverticulitis.

Top Fibre Choices

- Black beans, 1 cup cooked, 15 grams fibre
- Pinto beans, 1/4 cup dry, 14 grams fibre
- Chickpeas, 1 cup cooked, 13 grams fibre
- Kellogg's Kashi Go Lean Protein/High Fibre Cereal & Snack, 3/4 cup, 10 grams fibre
- Lentils, 1/4 cup dry, 9 grams fibre
- Nestlé Shredded Wheat, 11.8g fibre
- Raspberries, 1 cup raw, 8 grams fibre
- Frozen green peas, 1 cup, 7 grams fibre

The Thirty-Day Fibre Challenge

Here's a way to get you on the fibre bandwagon. It's simple. It will change your life and get you healthy.

It takes about thirty days for your gastrointestinal system to adjust to an optimum fibre intake. If you go too quickly, you'll experience diarrhoea, gas and bloating. In order to meet my HealthStyle Fibre Challenge Goals, you should begin by assessing your current fibre intake. Analyse your fibre intake for a typical day. Write down everything you eat – and the amounts – including all meals and snacks. (This is a great exercise, as it will help you focus on various aspects of your diet.) Once you have your day's food intake charted, find a reference on fibre amounts in foods. Here's a Web source that is quite complete: http://www.nal.usda.gov/fnic/foodcomp/Data/ SR17/wtrank/wt_rank.html. *Your Personal Nutritionist Fiber and Fat Counter* by Ed Blonz is also a helpful resource.

Once you know what your typical daily fibre intake is, it's time to increase it. Try to increase your fibre intake by 4 to 8 grams per week until you reach the goal of 45 grams daily for adult men and 32 grams daily for adult women. Choose one high-fibre food from each class in the list beginning on page 203. Some foods may cause digestive problems; others will not. At the end of four weeks you should have reached your fibre goal. You'll probably notice that you get full more quickly and that your normal regularity is enhanced.

- Pay attention to food labels. The labels of almost all foods will tell you the amount of dietary fibre in each serving.
- Choose whole-grain cereals for breakfast that have at least 3 grams of fibre per serving. Top with wheat germ, ground flaxseed meal, bananas, berries or raisins to increase fibre.
- Eat whole fruits instead of drinking fruit juices. Avoid peeling fruits or vegetables when possible.
- Replace white rice, bread and pasta with brown rice and whole-grain products. Snack on raw vegetables instead of crisps, crackers or chocolate bars.
- Substitute beans for meat two to three times per week in chilli and soups, and add beans to soups, stews and salads.
- Experiment with international dishes that use whole grains and legumes as part of a meal, as in Indian dals or in salads, for example, Middle Eastern tabbouleh.
- Read the following list of brand-name and whole foods that are top choices for high fibre.

It's important to understand exactly what a serving of whole grains is. The following are all considered one serving each: 1 small bran muffin, 1 slice of whole-grain bread, 1 oatmeal cookie, 5 whole-wheat crackers, 1 cup of popcorn, 1 cup cooked brown rice, 1 cup cooked oatmeal.

Top HealthStyle Fibre Choices

Cereals

- Kellogg's Kashi GoLean High Protein/High Fibre Cereal, 10 grams fibre per ¾ cup, 140 calories
- Kellogg's All Bran Bran Buds, 13 grams fibre per ½ cup, 70 calories
- Kellogg's Sultana Bran, 5 grams fibre/127 calories per serving, 13 grams fibre per ½ cup, 50 calories
- Kellogg's All Bran Original, 11 grams fibre, 110 calories per serving, 10 grams fibre per ½ cup, 80 calories
- Kellogg's Complete Wheat Bran Flakes, 5 grams fibre per ¾ cup, 90 calories
- Jordan's Wheat Germ, 2 grams fibre per 2 tablespoons (13 grams), 50 calories
- Quaker Oat Bran Hot Cereal, 6 grams fibre per ½ cup, 150 calories
- Simply Fibre, 14 grams fibre per 1 cup, 100 calories
- Check out Jordan's and Nature's Path products for other high-fibre options

Crackers and Crispbread

- Dr Karg Seeded Spelt Crisp Bread, 100 grams = 426 calories and 12.1 grams fibre
- Organic Finn Crisp, 100 grams = 18 grams fibre
- Ryvita Dark Rye whole-grain crispbread, 3 grams fibre per 2 slices, 70 calories (www.ryvita.com)
- Wasa Multigrain Crispbread, 2 grams fibre per 1 slice, 40 calories

Pizza

- A. C. La Rocca Pizza Company, multiple varieties, 3 to 8 grams fibre per serving

Fruits

- Mott's Organic Unsweetened Apple Sauce, 1 gram fibre per ½ cup, 50 calories

- Apple, 1 large with peel, 5.7 grams fibre, 125 calories
- Avocado, ½ cup medium, 4.2 grams fibre, 153 calories
- Blackberries, 7.6 grams fibre per 1 cup, 75 calories
- Blueberries, 3.9 grams fibre per 1 cup, 81 calories
- Dates, 3 grams fibre per 5 to 6 pitted Deglet Noor dates, 120 calories
- Figs, 2 medium, 3.3 grams fibre, 74 calories
- Kiwis, 5 grams fibre per 2 medium, 93 calories
- Orange, 3.4 grams fibre per 1 medium, 64 calories
- Papaya, 2.5 grams fibre per 1 cup cubes, 55 calories
- Pears, 4 grams fibre per 1 medium Bartlett, 98 calories
- Persimmons, 6.1 grams fibre per 1 large, 118 calories
- Pavich Organic Raisins, 2 grams fibre per ¼ cup, 120 calories
- Sunmaid Raisins, 2 grams fibre per ¼ cup (one small box), 130 calories
- Raspberries, 8.4 grams fibre per 1 cup, 60 calories
- Strawberries, 3.5 grams fibre per 1 cup, 46 calories
- Sweet potato, 3.7 grams fibre per 1 medium (4 ounces), 143 calories

Nuts (all listed per 1 ounce)
- Meridian Almond Butter, 7.4 grams fibre per 100 grams, 633 calories
- Almonds (24), 3 grams fibre and 160 calories
- Hazelnuts (20), 3 grams fibre and 180 calories
- Pecans (20 halves), 3 grams fibre and 200 calories
- Pistachios (49), 3 grams fibre and 160 calories
- Walnuts (14 halves), 2 grams fibre and 190 calories
- Peanuts (28), 2 grams fibre and 170 calories

Legumes
- Chickpeas, ½ cup cooked, 6.2 grams fibre, 135 calories
- Green peas, 8.8 grams fibre per 1 cup cooked, 134 calories
- Pinto beans, ½ cup cooked, 7.4 grams fibre, 117 calories

- Sainsbury's Organic Tuscan Bean Soup, 4 grams fibre per 100 gram serving
- Waitrose Perfectly Balanced Tuscan Three Bean Soup, 3.5 grams fibre per 100 gram serving, 33 calories

Vegetables
- Asparagus, 1 cup cooked, 2.9 grams fibre, 43 calories
- Broccoli, 1 cup cooked, 4.7 grams fibre, 44 calories
- Butternut squash, 3.5 grams fibre per ½ cup baked, 49 calories
- Cauliflower, 1 cup cooked, 3.3 grams fibre, 29 calories
- Spring greens, 5.3 grams fibre per 1 cup cooked, 49 calories
- Corn, 4.6 grams fibre per 1 cup cooked kernels, 177 calories
- Libby's 100% tinned pumpkin, 5 grams fibre per ½ cup, 40 calories
- Swiss chard, 3.7 grams fibre per 1 cup cooked, 35 calories
- Tomato, 2.5 grams fibre per 1 medium, 48 calories

Spring SuperFood Update
Tea

A source of:

- Flavonoids
- Fluoride
- No calories

SIDEKICKS: none
TRY TO DRINK: 1 to 4 cups daily or more

If you're not drinking tea regularly, you're missing out on an opportunity to give yourself a powerful health boost –

for no calories and very little cost. You probably have a few boxes of tea in your cupboard. If not, treat yourself to some of the new, flavourful teas that are now widely available. Next time you're relaxing on the sofa reading the paper, working at your desk, or sitting in the garden watching nature go by, make it a more healthful experience by sipping some tea. Iced or hot, tea is an all-season HealthStyle all-star.

Green tea, black, tea, oolong tea – they're all produced from the evergreen shrub *Camellia sinensis*, and they all are beneficial to your health in remarkable ways. It's the antioxidant flavonoids in tea that give it its health-promoting power. Green tea is particularly rich in flavonoids such as catechins, one of which, epigallocatechin-3-gallate (EGCG), plays an impressive role in fighting cancer.

Research has demonstrated that regular tea consumption is associated with:

- Lower blood pressure
- Cancer prevention
- Heart health
- Lower risk of stroke
- Lower risk of osteoporosis
- Lower risk of skin cancer
- Decreased sun-induced ageing of skin
- Cataract prevention, according to preliminary studies

In addition, tea is also recognized as being antiviral, anti-inflammatory and anti-allergy. And, finally, there's evidence that drinking tea is associated with beneficial changes in regard to obesity, periodontal disease, diabetes, longevity and neural function. Who could ask for more from an inexpensive, widely available flavourful drink?

Which tea is best: black or green, decaf or regular? Well, a cup of black tea has 268 mg of flavonoids; green, 316. Decaf tea has about 85 percent of the flavonoids found in regular tea. You can increase the flavonoid amounts in any tea by squeezing the bag after steeping for a few minutes. The amount of polyphenols is highest in freshly brewed tea and these decrease with time. Caffeine is a natural component of all teas. In general, a cup of tea contains less than half the caffeine of coffee. However, the actual milligrams of caffeine found in different teas are dependent on the specific brew strength and blends of tea leaves. Tinned, iced and powdered teas all have benefits, but the best bang for your money is from freshly brewed and then consumed tea.

Tea Update

Research into the power of tea is ongoing. Here are just a few highlights of what's been discovered recently.

Given the epidemic of hypertension today, it's excellent news that tea can play a beneficial role in reducing blood pressure. A study of more than 1,500 men and women who drank tea regularly for at least a year saw a considerable reduction in their risk of high blood pressure. Those who drank 1/2 to 21/2 cups a day saw a 46 percent reduction in risk while those who drank more than 21/2 cups saw a 65 percent reduction. This is an impressive result.

A UK study reported that green tea seems to inhibit heart cell death after a heart attack or stroke, and also that it appears to speed recovery from same.

An animal study suggests that eating black pepper at the same time as drinking green tea can significantly increase the amount of the cancer-fighting EGCG absorbed by your body. So, the next time you're drinking tea with a meal, grind some black pepper into your soup, salad or main course.

Green and black teas' ability to fight cancer has been amply demonstrated in study after study. Indeed, in the US the Chemoprevention Branch of the National Cancer Institute has even developed a project that will test compounds found in tea to study their cancer prevention abilities in human subjects. Interestingly, tea seems to help prevent cancer in a variety of ways: Its antioxidant ability has perhaps been most widely studied, but it also inhibits blood flow to cancer cells, thus starving them. Green tea seems to be able to shut off the growth-promoting genes in cancerous cells, thus encouraging the cancer cells to self-destruct. Tea also helps neutralize the cancer-promoting properties of certain environmental toxins.

One study showed that the polyphenols in green tea actually boosted the effectiveness of one of the most common cancer drugs – doxorubicin – by causing the cancer cells to retain the drug rather than repel it.

Given the alarming rise in the rate of diabetes worldwide, it's encouraging to learn that recent studies have shown that green tea is effective in improving insulin sensitivity. In one study, healthy subjects who consumed green tea were subsequently given glucose tolerance tests. The green tea actually increased the ability of the body to manage blood sugar effectively.

Finally, if there weren't enough good reasons to drink tea, here's a finding that sends most of my patients right to their kettles. In a recent study, it was found that green tea not only promoted cardiovascular health by reducing damage to LDL cholesterol and thus reducing plaque formation, it also reduced body fat. In the twelve weeks of the study, thirty-eight normal-to-overweight men who drank one bottle of green tea daily had significantly lower body weight, BMI, waist circumference, body-fat mass, and amount of subcutaneous fat compared with men who had consumed a bottle of oolong tea daily. It seems that the amount of catechin flavonoids made the difference. The green tea contained 690 mg of catechins while the oolong tea had just 22 mg of catechins.

The Tea in Your Life

As promising and indeed almost astonishing as some of these finds are, I really don't think anyone should drink tea with the single intention of, say, lowering blood pressure or losing weight. On the other hand, given the incredibly impressive ability of tea, particularly green tea, to promote health, I can't imagine why anyone wouldn't drink it regularly. I sip it often in the course of the day. When I travel, I tuck some green tea bags into my pocket for an in-flight beverage or something to sip in a hotel room (many hotel rooms have coffeemakers or kettles that will heat water for tea).

Here are some ideas for using tea, particularly green tea:

- Brew green tea with a few slices of fresh peeled ginger and lemon.
- Brew green tea in room-temperature water for a half hour and use in marinades, dressings, soups and sauces. Brewing at room temperature or in cool water will prevent bitterness.
- Mix brewed tea with fruit juice and pour over ice.

SPRING HEALTHSTYLE RECIPES
Sweet Potato, Tofu and Kale Frittata

Serves 5

This is delicious served hot, warm or cool. Frittatas make excellent sandwiches with crusty bread, lettuce and a little mustard. You can use any type of tofu for this frittata: Soft tofu is similar to a creamy cheese, and firm tofu is like a harder cheese. I enjoy it both ways. Most cookware, even those with plastic handles, can go into an oven preheated to 350°F. Check the instructions that came with your pan.

⅔ cup peeled and diced sweet potato
3 whole kale leaves, finely diced
4 large omega-3 eggs
3 large egg whites
½ cup diced soft or firm tofu
1 garlic clove, minced
½-inch piece fresh ginger, peeled and minced
2 tablespoons chives, minced
⅛ teaspoon sea salt
Olive oil spray

Preheat the oven to 350°F. Steam the sweet potato and kale with a little water in a covered pan to soften slightly, 5 to 7 minutes (or place in a bowl with a little water, cover, and microwave on medium for about 3 minutes). Whisk the eggs and egg whites. Stir in the tofu, garlic, chives and sea salt. Pour into a 9- or 10-inch nonstick pan sprayed with olive oil spray. Cook in the oven for 30 minutes, or until the centre is set. There is no need to turn the frittata over or grill the top unless you'd like to do so.

Calories: 114
Protein: 10 g
Carbohydrates: 7 g
Cholesterol: 148 mg
Total fat: 5.3 g
  Saturated fat: 1.2 g
  Monounsaturated fat: 1.5 g

Polyunsaturated fat: 1.7 g
  Omega-6 linoleic acid : 1.1 mg
  Omega-3 linoleic acid: 0.1 g
EPA/DHA: 0.44 g
Sodium: 150 mg
Potassium: 209 mg
Fibre: 7.6 mg

Strawberry, Kiwi and Banana Compote

Serves 6

The mixture of honey and orange creates a delicious sauce. You can toast the walnuts in a 300°F oven for about 10 minutes, or until fragrant and golden before stirring them into the other ingredients. I like this fruit compote on oatmeal in the winter and on pancakes all year round.

2 pints strawberries, organic
3 medium bananas, ripe
5 medium kiwis, ripe
2 medium oranges, zest and juice
2 tablespoons honey
¼ cup walnuts, crushed

Quarter the strawberries, slice the bananas and peel, core and dice the kiwis. Gently toss with the orange juice, zest and honey. Stir in the crushed walnuts. Allow to macerate at room temperature or in the fridge for at least 30 minutes. Serve over soy ice cream, frozen yogurt, or breakfast foods like oatmeal, whole-grain pancakes or waffles.

Calories: 202
Protein: 3.2 g
Carbohydrates: 41 g
Cholesterol: 0.0
Total fat: 4.4 g
  Saturated fat: 0.5 g
  Monounsaturated fat: 0.6 g

Polyunsaturated fat: 2.8 g
  Omega-6 linoleic acid: 2.1 g
  Omega-3 linoleic acid: 0.6 g
Sodium: 3 mg
Potassium: 707 mg
Fibre: 7.2 g

Sesame Noodles with Spinach and Courgette Sauté

Serves 4

Use buckwheat soba, udon, Chinese noodles, fettuccine or linguine in this dish. Toasted sesame oil, a rich dark brown in colour, is used as a flavouring.

1 pound noodles
1 tablespoon extra virgin olive oil
3 garlic cloves, minced
1 medium leek, halved and sliced, white and green parts
1-inch piece fresh ginger, peeled and minced, optional
3 small courgettes, halved lengthwise and cut into 1/2-inch-thick slices
2 tablespoons low-sodium soy sauce
⅔ cup brewed green tea
1 cup fresh or frozen green soybeans, shelled, or green peas
4 cups fresh baby spinach
1 medium lemon, zest and juice
2 teaspoons toasted sesame oil
2 tablespoons sesame seeds

Bring a large pan of water to a boil for the noodles. Note that Asian noodles usually have a higher salt content than Italian pasta, so salt the water accordingly, and they cook much faster than pasta. While the noodles are cooking, heat the olive oil in a large frying pan, add the garlic and sauté for a minute, then add the leek and sauté until softened and bright green, about a minute. Add the ginger, if using, and the courgettes and sauté until the courgettes are almost tender, about 3 minutes. Add the soy sauce, brewed tea and soybeans, and bring to a low boil. Add the spinach, lemon juice and zest, toasted sesame oil and sesame seeds, and stir once. Serve over drained hot noodles.

Calories: 538
Protein: 23 g
Carbohydrates: 103
Cholesterol: 0.0
Total fat: 9.4 g
  Saturated fat: 1.4 g
  Monounsaturated fat: 4.7 g

Polyunsaturated fat: 2.6 g
Omega-6 linoleic acid: 2.2 g
Omega-3 linoleic acid: 0.1 g
Sodium: 1,251 mg
Potassium: 1,018 mg
Fibre: 13.7 g

Flavourful Roasted Tofu

Serves 6

Even if you're a tofu novice, this tastes good. Roasted tofu is a versatile addition to a green salad, served over brown rice, or in place of cheese in a sandwich. Try it with avocado, tomato and lettuce on whole-wheat bread for a taste treat. Dice it up with some peas and corn and have it as a lettuce wrap.

3 garlic cloves
1- to 1½-inch piece fresh ginger, peeled
2 medium shallots, thinly sliced
1 teaspoon chilli powder
2 tablespoons any type of miso
2 tablespoons extra virgin olive oil
Freshly ground black pepper
1 cup low-sodium organic vegetable or chicken stock
1 large orange, zest and juice
1 pound firm tofu

Preheat the oven to 425°F. Finely mince the garlic and ginger in a food processor, or slice or mince with a knife, and add them to the chilli powder, miso, oil, pepper,

stock, orange zest and juice. Rinse the tofu, cut it into
½-inch-thick slices, and pat dry. Lay the tofu in a rectangu-
lar baking dish. Pour the marinade over the tofu and bake
immediately. (Alternatively, allow to marinate for an hour,
or even overnight, in the fridge before baking.) When most
of the liquid is evaporated and saucy, the tofu is ready, 30
to 40 minutes.

Calories: 133 *Polyunsaturated fat: 2 g*
Protein: 7.4 g *Omega-6 linoleic acid: 1.8 g*
Carbohydrates: 9.1 g *Omega-3 linoleic acid: 0.2 g*
Cholesterol: 0.0 *Sodium: 240 mg*
Total fat: 8.5 g *Potassium: 255 mg*
  Saturated fat: 1.2 g *Fibre: 1.6 g*
  Monounsaturated fat: 0.8 g

A Greener Salad

Serves 8

A refreshing salad that is a study in green with lettuces,
edamame, cucumbers and apple.

Dressing
1 medium shallot, minced
1 tablespoon any type of miso
1 tablespoon Dijon mustard
¼ cup red wine vinegar
2 tablespoons extra virgin olive oil

Salad
Black pepper
1 medium cucumber, sliced
1 medium Granny Smith apple, cored and sliced
1 pound green soybeans (edamame), cooked
  according to package directions

1 head romaine lettuce, torn into bite-sized pieces
2 heads Butterhead lettuce, torn into bite-sized
pieces

Whisk together the dressing ingredients and set aside. In a large bowl, toss the cucumber, apple and green soybeans with just enough of the dressing to coat. Add the lettuces with more dressing to coat. Divide among 8 salad plates.

Calories: 148	*Polyunsaturated fat: 2.2 g*
Protein: 8.9 g	*Omega-6 linoleic acid: 1.7 g*
Carbohydrates: 12.9 g	*Omega-3 linoleic acid: 0.3 g*
Cholesterol: <1 g	*Sodium: 83 mg*
Total fat: 7.8 g	*Potassium: 620 mg*
Saturated fat: 1 g	*Fibre: 4 g*
Monounsaturated fat: 3.6 g	

Sichuan Green Tea, Cauliflower and Tofu Stir-fry

Serves 6

Fermented black beans and black bean chilli sauce are available in the Asian aisle of most supermarkets. Keeping the chilli peppers whole makes it easy to remove them once the dish is cooked. If you prefer not to use sherry, add two more tablespoons of tea. Grapeseed oil is neutral in flavour and has a high smoking point, but extra virgin olive oil works just as well.

2 tablespoons grapeseed or extra virgin olive oil
2 garlic cloves, minced
2 medium shallots, minced
1-inch piece fresh ginger, peeled and minced
1 package firm tofu, cut into 1-inch squares and
dried

1¼ cups whole almonds
6 small chilli peppers
1 tablespoon fermented black beans, optional
1 head cauliflower, broken up into florets
2 tablespoons Chinese sherry or dark sherry
2 tablespoons low-sodium soy sauce
½ cup brewed oolong or green tea

Heat the oil in a frying pan set over medium-high heat. When hot, add the minced garlic, shallots and ginger. Sauté until fragrant, about a minute. Add the tofu and sauté until lightly golden, about 7 minutes. Add the almonds and whole chillies and sauté for several minutes more. Add the black beans (if using) and the cauliflower, and toss. Add the sherry, soy and tea and sauté until the cauliflower is crisp-tender. Divide among 6 plates and serve.

Calories: 326	*Monounsaturated fat: 12.6 g*
Protein: 17 g	*Polyunsaturated fat: 6.5 g*
Carbohydrates: 18 g	*Sodium: 288 mg*
Cholesterol: 0.0	*Potassium: 938 mg*
Total fat: 23.7 g	*Fibre: 8 g*
Saturated fat: 2 g	

Honey Green Tea Sparkler

Serves 10

This is a refreshing and healthy alternative to fizzy drinks. If using green tea bags, use twelve or more. You can make all sorts of variations. Use any type of green tea you like, and family favourite juices like cranberry, all-natural lemonade, peach, orange, grapefruit, pineapple and blueberry. Try black tea with cherry juice for a tasty quencher. Make some into ice cubes to use when chilling the tea. San Pellegrino mineral water from Italy is a natural source of calcium.

¼ cup honey
½ cup jasmine green tea leaves, or more to taste
2 pints ice cubes
1 cup white grape juice
Sparkling water

Heat 2 pints water to boiling. Remove from the heat and stir in the honey, then the green tea leaves. Allow to steep for 3 to 5 minutes, then strain into a large pitcher. Add the ice cubes and stir to melt. Add the grape juice. Pour over ice into glasses 3/4 full. Top off with sparkling water, stir once, and serve.

Calories: 14
Protein: < 1 g
Carbohydrates: 3.4 g
Cholesterol: 0.0

Total fat: < 1 g
Sodium: 3 mg
Potassium: 76 mg
Fibre: < 1 g

Summer: Season of Peace

At last, it's summer. The days are long. The weather invites you outdoors and makes it easier to be active and stick with your exercise goals. The luscious fruits and vine-ripened vegetables of summer are at their best and readily available. Farmers' markets abound with produce, and the opportunity to get fresh foods at their source is something we should all take advantage of. Healthy meals seem a snap: Salads and grilled fish can be a quick and welcome meal after a day's work or an afternoon at the beach. It seems that nature is conspiring to help you achieve optimum HealthStyle.

While nature gives you so much encouragement in so many aspects of your HealthStyle summer goals, now it's time to take a look at a facet of a healthy life that is too often ignored: the impact of your mind on your physical health. This fascinating topic, which has only recently found strong support in various impressive studies, covers spirituality, stress control and other techniques that are available to improve your health in ways never imagined before.

WHOLE MIND/WHOLE BODY HEALTH

You are more than the sum of your parts. You are an intensely complicated mechanism of bodily systems, mental states, whims and enthusiasms that react to the weather, the traffic, the noise and a loved one's caress in unique and profound ways. You have good days and bad. Sometimes you turn the key and your engine purrs; other days you get nothing but a backfire.

What am I getting at here? I'm introducing one of the oldest concepts in human health that's become one of the hottest topics in medicine and research: the mind/body connection. Wise men have long known that there is an intimate connection between your inner self and your physical state. They really can't be separated. It's time to look at what, for many people, is a new frontier in medicine.

HealthStyle is about whole body/whole mind health. One of my goals is to have you appreciate that achieving your best healthy self involves more than good nutrition, exercise and other activities that focus on you as a physical machine. True health involves the whole you: body, mind, spirit.

There is a new field of medicine that explores this relationship. It's called psychoneuroimmunoendocrinology (or PNIE). This describes the study of the unity of mental, neurological, hormonal and immunological functions – in effect, the combination of mind, body and spirit.

Here are some intriguing examples to illustrate this field of research:

A study of people who had suffered a heart attack found that *those suffering from depression had a threefold risk of dying in the year after the event.*

A four-year study of nearly one thousand people from Finland found that the group identified as 'high-hopelessness' experienced a 19 percent greater thickening of atherosclerotic plaque compared with the 'moderate or low-hopelessness' group. This indicates that *intensely felt negative emotions can actually promote the development of cardiovascular disease.*

A study of nearly thirteen thousand men and women found that anger was a significant risk factor for death from coronary artery disease, independent of other biological risk factors exhibited by these subjects. Indeed, several studies suggest that *risks are greater for emotional distress – depression, anger, grief, hostility, anxiety, frustration, resentment – as well as social isolation, than for conventional medical risks.*

One study found a *significantly increased risk of suffering a heart attack following the death of a loved one.* The elevated risk in the first twenty-four hours after the loss is fourteenfold higher than if the subject were in a normal state without the loss of a loved one. In the second twenty-four hours following a loss, the risk is eightfold. Over the ensuing month, the risk is two- to fourfold higher.

Another study reported that among more than one thousand adults with coronary artery disease, the patients who were depressed felt a greater burden from their symptoms, greater physical limitations, worse quality of life, and worse overall health. It's not a simple matter of attitude influencing symptoms: intensely felt negative emotions – including anxiety and fear, anger and rage, and grief and sadness – are all associated *with increased incidence of premature cardiovascular death in adulthood as well as greatly increased complications after heart attack.*

Don't you find this information powerful but also rather intuitive? In your heart, you've probably always known that your mental state affects your health. HealthStyle's important message is that you can and must do something about this connection *over and above recognizing it.* You can't separate your physical health from your emotional/

mental/spiritual health. If you truly want to achieve optimum HealthStyle, you must recognize the power of the mind/body connection and take whatever steps you can to improve on this often neglected aspect of robust health.

How We Got Here

Modern medicine is in constant transition. New findings topple old; time-honoured practices are discarded as new ones prove more effective. If you are reading this book, you've no doubt seen dramatic changes in health care. A more recent change has involved my particular speciality – the role of nutrition in disease. It wasn't so long ago that nutrition was virtually ignored by traditional medicine as a factor in precipitating disease. For a period of time, vitamins, sometimes in mega-doses, were seen as a solution to health. Today, we know that whole foods are the backbone of a healthy lifestyle and that appropriate supplementation is important but is never a substitute for a healthy diet.

One exciting frontier in nutrition and health involves the precise and delicate interaction of the nutrients in foods and our genes. One day we may be able to prescribe a diet based on your genetic makeup – one that will use foods to enhance protective genes and suppress ones that make you susceptible to certain diseases. Of course, at present we know that a SuperFood diet is your best chance of promoting health, whatever your genotype. We also know that adequate exercise is absolutely fundamental to a healthy lifestyle – not just to lose weight and not just to get strong, but to amplify every single aspect of good nutrition.

We're ready as health care consumers to move into the new frontier of stress reduction and 'mindfulness' as a health-promoting activity. To that end I'd like to introduce my HealthStyle version of achieving stress relief and promoting lifelong health: Personal Peace. But before I can explain the goals and practice of Personal Peace, you have to understand the role of stress in your everyday life and its effects upon your long- and short-term health.

Stress

If there's an opposite of Personal Peace, it's stress. Stress is as much a part of living as breathing, but it's something that we ignore at our peril. We all have a general idea of what it is, but it was first studied by Hans Selye, who defined stress as both a psychological and a physiological event. It was recognized that there are both good and bad stressors. A positive stress is a challenge; a negative one is overload. Words that define our reactions to a negative stress could include fear, anxiety, frustration, anger, depression and helplessness. Many of us find our days laced with these emotions. Many of us are unaware that these 'feelings' are affecting both our short- and long-term health.

When we feel stress – an unreasonable boss, a sick child, too many bills, sleep deprivation, a rude shop assistant – our body shifts into overdrive. Levels of the stress hormones adrenaline and corcortisol elevate and the body shifts into fight-or-flight response with increased metabolism, heart rate, respiration, blood pressure and muscle tension. In a twenty-first-century world, usually there's no actual physical fight or flight involved as a result of stress. Rather, usually a slow burn with a metabolism in high gear and no physical response that allows us to let off steam. Too many of us spend too much time all stressed up with no place to go. The end result is more than simple frustration. It's an actual physical disease. An estimated 75 to 90 percent of all adult visits to primary-care physicians are prompted by stress-related complaints. We now know that unresolved chronic stress can damage the immune and other systems. It is linked to the development of insulin resistance (a risk factor for diabetes) as well as hypertension, coronary heart disease, osteoporosis and other disorders. There's some evidence that it might even promote cancer. There's also evidence that chronic, unrelieved stress causes a variety of physical reactions that may not go away. Eventually, enough stress over a long period of time renders us unable to calm down physiologically. It's as if our engines are locked in overdrive.

Symptoms of Stress
- You eat more or less than normal.
- You feel tired constantly.
- You drink more alcohol, smoke more or use drugs more frequently.
- Your sleep habits change.
- You have aches and pains that are not the result of exercise.
- You feel more anxious, nervous or angry than usual.
- You have to use the bathroom more or less often than normal.
- You are more forgetful.
- You notice other changes in the way you behave.

Personal Peace

Personal Peace is your weapon against unrelieved stress. Personal Peace allows the ratcheting down of the fight-or-flight response into a state of serenity that actually has positive physiological and psychological benefits. Just as a constant stream of multiple antioxidants fights the unending onslaughts of free-radical damage on a cellular level, so the regular achievement of Personal Peace enables your body to recover from the inevitable daily onslaughts of stress. To achieve optimum health, you need Personal Peace as much as you need the nutrients provided by whole foods. Personal Peace will restore you to your whole mind, body and spirit.

Personal Peace isn't something that you achieve once and for all. Rather, it's a process, a mind-set, a habit of regularly retreating to a place of inner calm. This retreat has actual physiological benefits that can pay off in reducing risk of a host of chronic diseases. The notion of Personal Peace is not a new idea. It has always existed in the context of religious teachings. In Eastern cultures, it is an essential part of daily existence. The news about Personal Peace or mindfulness or spirituality is that it has measurable definable physiological effects that can benefit us all.

As I mentioned, *Personal* is a key aspect to this concept. There's no simple prescription for achieving this. It's not comparable to the basic recommendation of eating a cup of spinach daily or getting thirty minutes of exercise. *Personal* Peace is about you and your world. So many factors come into play that will affect how the mind and spirit can best achieve Personal Peace. There are vast cultural, religious and even geographic and gender differences that affect us. There are more elusive, almost inexplicable preferences that guide us in our choices and our achievement of pleasure and serenity. You must determine your best route to Personal Peace. All I can do is urge you to take active steps to achieve this goal as the evidence is truly overwhelming that it's a route to a healthier and happier life.

How do you achieve Personal Peace? My general recommendation is to select one or more stress-reducing practices from the list below and incorporate them into your daily life. I use a host of these practices, from the relaxation response to prayer to exercise to nature, at various times every single day to achieve my own Personal Peace. Consciously working on this aspect of coping with stress has changed my life, and I know you'll reap similar rewards when you achieve your own Personal Peace. Here are some common, proven approaches to Personal Peace that have demonstrated physiological benefits:

The Relaxation Response

When I left home for college, my mother told me that it was important to learn to relax, that it wasn't always something that just 'happened', and that learning to relax could help me fall asleep and help me cope with the stresses of school. She told me to lie down and let each part of my body relax until it felt heavy. What my mother was teaching me was progressive muscle relaxation, or the relaxation response.

Herbert Benson, a doctor at Harvard, wrote about the relaxation response in his book *The Relaxation Response*. Here is the simple technique:

- Sit or lie down quietly (if lying down, be sure you don't go to sleep!). Close your eyes, deeply relax all your muscles, beginning at your feet and ending at your face.
- Breathe through your nose and become aware of your breathing. As you breathe out, say a word. ('One' was what Benson suggested but any word will do.) Breathe in, breathe out (repeat 'One'), breathe in, breathe out (repeat 'One'), and so on. Breathe naturally and easily.
- Continue for ten to twenty minutes. You can open your eyes to check the time, but don't use an alarm. When finished, sit or lie quietly for a few minutes.
- Be passive. Ignore distracting thoughts.

Two good resources for coping with stress are *Power Over Stress*, by Kenford Nedd, M.D., and *Instant Emotional Healing: Acupressure for the Emotions*, by George Pratt and Peter Lambrov.

You should do the relaxation response once or twice daily. Don't do it within two hours of eating, as digestion seems to interfere with the effectiveness of the response. At first, you may find it difficult to achieve the relaxation response. You'll be distracted and your head might fill with unrelated thoughts. Try to gently ignore those distractions and focus on your breathing.

You might find it a challenge at first. Perhaps it will seem like a waste of time, but persevere and you'll begin to reap the rewards. People who regularly practise the relaxation response find they have:

- A better awareness of the tension levels in their bodies and thus a better ability to relax in any situation
- Improved concentration
- Reduced resting levels of the fight-or-flight portion of the autonomic nervous system

The Relaxation Response

	fight or flight	relaxation response
Metabolism	up	down
Heart rate	up	down
Blood pressure	up	down
Breathing rate	up	down
Muscle tension	up	down

Want a simple method to achieve Personal Peace? Keep a photograph of loved ones in your wallet or at your workplace. In one study, it was found that sheep who are temporarily isolated from their flock endure an increase in stress as measured by heart rate, changes in movements and vocalization, and hormone levels. But when the sheep were shown photos of other sheep, all symptoms of stress were reversed. Abstract face shapes and goat photos had no effect. This positive response can be extrapolated to humans, as it involves our highly complex ability to recognize and respond to familiar faces. Though we don't understand precisely how this mechanism works, we do know that the link between face recognition and physiological response is real.

Meditation

Similar in many ways to the relaxation response, meditation is a state in which the body is relaxed and the mind is calm and focused. Mindfulness, or meditation, is the method the Buddha taught as part of the means to end suffering. Meditation is the practice of paying attention to the breath and to sensations in the present moment rather than getting lost in random thoughts, whether memories of the past, commentary on the present, or anticipation of the future. Meditation has been demonstrated to ease chronic pain, depression, anxiety and stress, improve heart health, boost mood and immunity, and generally improve symptoms associated with many chronic ailments. Meditation is not difficult to learn, and those who meditate regularly are able to achieve a relaxed, meditative state very quickly. The greatest rewards of meditation come with practice and persistence.

Almost all techniques of stress reduction have similar components: repetition of a sound or word, phrase or prayer; image or physical activity and a passive disregard of everyday thoughts as they occur. For me, silently repeating my mantra 'Trust in God' has a 100 percent track record in pushing any negative thought or emotion out of my mind.

Meditation has measurable effects on health. One study showed a significant lowering of blood pressure and heart rate in black adults, as well as a reduction in atherosclerosis of the carotid artery, which supplies blood to the brain.

Another study showed that African American teenagers who meditated for fifteen minutes twice a day for four months were able to lower their blood pressure a few points. This is significant, because African Americans suffer disproportionately from hypertension, and if blood pressure can be reduced in teens, they are more likely to enjoy a reduced risk for hypertension as they age.

Scientific evidence shows that people who are meditating experience an increase of activity in the part of the brain that controls metabolism and heart rate. Studies on Buddhist monks show that meditation produces long-lasting changes in the brain activity in areas involving attention, working memory, learning and conscious perception.

A recent study recruited sixty-two 'stressed-out' volunteers and found that those who underwent 'mindfulness training' had experienced an average 54 percent reduction in psychological distress by the end of the three-month study. The control subjects had no such reduction. The trainees also reported a 46 percent drop in medical symptoms over the period of the study, compared with a slight increase in the control group.

Meditation involves focusing the mind on an object or word, consciously relaxing the body and repeating a word or phrase. It's ideal to practise meditating twice a day – in the morning and evening. As Gandhi stated, 'Meditation is the key to the morning and the latch of the evening.' Set aside ten to fifteen minutes to meditate. Find a quiet place and sit comfortably relaxed with eyes open or closed. Choose a phrase to repeat. Feel your body relax and if your mind wanders, return it to your chosen phrase. Remain in this state for ten to twenty minutes.

Persistent high levels of stress hormones impair memory in people of all ages by affecting brain areas involved in

cognitive processing. These stress hormones – glucocorti-
coids – are normally released in times of stress, and studies
show that both short- and long-term exposure to these hormones can have a negative effect on the memory and
cognitive processing in both children and adults. Older
adults who experience constantly high levels of stress hormones may also experience as much as a 14 percent
shrinkage of the hippocampus – the brain area involved in
emotion and memory.

Spirituality and Religious Practice: The Power of Prayer
There is increasing evidence that religious practice such as
prayer enhances health. Since antiquity, people of every
geographic area, culture, ideology, and religious belief
system have used prayer as a means to positively affect
their daily life and well-being. William James described
prayer as 'every kind of inward communication or conversation with the power recognized as divine'.

Scientific studies suggest that if you want to live longer,
frequent attendance at religious services may yield positive
health benefits. Even among individuals who attend religious services once a month or more, mortality rates
appear to be lower than among people who attend rarely
or not at all. These benefits accrue for both Judeo-
Christian and non-Judeo-Christian religions, and at least
one study demonstrates a positive outcome for people who
primarily and regularly practise their prayer in a
nonchurch/religious-facility setting.

We know that religiosity or spirituality is associated
with lower blood pressure and less risk of developing
hypertension. Blood pressure studies show a generally con-
sistent pattern connecting greater religious involvement to
lower blood pressure or a lower incidence of hypertension.
There is also evidence that religious activity is associated
with better blood lipid profiles, with lower LDLs and

229

higher HDLs among those who regularly participate in religious services. Finally, there's evidence that those who worship regularly also enjoy better immune function.

Multiple studies on religion and health indicate 'a trend toward better health and less morbidity across the board in the presence of higher levels of religiosity'.

If you do regularly practise a religion, you can be encouraged by the positive evidence that this habit enhances your health.

> People who are interested in developing their spiritual side may experience fewer hospitalizations and require less long-term care than their peers who are less spiritual. An interesting study found a connection between spirituality and health care needs. While it's unclear what the exact connection between spirituality and health is, evidence suggests that those who are inclined to develop their spiritual life may reap the rewards of better health.

Personal Peace in an Instant

Stress can appear at any time. While a regular habit of stress-relieving meditation or relaxation response is restorative, it's also very helpful to take full advantage of other simple stress-reducing techniques throughout the day. Many of you probably use one or more of these techniques automatically and unconsciously, but sometimes when you employ a stress-reduction technique consciously and deliberately, it can be more effective.

Here are some simple techniques to bring more peace into your life:

Breathe Deeply. Deep, diaphragmatic breathing can be an excellent stress reducer. Research has shown that slowing down and deepening our breath shifts us from the stress response to the relaxation response. Optimal breathing can not only help reduce stress levels, it can also improve performance. I often stop and take a few deep breaths to reduce stress in any situation. Here's how: Sit or stand comfortably and place your hands on your stomach. (Once you've practised, you won't need to do this.) Inhale slowly and deeply, letting your abdomen expand like a balloon. Exhale, letting your abdomen fall as you release all the air. Press the air out as you contract your abdomen, pulling it in. Repeat a few times. Relax!

Listen to Music. Music can be an excellent stress reducer. Music has been shown to increase emotional arousal and induce positive emotions. It activates reward centres in the brain and inhibits negative emotions. Anthony Storr states, 'Music exalts life, and gives meaning . . . Music is a source of reconciliation, exhilaration and hope which never fails . . . An irreplaceable and unreserved transcendental blessing.' Many surgeons, me included, listen to music while operating. A 1994 study of fifty male surgeons showed that listening to music can reduce the elevations in blood pressure and heart rate that often accompany performing tasks under pressure. And music, like photos, can remind us of pleasant events in our past. Have readily available relaxing, soothing tapes and/or CDs in your car, workplace and home. If you're in the habit of listening to talk radio while you drive, now and again switch to a classical or soothing jazz station and feel your body relax as you listen. Put on music that you enjoy while completing chores or while walking the dog. Be an 'active' listener and allow the music to alter your mood and relax you.

Optimism Keeps You Healthy
A study of 334 healthy men and women was conducted to see how their 'emotional style' related to their vulnerability to colds. All subjects were given nasal drops containing

cold viruses, but the subjects with a 'highly positive' emotional style developed fewer cold symptoms. People with negative styles didn't get sick significantly more than those with only slightly positive emotions, but those who did reported more discomfort than objective measures would have predicted. Positive thinking pays off.

Seek Fun and Friendship. It seems that positive events have a much stronger impact on the immune function than upsetting events have a negative one. Simple activities like a walk in the park, a quiet dinner with friends or a cuddle with the family dog or cat can have immediate results, such as strengthening the immune system and temporarily reducing blood pressure. Fill your life with pleasurable social events and brief moments of relaxing pleasures. Social contact is a mitigating factor against a host of diseases including hypertension and heart disease. Many studies substantiate that people who enjoy high levels of social relationships tend to live longer than those who do not. In one study, living alone led to a near doubling of the risk for recurrent heart attack or death in patients who had already experienced a heart attack. Make a point of developing and enjoying a strong social support network.

Embrace Nature. Nature is man's refuge from the stresses and complications of daily life. Retreat to nature whenever you can for restorative moments. Whether it's a walk in a park, time spent in the garden, a hike in the hills, or even just a moment spent watching a pigeon on a city street corner, nature brings us back to ourselves and can serve as a sort of meditation.

Mother Earth plays an essential role in our health and well-being, including:

■ The health-promoting natural pharmacy in whole foods

- The gentle caress of the wind and rain on our skin (massage therapy)
- The fragrant smell of flowers and our own pheromones (aroma therapy)
- The magnificent visual images of natural beauty that can be found by everyone each and every day
- The many pleasing and calming sounds of the natural world (music therapy)

> Surely there is something in the unruffled calm of nature that overawes our little anxieties and doubts: the sight of the deep-blue sky, and the clustering stars above, seem to impart a quiet to the mind.
> *– Jonathan Edwards*

Reduce Anger. Anger robs us of health. Too many of us experience anger regularly in our lives and we will ultimately suffer the penalty. In one study of over one thousand medical students, it was revealed that those with the highest levels of anger (determined by expressed or concealed anger, gripe sessions and irritability) were at significant risk of developing premature heart attacks versus those with lower levels of anger. A high level of anger not only serves as a potential trigger for a heart attack, but in this study it was a trigger for causing a premature heart attack. These students with excessively angry responses to stress appeared to initiate biochemical changes marking them for an early heart attack. Another study of 540 middle-aged Finnish men found that an increase in a measure of their anger expression was associated with an increase in their risk of hypertension. Neal Krause of the University of Michigan School of Public Health found that people who forgive easily tend to enjoy greater psychological well-being and have less depression than those who hold grudges. A Hawaiiian kupuna (elder) expressed it beautifully: 'You have to forgive three times. You must forgive yourself, for you will never be perfect. You have to forgive your enemies, for the fire of your anger will only consume you and your family. And perhaps most difficult of all, if you want to find pleasure in your living, you have to forgive your friends, for because they are friends they are close enough to you to hurt you by accident. Forgiving is the meaning of and making of friendship.'

> Consider how much more you often suffer from your anger and grief than from those very things for which you are angry and grieved.
>
> – *Marcus Aurelius Antoninus*

A New Summer SuperFood
Avocado

A source of:

- Monounsaturated fatty acids
- Fibre
- Magnesium
- Folate
- Vitamin E
- Carotenoids
- Glutathione
- Beta-sitosterol
- Chlorophyll
- Polyphenols
- Lutein

SIDEKICKS: asparagus, artichokes, extra virgin olive oil
TRY TO EAT: ⅓ to ½ of an avocado multiple times weekly

How about a buttery green fruit that you can spread on a sandwich, dice into a salad, or mash into a favourite dip? Avocados have been cultivated for thousands of years. A favourite of the Aztecs, they were native to Central America. If avocados were only delicious and versatile, they would still be a treat worth serving frequently. Recent research has demonstrated that avocados also offer some surprising and powerful health benefits. One of the most nutrient-dense foods, avocados are high in fibre and, ounce for ounce, top the charts among all fruits for folate, potassium, vitamin E and magnesium. Indeed, the very impressive health benefits of eating avocados regularly have encouraged me to adopt them as a new SuperFood.

The delicious healthy monounsaturated fat in the avocado is one of its biggest SuperFood health claims. The only other fruit with a comparable amount of monounsaturated fat is the olive. The monounsaturated fat in avocados is oleic acid, which may help lower cholesterol. One study found that after seven days on a diet that included avocados, there were significant decreases in both total and LDL cholesterol as well as an 11 percent increase in the 'good' HDL cholesterol. Half an avocado has a really excellent overall nutrient profile. At 145 calories it contains approximately 2 grams of protein, 6 grams of fibre, and 13 grams of fat, most of which (8.5 grams) is monounsaturated fat.

Avocados are also rich in magnesium. Magnesium is an essential nutrient for healthy bones, the cardiovascular system (particularly in the regulation of blood pressure and cardiac rhythms), prevention of migraines and prevention of type II diabetes. Ounce for ounce, avocados provide more magnesium than the twenty most commonly eaten fruits, with the banana, kiwi and strawberry in second, third and fourth place, respectively.

Among the twenty most commonly eaten fruits, avocado ranks number one for vitamin E, lutein, glutathione and beta-sitosterol.

Avocados are also rich in potassium, which is of special interest to all HealthStylers, because potassium is a critical nutrient that up until now has not got deserved attention. Potassium helps regulate blood pressure, and an adequate intake of this mineral can help prevent circulatory diseases, including high blood pressure, stroke and heart disease. For more information on potassium, see page 267.

Avocados are also a rich source of folate. One cup of avocado contains 23 percent of the daily value for folate. Various studies have shown a correlation between diets high in folate and a reduced risk of cardiovascular disease and stroke.

In addition to their other heart-healthy qualities, avocados are rich in beta-sitosterol, a so-called phytosterol. Along with peanut butter, cashews, almonds, peas and kidney beans, avocado is one of the best sources of beta-sitosterol from whole foods. A phytosterol is the plant equivalent of cholesterol in animals. Because beta-sitosterol is so similar to cholesterol, it competes for absorption with cholesterol and wins, thus lowering the amounts of cholesterol in our bloodstream. Beta-sitosterol also appears to inhibit excessive cell division, which may play a role in preventing cancer-cell growth. In both animal and laboratory studies, this phytonutrient helps reduce the risk of cancer.

Perhaps the most interesting research on avocados demonstrates that it is a powerful 'nutrient booster': Avocados actually improve the body's ability to absorb nutrients from foods. It's important to remember that it's not just the presence of nutrients in foods that matter, it's also our body's ability to absorb these nutrients. In one study, adding about half an avocado (75 grams) to a carrot/lettuce/spinach salad increased the absorption of the following nutrients in the subjects who ate the salad: alpha-carotene by 8.3 times, beta-carotene by 13.6 times, and lutein by 4.3 times compared with the absorption rate of the same salad without avocado. In a second study, adding a medium avocado (150 grams) to a serving of salsa increased the absorption of lycopene 4.4 times and the absorption of beta-carotene 2.6 times compared with eating the salsa without the avocado. Both studies concluded that the healthy monounsaturated fat in the avocado caused a significant increase in the absorption of the fat-soluble carotenoid phytonutrients in the meal.

Avocado has more soluble fibre – the best fibre for lowering cholesterol – than any other fruit.

Avocado can play a role in a weight-loss diet if eaten in moderate amounts. While high in calories – at 48 calories per ounce, avocados are equivalent to skinless roast chicken breast – avocados help fight obesity because they boost satiety. Satiety is the feeling of fullness that signals us to stop eating and thus helps us control our calorie intake. Perhaps more interesting, research suggests that exercise burns monounsaturated fat more rapidly than saturated fat. This means that even though an avocado is high in monounsaturated fat, this fat will be burned more quickly than saturated fat. The body prefers to burn this fuel over the saturated fat found in meat and dairy.

Interesting recent research shows that avocado seems to be a potent warrior in the fight against prostate cancer. Avocados contain the highest amount of the carotenoid lutein of all commonly eaten fruits. In addition, they contain related carotenoids, including zeaxanthin, alpha-carotene, and beta-carotene, as well as significant amounts of vitamin E. A very recent study showed that an extract of avocado containing these carotenoids and tocopherols inhibited the growth of prostate cancer cells. Interestingly, when researchers used lutein alone, the cancer cells were unaffected, thus demonstrating once again that it's the synergy of health-promoting nutrients in whole foods that makes the difference.

Research at Tufts University suggests that avocado can play an important role in optimizing brain health and function.

How to Buy and Eat an Avocado

An unripe avocado will have none of the delicious creaminess of a ripe one. When shopping for avocados, select fruit that is unblemished, without cracks or dark sunken spots. A ripe avocado will yield slightly to the touch when pressed, and this slight softness indicates it's ready to eat. It's often difficult to find a ripe avocado in the supermarket, but it will ripen at home in a few days in a paper bag or on the kitchen counter. Plan in advance so you'll have ripe avocados when you need them. Do not refrigerate avocados.

Guacamole is a favourite use for avocado and I've included a great 'guac' recipe. There are many variations on this basic recipe, the simplest probably being mashing a ripe avocado with a roughly equal amount of prepared salsa.

My favourite ways to eat avocado are:

- Spread on toasted whole-grain bread and topped with salsa
- As a garnish for turkey tacos
- Diced into any green leafy salad

If you're counting calories, that's no reason to exclude avocados from your diet. Just use them judiciously. For example:

- Spread a bit of mashed avocado on a sandwich in place of mayo.
- Chop and sprinkle avocado on top of a bean soup.
- Add to tofu and spices and blend to make a delicious, creamy dressing.

Barbara's Guacamole

Makes approximately 6 cups, or 12 servings

My friend Barbara Swanson shared her recipe with me and says, 'I think the reason most people like my guacamole is that I do not overpower it with either too much or too large chunks of onion. That's why it is important to *finely* mince the onion. All ingredients are approximate, start with less and add more to taste. The size of avocados varies, so adjust amounts accordingly. Also, if you are serving this with very salty chips, cut down on the salt.'

6 avocados
½ teaspoon extra virgin olive oil
1½ teaspoons lime juice
½ teaspoon (about 8 to 10 dashes) Tabasco
2½ tablespoons finely chopped onion
¼ to ½ cup chopped coriander
½ teaspoon seasoned salt
3 plum tomatoes, diced

Scoop the avocados into a bowl and add the ingredients in the order given. I mix with a fork after each addition (do not overmix) so that the guacamole remains chunky. Cover with clingfilm until serving time.

Blueberries

A source of:

- Synergy of multiple nutrients and phytonutrients
- Polyphenols (proanthocyanins, anthocyanins, quercetin, catechins)
- Salicylic acid
- Carotenoids
- Fibre
- Folate
- Vitamin C
- Vitamin E
- Potassium
- Manganese
- Magnesium
- Iron
- Riboflavin
- Niacin
- Phyto-oestrogens
- Low calories

SIDEKICKS: purple grapes, cranberries, loganberries, raspberries, strawberries, fresh currants, blackberries, cherries, and all other varieties of fresh, frozen or freeze-dried berries
TRY TO EAT: 1 to 2 cups daily

Blueberries are perhaps everyone's favourite SuperFood, and summer is a perfect time to take another look at this delicious fruit. Blueberries are such powerful health promoters that if you ate only three SuperFoods, blueberries, along with wild salmon and spinach, you would be ahead of the game. Amazingly rich in antioxidant phytonutrients, particularly one type known as anthocyanin, blueberries preserve cell health and help prevent many of the degenerative diseases that plague us as we age. Here's what you need to know about blueberries in a nutshell: Blueberries contain more powerful disease-fighting antioxidants than any other single fruit. They're absolute powerhouses in the world of health-promoting foods.

In brief, blueberry consumption is associated with:

- Brain health and preservation of cognitive ability; prevention of Alzheimer's disease
- Cancer prevention
- Cardiovascular health
- Diabetes prevention
- Vision/eye health
- Urinary tract health
- Decreased inflammation

The extraordinary power of blueberries derives from their rich supply of the antioxidant anthocyanins. Anthocyanins are the red/blue pigment in blueberries and their sidekicks, and they perform a range of impressive health-promoting functions that primarily help neutralize the effects of free-radical damage to cells and tissue. Anthocyanins also enhance the positive effects of vitamin C.

The berries also contain carotenoids, fibre, folic acid and vitamin C, each of which makes a major contribution to long-term health. Antioxidant carotenoids work to modulate your immune system, increase the UV protective capacity of your skin, decrease the redness of your skin after sun exposure, decrease the incidence of age-related macular degeneration, inhibit abnormal cell growth, and decrease the mutation rate of cells.

The most exciting news about blueberries is their effect on brain health. This benefit has been widely reported, but is no less exciting than when first discovered. Researchers have found that blueberries can help to protect the brain against oxidative stress, which may reduce the effects of age-related conditions such as Alzheimer's disease and dementia. Given that statistically nearly half of those persons reaching age eighty-five face the possibility of developing some sort of dementia, this is reason enough to eat blueberries frequently. In addition, oxidative stress can lead to cancer, atherosclerosis, cataracts, macular degeneration and other adverse effects of ageing. In animal studies, blueberries, even more than spinach and strawberries, slowed and in some cases reversed deficits in brain function, motor performance, and learning and memory abilities in old animals.

In an interesting study of nineteen male rowers, it was found that dietary supplementation of anthocyanin-rich chokeberry (or Aronia) juice limited the exercise-induced oxidative damage of red blood cells, most likely by enhancing their antioxidant defence system.

The other health benefits of blueberries are also extremely impressive. We know that blueberries contribute to cardiovascular health; we now know another reason why. In addition to anthocyanin, blueberries contain a compound called pterostilbene, which may be able to lower cholesterol as effectively as many drugs. In an experiment conducted on rats, researchers found that the pterostilbene activates a cell receptor that plays a role in lowering cholesterol and other blood fats. This effect is similar to the effect of the cholesterol-lowering drug ciprofibrate. It's not yet known how many blueberries one would have to eat to duplicate this effect, but it is further evidence of the power of this delicious fruit to promote health.

SuperSidekick

Don't forget about a blueberry SuperSidekick: cranberries. Cranberry consumption has been associated with protection against urinary tract infections, kidney stone formation, periodontal disease, and also genital herpes, among other benefits. A recent study reported that drinking one glass of light cranberry juice cocktail daily was associated with a 6.4 percent increase in heart-protective HDL cholesterol. It's not surprising that this cousin of the blueberry is so powerful. Cranberries contain among the highest levels of phenols of commonly consumed fruits. One study at Cornell University that compared the phenolic compounds in common fruits found that cranberries were richest in phenolics, followed in descending order by apple, red grape, strawberry, pineapple and banana.

Fresh cranberries are harvested in the autumn and are usually only available in markets from October to December. I always buy extra bags at this time of year to put into the freezer. When spring comes and my frozen cranberry supply dwindles down, I rely on dried cranberries to toss in oatmeal or yogurt or even on salads.

A warning on cranberries: If you take the blood thinner warfarin, you may need to avoid drinking cranberry juice, as it seems to amplify the effect of the drug. This can lead to serious bleeding issues.

Fresh Versus Frozen

New data on frozen berries yields some very interesting and encouraging news for those of us – probably most people – who can only get fresh berries for a short period of time. Indications are that frozen berries provide all the benefits of fresh. A European study compared two groups of healthy older men (age sixty) and found that those eating frozen berries daily had a 32 to 51 percent higher blood level of quercetin – a powerful anticancer, antioxidant flavonoid – than those who ate no berries. The results showed that eating even frozen berries can significantly boost your body's level of powerful disease-fighting flavonoids.

The Maine Paradox

Perhaps you've heard of the 'French paradox', a term that refers to the seeming ability of the French to experience less cardiovascular disease than would be expected given their penchant for rich cheeses and other high-fat foods. It's been speculated that the solution to this riddle is the French love of wine. Well, now we have another contender for a top cardioprotective food: blueberries. A recent study found that blueberries deliver 38 percent more free-radical-fighting anthocyanins than red wine. In one study, a 4-ounce drink of white wine contained 0.47 mmol of antioxidants, red wine contained 2.04 mmol, and a drink made from highbush blueberries delivered 2.42 mmol of these powerful antioxidants.

Enjoying Blueberries

Nothing is more delicious than a bowl of yogurt topped with fresh blueberries and perhaps a sprinkle of wheat germ. In the past, this was a treat that we'd enjoy only for a few months in the summer when blueberries are at their peak. Fortunately, there's been a revolution in blueberry availability, no doubt due to the publicity they've received as SuperFoods and the public clamour for them. Frozen blueberries, including those that are frozen organic ones, are available at very reasonable prices in a variety of shops. I always keep some in my freezer. Wild blueberries have even more antioxidants than commercial varieties and are often found in the frozen berry section of most super-markets. If fresh berries are unavailable, I put a cup or so of frozen berries in a container in the fridge to defrost overnight so I can sprinkle them on my cereal or yogurt the next morning. (When making a smoothie, I just use frozen berries.) You can toss berries while still frozen into pan-cake, muffin and quick bread batter. Don't forget purple grapes. Packed with disease-fighting phytonutrients, they're readily available and can be fresh, in 100 percent juice, or in jams. They're even delicious, believe it or not, straight from the freezer. Frozen grapes make a refreshing snack on a hot day.

Summer HealthStyle Focus

How to Avoid Alzheimer's Disease

There are few diseases more feared than Alzheimer's, no doubt because any mental disorder is frightening. Moreover, this affliction has become so common that many people find their lives touched by it. Of course, one of the tragedies of Alzheimer's disease is that entire families are affected, as they must bear responsibility for helping loved ones with this disease. In the US alone there are currently about 4.5 million people with Alzheimer's, and the number is expected to rise to 16 million by the year 2050. Women seem to be most at risk, although the precise reason for the development of Alzheimer's is still something of a mystery. The lifetime risk for Alzheimer's disease is reported to be 12 to 19 percent for women over age sixty-five and 6 to 10 percent for men of the same age. We do know that some cases are linked to genetic susceptibility, while others may be due to damage from tiny strokes and resulting decreased blood flow to the brain. It's also clear that cardiovascular risk factors, including obesity, high blood pressure and high cholesterol, are associated with the cognitive decline we recognize as Alzheimer's.

Alzheimer's disease is a form of dementia. Dementia affects about 10 percent of the adult population over age sixty-five and about 45 percent of those over age eighty-five. Alzheimer's disease is the most common form of dementia and it's generally defined as an irreversible progressive decline in memory, language skills, orientation in time and space, and ability to perform routine tasks.

Since it now stands that one out of two of us who are reading this are likely to develop Alzheimer's or some form of dementia, if we live long enough, efforts at prevention are certainly well advised.

Fortunately, there are steps we can all take to reduce our risk of developing Alzheimer's. Like all HealthStyle recommendations the positive changes you adopt to avoid Alzheimer's disease will also help you avoid a host of other chronic disabling conditions. Like most diseases, Alzheimer's begins decades before the onset of clinical symptoms – the brain changes very slowly – so you do have time to take steps now. Indeed, one study of 13,000 women from the Nurses' Health Study found that women who ate the most SuperFood vegetables, like spinach, broccoli and Brussels sprouts, in their fifties and sixties showed less cognitive decline in their seventies compared with women who ate less of these vegetables.

In general, a HealthStyle of abundant SuperFoods, adequate exercise, and stress control is the best defence against this disease. Overall, since the brain relies on optimum blood flow, adequate nutrients and the right balance of fats, those are the three areas that need special attention if we want to preserve optimum cognitive ability long into our senior years. We know for sure that a healthy cardiovascular system is the foundation for a healthy brain, and so that is the bedrock of an effective Alzheimer's defence.

Here are some guidelines for avoiding Alzheimer's:

- Eat fish, particularly fatty varieties like wild salmon, regularly. I recommend 3 ounces four times a week. Since omega-3 fatty acids, particularly DHA, one of the fats found in fish, is a primary component of brain cell membranes and is known to directly promote brain health, an adequate intake of fish – the best food source – is the cornerstone of any Alzheimer's-avoidance programme. In one study, people who ate one or more fish meals a week had 60 percent less risk of Alzheimer's than people who ate fish rarely or never. In this study, total intake of DHA fatty acids was inversely associated with risk: People in the top fifth of intake had a 70 percent reduction in risk compared with those in the lowest fifth. Remember, fish is not only for dinner: Think salmon salad sandwiches or salad of fresh greens topped with chunks of leftover grilled salmon. Don't forget high omega-3 eggs. You can put a chopped, hard-boiled egg on top of a salad for a great nonfish source of DHA. A recent study demonstrates that six DHA-enriched eggs a week supply a measurable bioavailable source of this important fat.

- Keep your blood pressure low – ideally below 120/80 or lower. We know that hypertension is a risk factor for developing Alzheimer's.

- Keep your weight at optimum levels. Obesity is another risk factor for Alzheimer's disease.

One exciting recent study showed that both green and black tea hinder the activity of two enzymes in the brain that have been associated with the development of Alzheimer's disease. The effects of green tea were longer lasting – a week – while the effects of black tea lasted only a day. Make both green and black tea part of your regular daily diet (see 'Tea', page 205).

- Feed your brain with SuperFoods. A constant supply of glucose is required, so look to complex carbohydrates – whole grains, fruits and vegetables – to provide a steady, healthy source of fuel. In one study, twenty-eight healthy elderly people who took 3.5 tablespoons of sugar enhanced recall and verbal fluency compared with a control group who took saccharin. Yet another study of Alzheimer's patients found that increasing blood glucose levels improved memory by 100 percent in some of the subjects. The point is not to increase your sugar intake, but rather to try to give your brain the steady supply of glucose that it needs from complex carbs. These studies also point to the biological plausibility that long-term low-carb diets might have a negative effect on the brain.

- Check your homocysteine levels. One study found that the presence of elevated homocysteine could nearly double the risk of developing Alzheimer's disease. If your levels are high, be sure to take a multivitamin with the RDA for all the B vitamins, especially folate, B6 and B12.
- Have a complete blood count (CBC) to be sure you're not anaemic, as low-iron stores are implicated in neurological deficits. Do not, however, take an iron supplement without consulting with your health care provider.
- Aim for a total cholesterol below 200 mg/d and an LDL-C of 70 mg. High cholesterol promotes atherosclerosis, or hardening of the arteries, and may also contribute to the brain plaques that are typical of Alzheimer's.
- Aim for a fasting glucose of less than 100 during your annual physical.
- Be wise about your alcohol intake. A study of older adults found that those who drank one to six alcoholic drinks per week were least likely to have dementia. (In the same study, those who had fourteen or more drinks per week were *more* likely to develop dementia than those who never drank.) Red wine contains polyphenols (antioxidants), which may have additional benefits to those of alcohol. Of course, you shouldn't start to drink to stave off Alzheimer's disease, but if you already do, keep within the range of one to six drinks per week. For abstainers, I suggest 4 to 8 ounces of purple grape juice daily.

- Exercise! Exercise increases blood flow to the brain and reduces the production of stress hormones, such as cortisol, that can have an adverse effect on the brain. Follow the HealthStyle ERA suggestions (see page 55) and try to get at least 30 minutes of physical activity daily.
- Socialize. Relationships with others seem to play a role in brain health. Seek out regular social interaction, especially as you age and might have less routine contact with others in work situations.
- Lower your risk of diabetes, as this disease is a risk factor in developing Alzheimer's (see page 97)
- Eat blueberries – one cup fresh or frozen – or its sidekicks daily. Blueberries are 'brain berries': They seem to have powerful effects on the preservation of cognitive ability.
- Eat avocado. Preliminary research suggests that this fruit works in a similar fashion to blueberries in promoting brain health.
- Avoid trans fats.
- Concentrate on a high dietary intake of vitamins C and E. Also consider taking a daily supplement of vitamins C and E. These vitamins may help lower your risk of Alzheimer's. If you take E supplements, be sure they contain all eight forms of vitamin E (four tocopherols and four tocotrienols). Take 100 to 200 IU of natural vitamin E and 200 to 500 mg of vitamin C daily.
- As there may be a relationship between low intake of dietary beta-carotene and cognitive decline, boost your intake of this important nutrient with the SuperFood pumpkin. Try pumpkin smoothies, pumpkin soups and pumpkin puddings. Spinach is also a good source of beta-carotene, and animal studies suggest that spinach prolongs normal cognition in older animals.
- Consider taking ginkgo biloba extract. Although the data is not clear, the *Cochrane Reviews* stated in 2002: 'Overall there is promising evidence of improvement in cognition and function associated with ginkgo.' There

is no established amount, but a typical dose is 120 to 240 mg per day, divided into two or three doses. Consult with your health care professional before using and don't take ginkgo biloba in conjunction with other blood thinners such as aspirin, as there is an additive effect.

- Consider taking acetyl-L-carnitine. This substance mimics the action of acetylcholine – a major neurotransmitter – in the brain. It may have efficacy in retarding the ageing of cellular mitochondria, the energy factory in the cells, and many feel that this is a key to increasing longevity. To date, acetyl-L-carnitine has been shown to slow the progression of Alzheimer's in at least two studies, though there hasn't been a published report on the effectiveness of this substance to prevent Alzheimer's. Take 500 mg twice a day.
- Spice it up. Preliminary data suggests that turmeric may play a role in preventing and/or treating Alzheimer's.
- Calorie restriction may prevent Alzheimer's disease and other ageing disorders.
- Increase your niacin intake. A recent study of 6,158 men and women age sixty-five and older reported an inverse association between Alzheimer's disease and age-related cognitive decline and dietary intakes of total niacin from food and supplements and also niacin from foods only. Excellent sources of niacin include turkey or chicken breast, tuna, wild salmon, sardines and halibut, peanut butter and vitamin-enriched cold cereals.

Summer SuperFood Update
Low-fat or Nonfat Yogurt

A source of:

- Live active cultures
- Complete protein

- Calcium
- B2 (riboflavin)
- B12
- Potassium
- Magnesium
- Zinc
- Conjugated linoleic acid

SIDEKICKS: kefir, soy yogurt
TRY TO EAT: 1 to 2 cups most days

Believe it or not, there was a time when yogurt was viewed as an exotic health food. Only one or two brands were available and the varieties offered were fairly basic. Times sure have changed. Today, yogurt can be found in whipped drinkable, custardy, frozen and low-carb versions.

Yogurt is still a health food – indeed, a topnotch SuperFood – but it does take careful shopping to get the best from this highly nutritious dairy product.

Yogurt is most commonly made from cow's milk, but it can also be made from goat, sheep or buffalo milk. Yogurt is, quite simply, milk that has been curdled. To make yogurt, pasteurized, homogenized milk is inoculated with bacteria cultures and kept warm while the lactose or milk sugar turns into lactic acid. This process thickens the yogurt and gives it its characteristic tart, tangy flavour. The process is very similar to that used when making beer, wine or cheese, in that beneficial organisms ferment and transform the basic food.

Many of the benefits of yogurt are due to the power of two substances – prebiotics and probiotics. You are probably seeing more about both these substances in the media today as food manufacturers are adding them to foods and beverages. Probiotics are live organisms – bacterial strains – that have certain proven health benefits. Prebiotics are, in effect, food for those beneficial probiotics. Prebiotics can

251

benefit the body by, for example, promoting the absorption of calcium.

> The typical adult human body harbours about 100 trillion bacteria from at least 500 species – ten times the number of human cells. Most of these 'friendly' bacteria perform biological functions that are important for survival. It's the proper balance of good bacteria versus bad bacteria that helps to maintain optimum health.

It's important to know that some of the health benefits of yogurt depend on the pre- and probiotics. Many yogurt products contain none. To be sure you're getting live active cultures, look for the 'live active cultures' seal on the yogurt container, which guarantees that the yogurt has at least 100 million cultures per gram. Many yogurt-covered sweets and yogurt-flavoured salad dressings do not contain live active cultures. Yogurt with live active cultures must be refrigerated and date-stamped to indicate their short shelf life. After the expiration date on the yogurt, the bacteria numbers go down.

Yogurt and Your Health

What can yogurt do for you? Like all the other SuperFoods, the components of yogurt work synergistically to promote health and fight disease. Some of the important components of yogurt include live active cultures, protein, calcium and B vitamins. Working together, they are responsible for mitigating the following conditions:

Cancer. There is evidence that yogurt consumption is helpful in reducing the risk for both colon and breast cancer. It seems that the probiotics neutralize mutagens that cause cancer. The probiotics also stimulate the immune system by both promoting immunoglobulin production and decreasing inflammation. By encouraging the proliferation of 'good' bacteria and limiting the growth of 'bad' bacteria, the probiotics also inhibit the growth of the intestinal microflora that promote the development of cancer. In one French study, people who ate the most yogurt had half as many precancerous colon polyps as those who ate no yogurt.

Lactose Intolerance. Some people lack the enzyme that enables them to digest the sugar (lactose) in milk. In America, primary lactose intolerance occurs in 53 percent of Mexican Americans, 75 percent of African Americans, and only 15 percent of whites. Lactose intolerance occurs in more than 50 percent of adults in South America and Africa, approximately 2 percent of Scandinavians, and about 70 percent of southern Italian adults. Lactose intolerance approaches 100 percent in some Asian countries. This can be a problem because it limits a source of highly bioavailable calcium in the diet. Yogurt solves this problem, since the probiotics in yogurt have already digested the lactose, allowing even those unable to digest milk to enjoy this calcium-rich food. As significant numbers of the lactase (the enzyme that 'digests' lactose) -producing bacteria survive for less than an hour after ingestion, it is important to consume probiotics frequently if you suffer from this malady.

Allergies. Keeping in mind that probiotics affect the entire skin surface – including every area that has contact with the outside world, such as the nasal passages and gastrointestinal tract – what could improve the digestive tract could also have an effect on, say, the nasal passages. There is evidence that the probiotics in yogurt can be helpful in relieving atopic eczema as well as milk allergy. Studies show that babies who are exposed to probiotics after the age of three months have a better probability of avoiding various allergies, particularly eczema, later in life.

Cholesterol Reduction. Interesting evidence points out that probiotics in yogurt reduce bile acids, which in turn decrease the absorption of cholesterol from the gastro-intestinal tract, thus reducing cholesterol levels. This effect is most apparent in those who already have elevated cholesterol. As an added bonus, yogurt helps lower blood pressure.

A small study in Japan found that yogurt could be helpful in fighting bad breath (halitosis). The participants ate yogurt twice a day for six weeks. Eighty percent of those who had had halitosis showed lowered levels of the sulphide compounds that contribute to bad breath compared with samples taken during a time when no yogurt was consumed. The people who had eaten yogurt also had less plaque and gingivitis, indicating that yogurt can make a real contribution to oral health when eaten regularly.

Inflammatory Bowel Disease. An important function of probiotics is to help regulate the body's inflammatory response. The probiotics in yogurt seem to be able to help maintain remission in those who suffer from IBD.

Diarrhoea. Yogurt helps to alleviate diarrhoea by stimulating the immune system and crowding out negative microflora in the intestines and also stimulating the growth of beneficial bacteria. Yogurt is particularly useful to those undergoing antibiotic therapy, as it helps to restore the beneficial flora in the digestive tract.

Vaginal Infections and Urinary Tract Infections. Again, we see that the probiotics in yogurt can work to help balance the bacteria in the urogenital system, crowding out the 'bad' bacteria and encouraging the proliferation of the 'good' bacteria.

Weight Control. The evidence has been mounting that yogurt can play a role in a weight-reduction diet. A recent study showed that obese people on a low-calorie diet who included three 6-ounce servings of nonfat yogurt daily for twelve weeks lost 22 percent more weight than dieters who ate little or no dairy foods. Perhaps more important, they lost 60 percent more body fat and maintained more lean muscle mass. It does seem that calcium-rich foods are helpful in reducing or controlling weight. Nonfat yogurt is a low-calorie, high-protein, high-calcium food that may make a significant contribution to your efforts at weight control.

Helicobacter pylori. Infection with *H. pylori* has been reported to play a role in chronic gastritis, peptic ulcer disease, gastric (stomach) cancers and duodenal ulcers. Although the data is somewhat preliminary, probiotics (and cranberries) seem to increase the eradication rate of *H. pylori.*

In addition to the significant abilities of yogurt to fight disease as outlined above, another important contribution that yogurt makes to a healthy diet is as a source of calcium. It's amazing to me that so many people – nine out of ten women and seven out of ten men in the US – don't get sufficient calcium each day. As milk consumption has gone down and has too often been replaced by soft drinks, children and teenagers are failing to get adequate supplies of calcium. Yogurt can help make up for this deficit. Just a single cup of yogurt has 414 mg of readily absorbed calcium, or 40 percent of your daily requirement. In comparison, a similar amount of nonfat milk has only 300 mg of calcium.

Yogurt is also an excellent source of readily digestible protein. With double the protein of milk, yogurt is a powerful weapon in building and maintaining strong bones and thus preventing osteoporosis.

Yogurt in the Kitchen

When buying yogurt, always check the label to be sure there are live active cultures. Most yogurts contain *L. acidophilus* and *S. thermophilus*. But some yogurts contain more cultures, including *L. bulgaricus*, *B. bifidus*, *L. casei*, and *L. reuteri*. Seek out yogurts that contain the best variety of cultures, as all make different, important contributions to your health. I always buy yogurt with fruit on the bottom for the taste which permeates the yogurt. I leave the fruit and syrup alone, thus reducing the calories and sugar I consume. On the other hand, if you buy nonfat or low-fat plain yogurt and add your own fruit as well as nuts, you'll have a lower-calorie, less sugary and less expensive food.

Here are a few ideas to get yogurt into your daily diet:

- Use yogurt to make healthy dips to keep in the fridge to enjoy with baby carrots, celery stalks and pepper strips. Mix yogurt with fresh herbs, freshly ground pepper, some chopped garlic, or some chopped jalapeño pepper. Process the yogurt and spices in a blender or food processor for a few seconds and store in the fridge. Put the dip out for an after-school snack, while watching TV, or before dinner when everyone is 'starving'.
- Make thick yogurt 'cheese' by draining non- or low-fat yogurt in a sieve lined with a coffee filter and placed over a bowl, and put in the fridge. The longer it drains, the thicker it becomes, yielding a healthy substitute for mayo on sandwiches or in dips. Use it as a dressing on fruit.

- Add yogurt to smoothies. A half cup or so of yogurt added to some frozen banana slices, frozen pineapple chunks, blueberries and a splash of orange juice is an excellent start to your day.
- My all-time favourite way to eat yogurt is as a quick, healthy breakfast. I like nonfat yogurt with fresh fruit – berries, sliced oranges, whatever is in season – sprinkled with some wheat germ, some crushed nuts and a drizzle of honey. It's the perfect mix of healthy protein, fibre, and a host of health-boosting nutrients.
- Yogurt makes a great salad dressing. Use yogurt cheese or yogurt right from the container. Blend it with fresh herbs and spices or make a sweet dressing to use on fruit. For the latter, blend yogurt with honey, orange or lemon zest, and perhaps a dash of ground coriander.
- A cooling salad of diced cucumber and yogurt is a refreshing summer side dish. Add diced red or green onion and fresh chopped herbs like dill or coriander.
- Use fat-free yogurt as a healthy substitute for sour cream. When adding it to hot mixtures, stir it in at the very end of cooking and warm it only briefly so it won't separate and curdle.

Yogurt Coriander Topping

This is great on a baked sweet potato, grilled turkey breasts or turkey tacos.

1 cup nonfat or low-fat plain yogurt
¼ cup chopped fresh coriander leaves
2 tablespoons minced spring onions or red onion
2 teaspoons fresh lime juice

Whisk all the ingredients together in a small bowl. Refrigerate, covered, for a couple of hours to let the flavours develop. If you make this with yogurt cheese, it will be thicker.

Syndrome X or Metabolic Syndrome

In America at least sixty-four million people – nearly a third of adults age twenty and older – suffer from a condition known as metabolic syndrome, called by its discoverer Dr Gerald Reaven 'Syndrome X'. The rate of those who probably meet the federal government's criteria for the syndrome approaches 50 percent among the elderly. It also turns up in people who are not obese but have recently put on a lot of weight around their middles and, alarmingly, in an increasing number of overweight children. Researchers speculate that metabolic syndrome is caused by a fundamental malfunctioning of the body's system for storing and burning energy. Contributing to the syndrome are genetics; a sedentary lifestyle; a Western diet high in refined carbohydrates, low in fibre, and high in saturated fat; smoking, and progressive weight gain.

Metabolic syndrome is really a cluster of risk factors that, taken individually, have negative health consequences but, when appearing together, exponentially increase the risk of various health problems, notably heart disease, diabetes, and possibly certain types of cancer. It's the synergy of the multiple factors that increases the risk of disease and death. Like the synergy of good factors that we've been exploring in the nutrients in whole foods, the synergy of negative factors present in metabolic syndrome can create a danger much greater than one risk factor alone.

Do you suffer from Syndrome X? If you have three or more of the following risk factors you do have it, and you must begin right now to reverse your risk with diet and exercise. It's important to remember that you don't need to be obese to suffer from Syndrome X: Many people who have three or more of the risk factors ignore them because they think that obesity is a crucial factor in the syndrome.

This is not the case and it's dangerous to go for a long period of time without any treatment for the syndrome as your risk of developing a serious, if not fatal, ailment increases.

- Waist: more than 40 inches for males, 35 inches for females
- Serum triglycerides: greater than 150 mg/dl
- HDLs: less than 40 mg for males and less than 50 mg for females
- Blood pressure: greater than 130/85
- High fasting glucose, or blood sugar, of at least 110 mg/dl of blood

If you do have three or more of these risk factors, discuss Syndrome X with your health care provider to see if you should pursue a course of medication in addition to the HealthStyle recommendations concerning diet, exercise and stress control.

In general the following steps should be taken if you have metabolic syndrome:

- Lose excess weight.
- Increase physical activity.
- Eat a SuperFoods diet of whole foods with plenty of vegetables and fruits.
- Avoid a very low-fat diet. Any diet that has less than 20 percent of calories from fat could exacerbate metabolic syndrome. Usually, eating very little fat means an increase in carbohydrate consumption and too many carbs, and can cause both triglycerides and blood glucose to rise, worsening metabolic syndrome.
- Pay attention to your cholesterol levels. Consult with your health care professional, and if diet and exercise don't get your blood lipid levels into line, consider taking medications.

- Pay attention to your blood pressure (see 'Hypertension', page 327). Have it checked regularly and take steps to reduce it if it is high.
- Practise stress control. See 'Whole Mind/Whole Body Health', page 219.

> There may be an association between HDL cholesterol typical of metabolic syndrome and breast cancer. A study of older, overweight women with metabolic syndrome revealed that those who had the lowest levels of HDL had the highest risk of breast cancer. Future studies will reveal the complex nature of the connection between metabolic syndrome and chronic diseases such as cancer.

Summer SuperFood Update
Wild Salmon

A source of:

- Marine-derived omega-3 fatty acids
- B vitamins
- Calcium (when tinned with bones)
- Selenium
- Vitamin D
- Potassium
- Protein
- Carotenoids

SIDEKICKS: Wild halibut, tinned albacore tuna, sardines, herring, trout, sea bass, oysters and clams
TRY TO EAT: 3 to 4 ounces 2 to 4 times per week

Salmon has received a great deal of attention lately because of its health-promoting benefits. It is recognized as a SuperFood and research continues to highlight the wisdom of including salmon and its sidekicks routinely in your diet. While salmon is rich in protein, B vitamins, potassium and other important minerals, it's the ample supply of omega-3 fatty acids that makes it such a standout among health-promoting foods.

The story of omega-3 fatty acids in the diet is an interesting one. First, a little very simplified chemistry: There are two fatty acids – essential because the body can't manufacture them and must rely on dietary supplies – that are vital to health. They are omega-3 fatty acids and omega-6 fatty acids. Both of these fatty acids are similar enough in molecular structure that they compete for entry into the cell membranes around each cell in our body. Once upon a time, about a century ago, we got a significant percentage of our dietary fat from free-range animals. This source of fat had high levels of omega-3 fatty acids. A century later, two important changes in our diets have resulted in a dramatic shift in our essential-fatty-acid balance. Our meats are much lower in omega-3 fatty acids. Since these animals are no longer primarily free range, their diets are now rich in omega-6s and thus so are the meats they produce. Moreover, our packaged foods are high in omega-6 fatty acids, due to the increasing use of corn, safflower, cottonseed and sunflower oils that are used to produce them.

The end result of these two critical changes is that crucial health-promoting omega-3 fatty acids have been crowded out of our diets. Researchers speculate that due to this gradual change in the source of fatty acids the effect on both our mental and physical health could be seismic. For one thing, the body relies on a rich source of omega-3 to build flexible and efficient cell membranes. A cell membrane that is deficient in omega-3s will function poorly and will put you at risk of a host of diseases including stroke, heart attack, cardiac arrhythmias, some forms of cancer, insulin resistance, asthma, hypertension, age-related macular degeneration, chronic obstructive lung disease (COPE), autoimmune disorders, attention-deficit/ hyperactivity disorder and depression. Dr William S. Harris has said: 'In terms of its potential impact on health in the Western world, the omega-3 story may someday be viewed as one of the most important in the history of modern nutritional science.' There's little doubt that if you want to preserve your health, you should include increasing amounts of food sources of omega-3 fatty acids in your diet, while at the same time decreasing your intake of omega-6s.

Increasing your intake of omega-3s can play an important role in promoting cardiovascular health. Omega-3 fatty acids promote the production of anti-inflammatory hormonelike substances known as prostaglandins. These prevent platelets from sticking together and thus promote blood flow. Omega-3s also improve the ratio of good to bad cholesterol and lower triglycerides (another form of fat that may be more dangerous than elevated cholesterol). Omega-3s also stabilize your heartbeat, thus preventing cardiac arrhythmias that can lead to sudden death.

Tips for increasing your intake of omega-3 fatty acids:
- Use omega-3 enriched eggs.
- Cook with extra virgin olive oil rather than corn or safflower oil.
- Eat walnuts and soy nuts, pecans and pumpkin seeds.
- Sprinkle wheat germ and/or ground flaxseed meal on cereal and yogurt; add a tablespoon or two when baking.
- Eat salmon or its sidekicks two to four times per week.
- Look for salad dressings that contain some soybean or extra virgin olive oil.
- Use walnut oil in homemade salad dressings.
- Add ground flaxseed when baking muffins, breads and pancakes.
- Avoid processed foods, including packaged cakes, biscuits and baked goods.

Omega-3s are also important players in the effort to reduce elevated blood pressure. Evidence has shown that the more omega-3 fatty acids you consume, the lower your blood pressure, so this should be reason enough to make fish a regular part of your diet.

Salmon and its sidekicks also promote heart health by possibly lowering the risk of atrial fibrillation – one of the most common types of heart arrhythmias. In a twelve-year study of 4,815 people over age sixty-five, it was found that eating tinned tuna or other grilled or baked (not fried) fish one to four times weekly yielded a 28 percent lower risk of atrial fibrillation. Those who ate even more fish – five times weekly – enjoyed a reduced risk of 31 percent.

Finally, in terms of cardiovascular health, a meta-analysis of eight studies found that the risk of ischemic stroke – the type caused by a lack of blood to the brain – drops in inverse relation to fish consumption. Those who ate the most fish enjoyed the most reduced risk; eating fish five times a week yielded a 31 percent reduced risk of ischemic stroke.

A fascinating body of research has shown that omega-3s can promote mental health. When you consider that your brain is 60 percent fat, it makes sense that the type of fat could affect its functioning. Perhaps the most intriguing research on omega-3 fatty acids has suggested that the plague of mental health problems witnessed in the twenty-first century, including depression, attention-deficit/hyperactivity disorder, dementia, schizophrenia, bipolar disorder and Alzheimer's disease, could be due in part to the lack of sufficient omega-3s in our diet.

Various recent studies have highlighted the role of salmon and its sidekicks in promoting better mental health. One fascinating study found a relationship between the consumption of fish rich in omega-3s and the 'hostility score' in 3,581 young urban black and white men. These young adults were enrolled in the CARDIA (Coronary

Artery Risk Development in Young Adults) study, which is trying to determine the factors that promote the development of heart disease. As high hostility levels are associated with the development of coronary artery disease, the researchers were interested to find that the young adults with the highest intake of omega-3 fats were 18 percent less likely to exhibit high hostility compared with those who did not eat fish high in omega-3s.

Another interesting recent study found that for people over the age of sixty-five, eating at least one fish meal a week could reduce their risk of developing Alzheimer's disease. The study involved 815 residents of Chicago. Those who ate fish at least once a week had a 60 percent lower risk of developing Alzheimer's compared with those who never or rarely ate fish. Researchers noted that some participants in the study also saw a decreased risk for Alzheimer's after eating vegetables and nuts rich in omega-3 fatty acids.

It's not only young adults and older people who benefit from salmon and its sidekicks when it comes to mental health and performance. One study found a correlation between salmon and tuna and mental performance in midlife. The five-year study of 1,613 people found that eating fish high in omega-3 fatty acids several times each week reduced the risk of impaired overall cognitive function by almost 20 percent. Those who ate a diet high in cholesterol, by contrast, were found to have a 27 percent greater risk of impaired memory and mental flexibility.

Pregnant or nursing women, women of childbearing age and children should look at the FDA website (www.epa.gov/mercury/fish.html) before consuming tuna.

A Fish Story

Though more and more people are aware of the benefits of eating salmon and its sidekicks, there's much confusion on the safety of seafood. Scares about mercury in fish and environmental dangers of farmed fish have made consumers skittish about eating fish. There are two issues to consider: the environmental issue of how fish are caught and raised and the health issue of what contaminants and nutrients are in various types of fish.

One of the big environmental issues has to do with farmed fish. Farmed fish have come to dominate many sectors of the seafood market. You've no doubt noticed a wide variation in the price of salmon, from very inexpensive farmed salmon to very expensive fresh wild salmon. Many environmental groups are opposed to farm-raised salmon, and there is some controversy about the omega-3 content of this salmon, as they're not always fed the marine diet that produces high amounts of omega-3 fatty acids.

Other heart-healthy, environmentally safe seafood choices include the following: Clams (farmed), crab (Dungeness), crayfish, halibut, mahimahi, mussels (farmed), sablefish, sardines, scallops (farmed), striped bass, tilapia (farmed) and herring.

For up-to-the-minute information on choosing seafood, check the following websites:
www.audubon.org (888-397-6649)
www.environmentaldefense.org (202-387-3525)
www.mbayag.org (831-648-4800)

Tinned wild salmon is an excellent choice. Tinned sockeye salmon has 203 mg of calcium – 17 percent of your daily requirement – if it's tinned with the bones. This is over and above all those good omega-3s. Tinned tuna (minus the calcium boost) is another excellent and very popular choice. You can make delicious burgers from tinned tuna or salmon. Tinned sardines are another great source of omega-3s. Like some tinned salmon, they also offer the calcium benefit from the hidden soft bones. Sardines packed in olive oil taste best, but the ones packed in tomato sauce are excellent and also offer the benefit of the lycopene in the tomato.

What About a Supplement?

I have patients who won't or can't eat fish. While I always advocate whole foods as a source of nutrients, I do believe that getting adequate omega-3s is important enough to argue for taking a supplement if you can't get them any other way. If you must rely on a supplement, take at least a gram of EPA/DHA per day with food. I take a supplement if I'm not having appreciable dietary omega-3s on a given day. In those instances, I take 500 mg of EPA/DHA with two of my meals. Look for fish oil that lists a small amount of d-alpha tocopherol (vitamin E) or other antioxidant on the label. This helps to keep the fish oil fresh. Be sure to store fish oil in the fridge, as it can deteriorate quickly. My favourite fish oil supplement is wild sockeye salmon oil from www.vitalchoice.com, which contains all thirty-two fatty acids as they are found in this fish and which is preserved with the astaxanthan found in the salmon flesh. If you burp up a fishy taste when first trying fish-oil supplements, persevere. Take the soft gel capsules with a meal and in almost all cases the fishy burps will stop within a week.

Tinned tuna is a convenient way to get omega-3s into your diet. Here's what you need to know about eating tinned tuna:
- Always buy water-packed, low-sodium albacore tuna (higher in omega-3s) or chunk light tuna.
- Adults shouldn't eat more than one tin of tuna weekly.

Salmon in the Kitchen

Many people initially think that having a few fish meals a week can be a real challenge. Yes, it's true that finding good fresh fish is not always easy, but you can rely on tinned fish or even frozen fish to get the powerful health benefits of omega-3s. Salmon or tuna burgers are a great way to boost your family's omega-3 intake. They're easy to make, cook quickly, and can be spicy or mild to suit your family's taste. Put grilled fresh salmon or tuna on a bed of greens with cut-up vegetables. Dress the salad lightly, and you have a healthy warm-weather meal. You'll find the best local seafood by befriending your fishmonger. Don't be shy about asking about the freshness of the fish and don't hesitate to give it a sniff test; if it doesn't smell like the sea, don't buy it. A 'fishy' smell is really the sign of seafood that is past its prime.

You don't think you can get your family to eat fish two or three times a week? Don't give up: A study involving more than twenty thousand male physicians in the US showed that as little as one serving of fish a week resulted in a significantly reduced risk of total cardiovascular death after eleven years. Some is better than none!

POTASSIUM POWER

You probably know that if you've been diagnosed with hypertension, or high blood pressure, you should cut down on the sodium in your diet (see page 327-8). Limiting sodium is an important step that everyone should take to preserve health. There's another simple but important dietary modification that you should consider, which unfortunately, few people know about: increase your potassium intake. Potassium is a mineral – an electrolyte – that helps to balance the acidity/alkalinity of the body's fluids as it also helps control blood pressure. Too much fluid increases blood pressure and potassium plays a crucial role in maintaining optimum fluid levels.

Before the emergence of agriculture, humans consumed a diet that was high in potassium and low in sodium. Lately, with the increase in the popularity of processed foods along with a reduction in the consumption of fruits and vegetables, most of us have decreased our potassium intake as we've increased our sodium intake. While deficiencies of potassium are rare because potassium is widely available in a variety of foods, it's my strong belief that a large percentage of those eating a Westernized diet suffer from a discrete but important deficiency of potassium. In the developing world, where diets are rich in potassium and low in sodium, high blood pressure is virtually nonexistent.

> Highly refined wheat flour contains less than half the potassium level of whole-grain flour.

Why is a rich supply of potassium important? Research has now established that a high intake of potassium plays a protective role against hypertension, stroke, cardiac dysfunction, including arrhythmias, as well as kidney damage and osteoporosis. The DASH (Dietary Approaches to Stop Hypertension) diet recommends a rich intake of potassium foods and has shown a marked ability to lower blood pressure.

> In an epidemiologic study of 84,360 American women over a six-year period, a high intake of potassium was associated with a lowered risk of developing diabetes mellitus.

We should be getting *three to five times* the amount of potassium as sodium in our diets: unfortunately most of us get about half that amount of potassium; some of us even get less potassium than sodium. In the US, new government guidelines recommend that you consume at least 4,700 mg of potassium daily; my own recommendation is that you aim for 8,000 mg daily. It's not difficult to reach that goal when you appreciate that green, leafy vegetables, citrus fruits and beans are rich in potassium. Other good choices include dairy products, fish and nuts.

Good Sources of Potassium
    Potato, 1 medium baked, 926 mg, 161 calories
    Sweet potato, 1 cup cooked, 950 mg, 180 calories
    Clams, 6 cooked, 705 mg, 166 calories
    Butternut squash, 1 cup cooked, 582 mg, 82 calories
    Figs (dried), 4 large, 541 mg, 194 calories
    Prune Juice + Lutein, 1 cup, 540 mg, 170 calories
    Libby's Tinned Pumpkin, 1 cup, 505 mg, 83 calories
    Salsa with mesquite kettle chips, 1 oz, 495 mg, 140 calories
    Cantaloupe, 1 cup, 494 mg, 60 calories
    Lentils, 1/2 cup cooked, 475 mg, 115 calories
    Orange juice, 8 oz, 473 mg, 118 calories
    Oysters, 6 medium, 453 mg, 245 calories
    Avocado, 1/2 avocado, 439 mg, 145 calories
    Soy Milk, 1 cup, 440 mg, 130 calories
    Pomegreat Juice, 8 oz, 430 mg, 140 calories
    Banana, 1 medium, 422 mg, 105 calories
    Spinach (cooked), 1/2 cup, 419 mg, 21 calories
    Salmon (wild), 3 oz, 369 mg, 118 calories
    Dried plums (prunes), 6 uncooked, 366 mg, 120 calories
    Oats, 1/2 cup, 335 mg, 302 calories
    Spinach, 2 cups raw, 334 mg, 14 calories
    Tomato paste (purée), 2 tablespoons, 324 mg, 26 calories
    Dates, 6 dates, 324 mg, 138 calories

Wild salmon (tinned), 3 oz, 320 mg, 130 calories
Raisins, 1/4 cup, 309 mg, 123 calories
Soymilk, 1 cup, 300 mg, 100 calories
Pinto beans, 1 1/2 cup tinned, 292 mg, 103 calories
Blackberries, 1 cup, 282 mg, 75 calories
Strawberries, 1 cup, 252 mg, 46 calories
Turkey (skinless breast), 3 oz, 248 mg, 115 calories
Apricots (dried), 6 halves, 246 mg, 48 calories
Orange, 1 medium, 237 mg, 64 calories
Broccoli (cooked), 1/2 cup, 228 mg, 44 calories
Tofu, 1/2 cup, 221 mg, 183 calories
Chickpeas, 1/2 cup, 207 mg, 143 calories
Tomatoes (raw), 1/2 cup, 200 mg
Almonds, 1 oz, 198 mg
Peanuts, 1 oz, 191 mg
Apple sauce (unsweetened), 1/2 cup, 183 mg, 50 calories
Flaxseed, 2 tablespoons, 164 mg, 118 calories
Figs, 1 large (1 1/2-inch-diameter), 148 mg, 47 calories
Wheat germ, 2 tablespoons, 134 mg, 52 calories
Walnuts, 1 oz, 124 mg, 183 calories
Nestlé Carnation Evaporated Fat Free Milk, 2 table-
spoons, 110 mg, 25 calories

A New Summer SuperFood
Garlic

A source of:

- Organosulphur compounds (75 total, with allicin the most active)
- Saponins
- Polyphenols
- Selenium
- Arginine
- Vitamin C
- Potassium

SIDEKICKS: spring onions, shallots, leeks, onions
TRY TO EAT: 'to taste' multiple times per week

Garlic, a small and humble-looking vegetable, plays a huge role in the major cuisines of the world. It's hard to imagine Italian, French or Asian cooking without garlic. The big news on garlic isn't its ability to flavour a dish, but rather its considerable role as a health promoter. Indeed, recent findings on the power of garlic to fight cancer and cardio-vascular disease, as well as its anti-inflammatory and antiviral properties, give garlic the bona fides to elevate it to SuperFood status.

Garlic, a member of the lily, or *allium*, family, traces its origin to Central Asia. Garlic is a major flavouring agent, particularly in Mediterranean cuisine, but as far back as 2600 BC, it was used by the Sumerians as medicine. One of the oldest cultivated plants in the world, garlic was recognized by early civilizations as a source of strength and was mentioned in the Bible. Indeed, throughout the history of civilization, the medicinal properties of garlic have been prized, and it's been used to treat ailments, including atherosclerosis, stroke, cancer, immune disorders, cerebral ageing, arthritis and cataract formation.

Garlic's power as a heath promoter comes from its rich variety of sulphur-containing compounds. Of the nearly one hundred nutrients in garlic, the most important in terms of health benefits seems to be the sulphur compound allicin – an amino acid. Allicin is not present in fresh garlic, but it is formed instantly when cloves are crushed, chewed or cut. Allicin seems to be responsible for the superbiological activity of garlic as well as its odour. In addition to allicin, a single clove of garlic offers a stew of compounds with potential health benefits, including saponins, phosphorus, potassium, zinc, selenium, polyphenols and arginine. In addition to these compounds, garlic is a good source of vitamin B6 and also of vitamin C. As with most whole foods, garlic's antioxidant and anti-inflammatory abilities are probably due to the sum of the whole rather than a single agent.

Garlic and Cardiovascular Disease

A number of studies have shown that garlic has an important impact on risk factors for cardiovascular disease. It has been demonstrated that those who make garlic a regular part of their diets enjoy lowered blood pressure and decreased platelet aggregation, as well as decreased triglycerides and LDL ('bad') cholesterol. Garlic also may increase HDL ('good') cholesterol. Consuming one half to one clove of garlic daily lowers LDL cholesterol levels by approximately 10 percent, partially by decreasing cholesterol absorption. Garlic extracts have also been shown to decrease blood pressure: In one study, a 5.5 percent decrease in systolic blood pressure and a slight decrease in diastolic pressure were noticed. While these are modest decreases, they could still lead to a significant lessening of the risk for stroke and heart attack. The end result of all of these benefits is a lowered risk of atherosclerosis and heart disease as well as a reduced risk of heart attack and stroke. Garlic oil has been shown to decrease total and LDL cholesterol and triglyceride levels.

Garlic's primary positive effect on cardiovascular disease comes from its sulphur compounds, but the effects of vitamin C, B6, selenium and manganese can't be ignored. Garlic's vitamin C – the body's primary antioxidant defender – protects LDL cholesterol from oxidation. It's the oxidation of LDL cholesterol that begins the process that damages blood vessel walls. Vitamin B6 lowers levels of homocysteine, a substance that can directly damage blood vessel walls. The selenium in garlic fights heart disease, while it's also working to protect against cancer and heavy metal toxicity. Manganese works on a variety of antioxidant defences, and studies have found that adults deficient in manganese have lowered their levels of the 'good', or HDL, cholesterol.

Garlic and Cancer

A number of studies have reported on garlic's ability to fight cancer, although further research is needed to clarify the precise role of garlic in this battle. Several population studies have shown a link between garlic in the diet and a decrease in the risk for colorectal and gastric cancer, and one clove of garlic daily may decrease the risk of developing prostate cancer. Recent reviews of more than thirty-five studies report some protective effect against cancer in about 75 percent of the published articles.

Garlic as Antibiotic

Two recent studies have shown that garlic can be a potent antibiotic. Particularly impressive was that garlic was effective against strains of pathogens that have become resistant to many drugs. One study showed that garlic juice showed significant antibacterial activity against a host of pathogens, even including antibiotic-resistant strains such as ciprofloxacin-resistant staphylococci. The second study, conducted on mice, found that garlic was able to inhibit a type of staph infection that's become increasingly resistant to antibiotics and increasingly common in hospitals. This type of staph infection has become a potential danger for health care workers, as well as for people with weakened immune systems. Sixteen hours after the mice were infected with the pathogen, garlic extract was fed to them. After twenty-four hours, garlic was found to have been protective against the pathogen and to have significantly decreased the infection.

The Best Source of Garlic

Although garlic is available in supplements, I believe that fresh garlic is the far better choice. There is variation among garlic products and some odourless garlic preparations may not contain active compounds.

Here's an interesting example: A dose of 600 mg of garlic extract typically produces 3,600 mcg (micrograms) of allicin. A dose of fresh garlic – about one clove – typically produces approximately 18,300 mcg of allicin. Obviously, the whole-foods version is more powerful. Moreover, you're more certain of getting the complete package of health boosters that garlic has to offer.

If you do, however, decide to try garlic powder, a reasonable dose is 300 mg of garlic powder, three times a day.

Buying and Using Garlic

Garlic in its fresh form seems to provide the most health benefits. This is good news for cooks and those who love the delicious flavour punch that garlic adds to food. When shopping for garlic, look for cloves that are plump and without blemishes. Avoid cloves that are soft, shrivelled or mouldy or that have begun to sprout. Store your whole garlic heads in a dark, cool place, keeping them away from dampness and sunlight. Once the head of garlic is broken, however, its shelf life is reduced, so keep cloves whole until needed.

It's easy to separate individual cloves of garlic from the head, but some cooks find peeling them a challenge. The most effective way is to place a garlic clove on a cutting board and press down on it with the flat side of a knife. The skin will break and be easy to remove. The green shoot in the centre can be bitter, so remove it with the point of a knife.

Here are just a few ideas for incorporating garlic into your diet:

- Add chopped garlic when sautéing greens such as spinach, kale or broccoli.
- Add chopped garlic to soups, stews and pasta sauces.
- Roast potatoes and whole cloves of garlic and puree them together with a bit of olive oil for garlic mashed potatoes.
- Add a bit of finely minced garlic to salad dressings.

Raw Garlic

You'll get maximum effect of the phytonutrients by including raw garlic in some of your dishes. The trick here is not to overdo. Just one clove, or even a half clove, of finely minced raw garlic in dressings, dips and guacamole adds great flavour without overpowering the dish.

New Vegetable Tip

Sauté a couple of minced cloves of garlic in a tablespoon or two of extra virgin olive oil, and then add broccoli, carrots or other vegetable and give the pan a shake. Add a few tablespoons of stock or water and allow the vegetables to steam until tender.

Summer SuperFood Update
Extra Virgin Olive Oil

A source of:

- Monounsaturated fatty acids
- Vitamin E
- Carotenoids
- Polyphenols
- Phytosterols

SIDEKICKS: canola oil
TRY TO EAT: about 1 tablespoon most days

If you were to make one change in your kitchen – one single simple adjustment – to promote health and gain substantial benefits in countless ways, it would be: Use extra virgin olive oil in place of other fats. So many studies have verified the health-promoting qualities of extra virgin olive oil that the European Union has embraced it as the oil of choice, and is investing more than thirty-five million euros to promote consumption in its member states. In the US, the FDA, for only the third time, granted a qualified health claim for conventional foods containing olive oil. These foods are allowed to carry labels saying they may reduce the risk of coronary heart disease.

Olive oil – made from the crushing and pressing of one of the oldest-known foods, olives – has been enjoyed since as early as 3000 BC. It is a staple of the extraordinarily healthy Mediterranean Diet, and it is now believed that the consumption of olive oil is a prime reason for the positive aspects of this particular diet.

It seems that the heart-healthy effects of olive oil are due to a synergy of health-promoting compounds. The monounsaturated fat in olive oil has various impressive health benefits. In addition to healthy fat, olive oil is a good source of vitamin E. One ounce of extra virgin olive oil contains 17.4 percent of the daily value (DV) for vitamin E. Interestingly, part of the nutrient synergy of extra virgin olive oil is that the abundant polyphenols not only provide their own health benefits, they also protect and preserve the accompanying vitamin E.

The powerful synergy of all the cooperating compounds in extra virgin olive oil seems to have beneficial effects on health, and a wide range of studies has demonstrated that adding olive oil to your regular diet could:

- Reduce your risk of breast and colon cancer
- Lower your blood pressure
- Improve your cardiovascular health

Olive Oil Fights Oxidative Damage

One of the most interesting studies on olive oil suggests what a protective role it can play in preventing cancer and cardiovascular disease. In this study, healthy men consumed 25 ml (millilitres) a day of olive oil (a dose similar to what is consumed in the Mediterranean Diet), and after only four days of olive oil intake, beneficial changes were seen in their blood plasma. The ingestion of the olive oil increased the vitamin E and phenolic content of their blood lipids, thus protecting them from oxidative damage that could lead to cardiovascular disease and the development of certain cancers. Interestingly, this is the first study to show the effect of olive oil on DNA. It's significant that following the consumption of the olive oil, there was less oxidation of the DNA. Oxidation of DNA is linked to the development of diseases such as cancer and even to ageing itself.

Olive Oil and Blood Pressure

Perhaps you've heard of the Mediterranean Diet. This name refers to the traditional diet eaten by people in Crete. First studied in the 1950s and '60s, the Mediterranean Diet was recognized as a particularly healthy eating pattern – one that seemed to promote long life expectancies and low rates of heart disease and some cancers. The Mediterranean Diet consists largely of plant-based foods – fruits, vegetables, coarsely ground grains, bread, beans, nuts and seeds – as well as olive oil. Fish, poultry and red meat are rare, special-occasion foods.

Remember that olive oil is a fat. It has 120 calories per tablespoon. If you eat too much of it, you will gain weight. For most people, as a SuperFood it's best used as a substitute for other, less healthy fats, such as butter.

People who ate a Mediterranean diet seemed to enjoy generally low blood pressure. Of course, the question remained: Was the low pressure a result of other components of the diet? What particular role did olive oil play? To learn the answer, a team from the University of Athens studied more than twenty thousand Greeks who were free of hypertension when the study began. At the end of the study, data confirmed that, overall, the Mediterranean Diet was consistently associated with lower blood pressure. When the effects of olive oil and vegetables were compared, olive oil alone was found to be responsible for the most beneficial effect in lowering blood pressure.

It seems that olive oil has a beneficial effect on the vascular endothelium, the cells lining the blood vessels. A study in Spain found that subjects who used olive oil for four weeks reported both systolic and diastolic blood pressure to drop approximately 8 mm. Another very interesting study found that not only did olive oil lower blood pressure, it also rendered medication less necessary for the participating subjects.

Olive Oil and Cardiovascular Disease

There's no doubt that olive oil is a rich source of antioxidants and other phytochemicals, and it's likely that the lower rates of coronary artery disease in Mediterranean countries are at least partly due to olive oil consumption. There is ample and impressive research evidence that demonstrates that olive oil can play a role in promoting cardiovascular health over and above its ability to reduce blood pressure. We know that diets rich in olive oil have been shown to be effective in lowering total cholesterol and LDL cholesterol. Certainly, olive oil is one of the significant constituents that contribute to the cardio-protective ability of the Mediterranean Diet. For example, we know that the polyphenols in olive oil are potent antioxidants that help protect LDL from oxidation. Moreover, the presence of monounsaturated fatty acids help biologic membranes, like those of our cell walls, better resist oxidative damage. We know that the oxidation of LDL plays a fundamental role in the progress of arteriosclerosis. In one study, when olive oil was added to the diet of healthy males, it significantly reduced the vulnerability of their LDL to oxidative damage.

Olive Oil and Cancer

There is reason to believe that extra virgin olive oil could play a significant role in preventing cancer. It's been estimated that up to 25 percent of the incidence of colorectal cancer, 15 percent of the incidence of breast cancer, and approximately 10 percent of the incidence of prostate, pancreas and endometrial cancers could be prevented if the populations of Western countries would consume the traditional Mediterranean Diet. Of course, this would mean an increase in fruit and vegetable intake as well as the substitution of olive oil as a main source of fat in the diet. While we don't know exactly what it is in olive oil that provides this protection against cancer, we do know that once again it seems to be the synergy of the whole food.

There has been great interest in the role of olive oil in the development and prevention of breast cancer. The role of fat in the diet and its effect on breast cancer is controversial, and a number of studies have been published with conflicting findings. In case-control studies, consumption of olive oil has been shown to reduce the estimated relative risk of breast cancer in Spain and Greece. Moreover, in animal studies, olive oil seems to have an antitumour effect. Interesting research points to the possible ability of olive oil to reduce breast cancer risk. It seems that oleic acid, the monounsaturated fat found in olive oil, may have the ability to inhibit the growth of certain types of breast cancer cells by inhibiting a gene that stimulates their growth.

There is some evidence that olive oil can play a role in the prevention of colon cancer as well as breast cancer. In one large European study, olive oil consumption was negatively associated with the incidence of colorectal cancer. Evidence suggests that compounds such as phenolics in olive oil act directly in the colon to reduce oxidative or free-radical damage in the colon. This reduction of free-radical damage would ultimately have a chemoprotective result. There's also evidence that substances in olive oil inhibit the formation of amines – cancer-causing compounds that form during the cooking of meat. This would indicate that a marinade that contains extra virgin olive oil may lessen cancer risk, as it would inhibit these cancer-promoting amines from forming in the first place.

Olive Oil in the Kitchen

The key to obtaining health benefits from olive oil is to use it as a substitute for corn, safflower and sunflower oils. Remember that the SuperFood recommendation is about one tablespoon a day: That isn't a lot of oil, so use it judiciously.

When shopping for olive oil you should know that there are different grades, depending on the processing method:

Extra virgin olive oil, which because of its higher polyphenol content is considered a SuperFood, is derived from the first pressing of the olives. It has a low acid content. In addition to its considerable health-promoting qualities, it has the most delicate flavour.

Virgin olive oil is from the second pressing of the olives. It has a higher acid content than extra virgin oil.

Fino is a blend of extra virgin and virgin oils.

Refined oil is made by using chemicals to extract the oil from the olives. It is often a blend of a variety of oils.

Cold-pressed extra virgin olive oil is the kind to buy, as it will provide the most health benefits as well as the most subtle taste. One study indicates that virgin olive oil (most studies do not differentiate the type of olive oil) provides greater protection against free-radical damage to LDL cholesterol – a first step in the development of atherosclerosis – than other oils. I always look for greenish-coloured extra virgin olive oil, since the colour indicates a high level of polyphenols. Different types of olive oil – from Spain, Greece, and even California – have different, interesting tastes.

Extra virgin olive oil is quite perishable. Buy no more than you'll use in two or three months. Decant some oil from the original container into an opaque bottle or tin and keep it away from the light; store it in a cool, dark place in your kitchen. Don't keep it near the stove! Store the rest of the oil in the fridge, where it will solidify slightly. Cold olive oil will quickly liquefy when brought to room temperature.

It's easy to use sufficient olive oil in your diet to get its considerable health benefits.

- Make salad dressing with 3 parts extra virgin olive oil and 1 part balsamic vinegar or lemon juice. You'll avoid the high sodium levels in most prepared dressings. Add finely chopped garlic or shallots and fresh herbs plus ground pepper, and use a salt substitute.
- Drizzle vegetables and sautéed greens with a bit of extra virgin olive oil before serving.

- Add extra virgin olive oil and roasted garlic to make delicious mashed potatoes.
- Drizzle asparagus, beetroots, red and white potatoes, turnips or carrots with extra virgin olive oil. Roast in a 400°F oven until crisp-tender.

SUMMER HEALTHSTYLE RECIPES
Maple Cashew Butter

Serves 10

Use this cashew butter to top pancakes or desserts. Whisk in the yogurt to create a thinner sauce.

1½ cups raw cashews
⅓ cup maple syrup
1 cup brewed green tea
1 cup low-fat yogurt, optional

Soak the cashews in clear water to cover for 8 hours or overnight. Drain well, and place cashews and maple syrup in a food processor or blender. Add about ¼ cup of the tea and blend until smooth, adding more tea as necessary to create a thick, creamy texture.

To make a more liquid sauce, whisk in the yogurt, if using.

Maple cashew butter (without yogurt)

Calories: 146	Total polyunsaturated fat: 1.6 g
Protein: 3.2 g	Omega-6 linoleic acid: 1.6 g
Carbohydrates: 14 g	Omega-3 linoleic acid: < 0.04
Cholesterol: 0.0	n-3s
Total fat: 9.6 g	Sodium: 5 mg
Saturated fat: 1.9 g	Potassium: 146 mg
Monounsaturated fat: 5.6 g	Total fibre: < 1 g

Calories: 161
Protein: 4.4 g
Carbohydrates: 15.6 g
Cholesterol: 1.5 mg
Total fat: 9.9 g
  Saturated fat: 2.1 g
  Monounsaturated fat: 5.7 g

Polyunsaturated fat: 1.6 g
Omega-6 linoleic acid: 1.6 g
Omega-3 linoleic acid: < 0.04 g
total n-3
Sodium: 22 mg
Potassium: 204 mg
Fibre: <1 g

Garlic and Black Pepper 10-Minute Marinated Salmon

Serves 4

Serve hot or chilled for sandwiches and salads. If there are any leftovers, stuff cold salmon into pitta bread with plenty of lightly dressed lettuce and sliced cucumber.

3 minced garlic cloves
½ cup nonfat plain yogurt
½ teaspoon black pepper
1 tablespoon paprika
2 tablespoons Dijon mustard
¼ teaspoon cayenne, optional
Four 5- to 6-ounce pieces wild salmon

Whisk together the garlic, yogurt, black pepper, paprika, mustard, and cayenne, if using. Arrange the salmon in a dish, coat each piece with the sauce, and allow to marinate for 10 minutes. Shake off any excess sauce and grill. Depending upon the thickness of the fish, it will take anywhere from 5 to 8 minutes to cook through.

Calories: 208
Protein: 32.7 g
Carbohydrates: 4.6 g
Cholesterol: 79 mg
Total fat: 6 g
  Saturated fat: 0.9 g
  Monounsaturated fat: 1.5 g
  Polyunsaturated fat: 2.2 g

Omega-6 linoleic acid: 0.2 g
Omega-3 linoleic acid: 0.1 g
EPA: 0.6 g
DHA: 0.9 g
Sodium: 228 mg
Potassium: 625 mg
Fibre: <1 g

Blueberry and Cranberry Brown and Wild Rice

Serves 8

Use your favourite method of cooking rice. This works well in a rice cooker or a good heavy pan with a tight-fitting lid. For an al dente crunch, bring the rice to a boil, cover, reduce the heat, simmer, then remove from the heat and let it stand, covered. For a creamier texture, experiment by adding ¼ to ⅓ cup water until you achieve the texture your family most enjoys.

1⅓ cups brown rice
¾ cup wild rice
1 tablespoon white miso
¾ cup dried cranberries
1 cup fresh or frozen blueberries
2 tablespoons maple syrup

Cook the brown and wild rices, along with the miso and cranberries, in about 4 cups water until the rice is tender, about 25 minutes. Remove from the heat and let stand for about 20 minutes, covered. Gently stir in the blueberries and syrup. Serve warm or cool.

Calories: 238
Protein: 5 g
Carbohydrates: 52.7 g
Cholesterol: 0.0
Total fat: 1.2 g
  Saturated fat: <1 g
  Monounsaturated fat: <1 g

Polyunsaturated fat: <1 g
  Omega-6 linoleic acid: 0.4 g
  Omega-3 linoleic acid: 0.1 g
Sodium: 66 mg
Potassium: 195 mg
Fibre: 3.9 g

Cedar Plank Salmon with Garlic Orange Glaze

Serves 4

Slow cooking on a cedar plank results in deliciously moist salmon with a slightly smoky flavour. You can buy individual cedar planks at kitchenware shops, or get untreated cedar planks at a lumber yard. If there is only one control for the grill, set it to low. If using a charcoal grill, let the coals die down to pinkish-grey, then push them to the outside and cook over indirect heat.

Olive oil spray
¾ cup orange preserves, 100% fruit
2 garlic cloves, minced
1 medium chilli pepper, minced, optional
⅓ cup brewed green tea
1⅓ pounds wild salmon
1 tablespoon sesame seeds
Freshly ground black pepper

Soak the cedar planks in water for at least 3 and up to 24 hours. If grill has two burners, set one side only to medium-high. Spray the top of the planks with oil. Place the planks on the cool side of the grill (indirect heat). In a small saucepan, warm the preserves, garlic, chilli pepper (if using), and green tea just to melt the preserves. Place the

285

salmon on the planks and brush with the sauce. Sprinkle sesame seeds and black pepper on top. Grill for 12 to 25 minutes, checking every 10 minutes. Salmon is done when just firm, but some like it more well done. When grilling a large fillet, the tail end will be more well done, while the thicker end is nicely tender, providing something for everyone.

Calories: 329	*Omega-6 linoleic acid: 0.8 g*
Protein: 34 g	*Omega-3 linoleic acid: 0.3 g*
Carbohydrates: 23.6 g	*EPA: 0.7 g*
Cholesterol: 68 mg	*DHA: 1.0 g*
Total fat: 10.4 g	*Sodium: 306 mg*
Saturated fat: 2.0 g	*Potassium: 724 mg*
Monounsaturated fat: 3.7 g	*Fibre: 1.5 g*
Polyunsaturated fat: 3.6 g	

Poached Salmon Poke

Serves 6

In the Hawaiian language, poke (pronounced po-*kay*) was originally a verb meaning to cut crosswise into pieces. Over time, the word has become a culinary noun used to describe a variety of chopped seafood salads seasoned typically with soy sauce and spring onions.

Ponzu is available at many supermarkets or online grocers. If you can't find ponzu, combine 2 tablespoons low-sodium soy sauce mixed with 1 tablespoon orange juice and 2 tablespoons water instead.

Salmon poke looks inviting when served in half an avocado or papaya. Or omit the cherry tomatoes and serve the salad on sliced heirloom tomatoes.

1 lemongrass stalk, optional
2 medium bay leaves

5 whole green tea bags
2 pounds wild salmon

Poke
1 tablespoon minced fresh ginger
1 garlic clove, minced
⅔ cup sliced spring onions
1½ cups quartered cherry tomatoes
¼ cup ponzu (or the orange juice, soy sauce and
    water mix)
1 tablespoon extra virgin olive oil
2 tablespoons minced coriander, optional
Black pepper

Garnish
¼ cup macadamia nuts, ground and toasted
1 medium mango
1 medium lime wedge
Lettuce

In a wide, covered pan, bring 4 pints water to a boil with the lemongrass (if using) and the bay leaves. When the water boils, reduce the heat to a simmer and add the green tea bags. When the broth gets nicely green after a minute or two, add the salmon and cover. Leave the heat on for 2 minutes, then turn off the heat and allow the salmon to poach for 5 to 7 minutes. Check for doneness with the point of a knife. Using a slotted spoon, remove the salmon to a platter and chill. Don't worry if it breaks up a bit when you're taking it out of the water. Meanwhile, combine all the poke ingredients and chill. Crush the macadamias, spread on a small baking sheet, and toast in a preheated 300°F oven until just golden, 10 to 15 minutes. Peel the mango, slice it, and squeeze a little lime on it. When the salmon is chilled, break it into large chunks and add to the poke; toss gently to coat. Serve on a bed of lettuce with mango slices on the side, and top with the ground macadamias.

Calories: 328	*Omega-6 linoleic acid: 0.4 g*
Protein: 35 g	*Omega-3 linoleic acid: 0.3 g*
Carbohydrates: 12.3 g	*EPA: 0.7 g*
Cholesterol: 68 mg	*DHA: 1.0 g*
Total fat: 16 g	*Sodium: 285 mg*
Saturated fat: 3 g	*Potassium: 981 mg*
Monounsaturated fat: 8.5 g	*Fibre: 2.3 g*
Polyunsaturated fat: 3.4 g	

Avocado Goddess Crunch Salad

Serves 6

This salad can be a stand-alone meal, or an accompaniment to poached, grilled or roasted wild salmon. If you don't like the anise flavour of tarragon, substitute basil, coriander, dill or marjoram. Substitute white or champagne vinegar for the tarragon vinegar if you like.

Dressing
2 tablespoons flaxseed oil
2 large ripe avocados
1 cup nonfat yogurt
1 medium shallot
2 tablespoons flat-leaf parsley
1 tablespoon chopped fresh tarragon, optional
3 tablespoons tarragon vinegar, or more
Salt and pepper
1 tablespoon Worcestershire sauce, optional

Salad
1 medium red onion
1 medium green pepper

1 medium orange pepper
1 medium red pepper
2 medium endive
1 large cucumber
1 medium jicama or waterchestnut
1 medium yellow squash or courgette
⅓ cup sunflower seeds, roasted

Combine all the dressing ingredients in a food processor or blender and blend until smooth. Add more vinegar if necessary to thin. Cut the onion into quarters and thinly slice. Soak the slices in ice-cold water for about 10 minutes. Drain and place in a salad bowl. Cut the peppers into 1/4-inch strips. Slice the endive into 1/4-inch slices on the diagonal, to get longer slices. Cut the remaining vegetables into julienne strips, about 1/4 inch by 2 inches – similar in size to the pepper strips. Toss the vegetables in the salad bowl with just enough dressing to coat. Garnish with a small dollop of dressing and top with sunflower seeds.

Calories: 250

Protein: 7 g

Carbohydrates: 19.4 g

Cholesterol: < 1 g

Total fat: 18 g

  Saturated fat: 2.4 g

  Monounsaturated fat: 8 g

Polyunsaturated fat: 6.5 g

  Omega-6 linoleic acid: 3.5 g

  Omega-3 linoleic acid: 0.1 g

Sodium: 72 mg

Potassium: 940 mg

Fibre: 6.6 g

Lemon Yogurt Cornbread

Serves 8

Brush the top of the bread with a little honey, hot from the oven, for a sweet glaze.

1 cup whole-wheat flour
1 cup white or yellow cornmeal
1 tablespoon brown sugar
2 teaspoons baking powder
1 teaspoon baking soda
Pinch of salt
¾ cup low-fat lemon yogurt
⅔ cup skimmed milk, or soymilk
2 large omega-3 eggs
1 medium lemon, zest and juice
1 tablespoon extra virgin olive oil
Olive oil spray for the baking tins

Heat the oven to 400°F. Whisk to combine the dry ingredients in a large bowl. In a smaller bowl, whisk together the wet ingredients. Fold the wet ingredients into the dry. Pour the mixture into sprayed muffin tins, loaf pan or preheated 10-inch cast iron frying pan. Place the tins or pan in the upper portion of the oven. Reduce the heat to 350°F. Cook for 30 to 40 minutes, or until a tester comes out clean.

Calories: 174
Protein: 6.5 g
Carbohydrates: 29.2 g
Cholesterol: 48 mg
Total fat: 4.5 g
  Saturated fat: < 1 g
  Monounsaturated fat: 1.7 g

Polyunsaturated fat: 1.3 g
  Omega-6 linoleic acid: 1.0 g
  Omega-3 linoleic acid: 0.2 g
  EPA: 0.1 g
Sodium: 262 mg
Potassium: 221 mg
Fibre: 3.8 g

Autumn: Season of Transition

It seemed that summer would last for ever, but of course it never does. One evening in late August, you notice that the sun is going down sooner and the morning air smells a bit different. There are still some hot days ahead, but change is in the air. Change is really the theme of autumn. Winter is winter all season long, but autumn begins as a wisp of leaf smoke on a warm golden day and ends as a cold night with moonlight through the leafless trees. We can wake up to an Indian summer day of intense heat and a few days later find ourselves searching for our warmest sweaters and jackets and hauling out the soup pot as a raw chill seeps through the windows. It's a season of transition for nature and for us and, like all transitions, it's not always smooth, and it's never seamless.

Those summer/autumn transition days are always bittersweet. It's the end of the joy of summer, the beginning of the more sombre months of winter. It's a perfect time to seize the opportunity to reassess our lives, our goals, our hopes for the future. The associations of autumn are indeed powerful: the end of the carefree days of summer (even if you've been working in a high-rise office, you never shrug off the illusion that summer is all about no school and fireflies and sticky beach afternoons), the beginning of a 'new' year. Each year, as time becomes ever more precious, autumn inspires us to pause and reorganize our lives and clean our mental closets. We do tend to think of autumn as a kind of beginning. Chalk that up to all the new pencils and notebooks and backpacks of our youth when we prepared for another year of school.

Autumn is a season of excitement, new beginnings and opportunity. It's the perfect time to think about health and fitness and personal improvement – all the topics of HealthStyle. Most of us already have the right mind-set to start anew in all our efforts. We're ready to wash away those lazy days of summer, brush the sand out of our shoes, and get down to business! The cooler air gives us renewed energy. We're ready to change our exercise programme or perhaps adopt one for the first time. We may have to be more organized on weekends to face shorter but busy weeknights.

This season, we'll look at a neglected subject – sleep – and how it affects our health and vitality in little-known ways.

The SuperFoods of autumn will be a special focus this season. Nuts, turkey, broccoli and pumpkin all have amazing health benefits and are appropriate to this time of year. We'll also look at some autumn fruits such as apples and pomegranates.

The fresh late-season produce that's available is drawing us into the kitchen. We're a little tired of 'toss something on the grill' cooking and ready to try something different. It's fortunate that the bounty of the harvest gives us lots of opportunities for wonderful healthy meals.

From the warm days of Indian summer to those chilly mornings of early winter, HealthStyle will keep you motivated with tips on how to combat the autumn villains of good health: less time and cooling weather.

SLEEP: THE LINCHPIN TO TWENTY-FIRST-CENTURY HEALTH

You do it every night but maybe not enough. Or at least not enough for your health.

As daylight grows short, you may well find your own days growing longer. Too often autumn is a time of increased workload, family responsibilities and household demands. Everything seems to need attention at once, whether it's health care appointments, homework supervision, travel plans, school forms, and even chimney cleaning. Everything that we might have put off over the carefree summer has come home to roost and it's overwhelming. The temptation is to burn the candle at both ends – stay up late to finish a project and get up a bit earlier to pack yet one more thing into the day. It's a good time to take a look at the dramatic effects of sleep loss on our health. Believe it or not, there's impressive evidence supporting the argument that the amount of time you sleep – even more than whether you smoke, exercise, or have high blood pressure or cholesterol levels – could be *the most important predictor of how long you'll live.*

Sleep. It's the most overlooked factor in achieving optimum health in the twenty-first century. We all know we should eat well and exercise. For many of my patients, even those committed to a healthy lifestyle, sleep is seen as a kind of luxury. Indeed, many people who follow sound diets and who routinely exercise are unwittingly sabotaging their efforts by depriving themselves of a pleasurable, satisfying, easy and inexpensive way to insure optimum health – sleep!

Feel yourself nodding off? You're not alone. A 2000 poll by the National Sleep Foundation found that sleep debt is a problem for more than 50 percent of American workers.

Data suggests that in the last century we've reduced the average amount of time we sleep by 20 percent.

It's easy to put sleep at the bottom of your to-do list. For one thing, our culture encourages it. We live in a 24/7 world where night and day dissolve into one long stretch of work and family obligations. Get up early to beat traffic and get a few phone calls in, stay up late after squeezing in some family time, so you can send a batch of e-mails and do some paperwork. Awake in the middle of the night? Look at it as a bonus to catch up on a little reading. And if you are up at 3 a.m. scanning magazines, you're likely to read about successful executives who boast about getting by on four or five hours of sleep a night. The implicit message is that sleep is for the weak and undisciplined.

The alarming truth is that sleep deprivation is taking a serious toll on our overall health. Chronic lack of sleep affects daily performance, overall productivity, and now, most significantly to HealthStyle, long- and short-term health. Sound far-fetched? Well, you may be surprised to learn that the sleep debt of only three to four hours that many of us routinely rack up in the course of a busy week can provoke metabolic changes that mimic a prediabetic state and hormonal changes that compare with those experienced by someone suffering from depression.

In a nutshell the amount of sleep you get has a direct bearing on the following:

- Obesity
- Coronary heart disease
- Hypertension
- Diabetes
- Immune function
- Cognitive performance
- Longevity

Sleep and Your Health

There's no question that sleep and health are intimately intertwined. Up until relatively recently, however, even though it was known that sleep affects performance in humans and sleep deprivation in rodents results in actual death, little attention was paid to the effect of sleep deprivation on human health. We now know that while the main function of sleep seems to be the refreshing of our brains, sleep and its lack affect many bodily systems, including our metabolism, our hormones and our immune function.

The important news, and one of the major messages of HealthStyle, is that chronic sleep deprivation is doing more than just making us tired and reducing our ability to perform at optimum levels. The big news on sleep is twofold: Many of us who think we're getting enough sleep really aren't, and our performance is affected even though we're unaware of our diminished abilities. Moreover, and most significantly, the lack of sleep that many of us endure routinely has now been conclusively linked with diabetes, metabolic syndrome and obesity – all increasingly common conditions that are taking a serious toll on our overall health.

Total sleep deprivation suppresses the immune system and even partial sleep deprivation has an effect on this important protective system. Even smaller amounts of partial sleep deprivation reduce natural killer cell activity and diminish the effectiveness of communication between our pituitary gland and our adrenal glands. This results in altered stress hormones, which in turn play a role in memory and glucose tolerance.

The summer is a time of no teachers, no books, and, for many children, no schedule. It's fun and flexible and allows for travel and visitors and catching fireflies. However, suddenly facing the first day of school without sufficient sleep can make the adjustment to a new teacher and a new classroom all the more difficult. Sleep deprivation in children affects mood, cognitive ability, memory, decision making, creativity – everything a child needs for good academic performance. Don't wait until the night before school starts to get the children back into a school sleep schedule. You should start at least a week in advance with earlier bedtimes and earlier risings. A six- to twelve-year-old will need between 10^1/$_2$ and 11^1/$_2$ hours of sleep a night. Get them into a good bedtime routine – say, dinner, bath, reading, bed – which they can follow for the full school year. A regular bedtime is critical. Our internal clocks are powerful and we sleep best if we fall asleep and wake up at the same times daily. If children have a week or two of restful sleep in advance of the start of school, they'll be better able to handle any night-before-the-first-day jitters and catch up on needed sleep quickly.

One fascinating area of research is discovering causative links between lack of sleep and diabetes and obesity. In one study, curtailing sleep to four hours per night for six nights impaired glucose tolerance and lowered insulin secretion in healthy well-rested young men. This condition was entirely reversed when these men made up their sleep debt with adequate rest.

The important message for all of us is that you don't have to lose huge amounts of sleep before it takes a toll. Partial sleep deprivation has a substantial effect on sleepiness, as you might guess, but also on motor and cognitive performance and mood.

From a very general standpoint, one study found that sleeping less than four hours per night was associated with a 2.8 times higher rate of mortality for men and a 1.5 times higher rate for women. The author of this study also found that length of sleep time was a better predictor of mortality than smoking, cardiac disease or hypertension. One other study found that people who slept six hours or less a night had a 70 percent higher mortality rate over a nine-year period than those who slept seven to eight hours a night.

It's not only long-term health that's affected by lack of sleep. Did your grandma ever tell you that you'll get sick if you don't get enough sleep? She was right. Studies have shown that people who suffer from acute and chronic sleep deprivation also experience immune changes, including a decreased number of protective natural killer cells and reduced activity of those natural killer cells. This reduced ability of our body to fight invaders on a cellular level will inevitably make us more vulnerable to colds and infections.

You're not only in danger of getting a cold if you don't get enough sleep, you're also at greater risk of developing chronic health problems including diabetes, metabolic syndrome and even obesity. While the links between these ailments and sleep deprivation are only emerging, we know for certain that loss of sleep affects hormone function as well as glucose tolerance and insulin resistance.

Attention Athletes

There is research evidence that most of the improvement of a motor skill depends on sleep. Improvement of a perceptual or motor skill continues after training has ended, and sleep is very important to maximize this improvement. The sleeping brain does a reprocessing of recent memory patterns involving motor skills. In addition, numerous studies support the idea that sleep is essential for brain memory function.

Sleep and Performance

You might have guessed that sleep deprivation takes a toll on performance. This is certainly true. One study showed that sleep restriction of six hours or less per night produced cognitive performance deficits that mimic the loss of two full nights without sleep. This is actually a relatively moderate sleep debt – many people experience it regularly – never imagining that it could seriously impair their waking neurological functioning. This same study, which involved forty-eight healthy adults aged twenty-one to thirty-eight, also reported (and this is critical information) that the study subjects were *largely unaware of their increasing cognitive disability*. Other reports corroborate this finding: We're tired, we're not performing well, and we're oblivious to the fact. Most people believe that they function normally despite being sleep deprived. No doubt this helps to explain why sleep deprivation has become a common condition.

We not only perform less well when sleep deprived, we try less. One study of college students who were sleep deprived found that on the day following their sleep loss they not only, as you might guess, were sleepy, fatigued, and had longer reaction times, but they also selected less difficult tasks than the control group. The selection of the least demanding option in a complex situation has obvious implications for the safety, reliability and effectiveness of workers.

Nearly 25 percent of the population, including night-shift workers and junior doctors, are particularly sensitive to sleep loss. A recent study of medical interns showed a clear relationship between the hours slept per day and the number of 'attentional failures' during night-shift work. Most significant, this study examined the work performance of a highly motivated, intelligent segment of the population, and clearly their sleep restriction had a significant effect on their ability to perform work. Another study of medical interns reported that those following a traditional schedule (little sleep and long hours) made 35.9 percent more medical errors than a group following a so-called intervention schedule (more sleep and reduced work hours). Another interesting study compared performance after being awake thirty minutes to five hours longer than the subjects' normal sleep time versus measured amounts of alcohol intake in the same subjects. The authors concluded that the magnitude of the behaviour impairment observed when the subjects were performing tasks just a few hours after their normal time of sleep onset exceeded that observed following a legally intoxicating dose of alcohol in these same subjects. The fatigue of sleep deprivation is an important factor that is very likely to compromise performance accuracy and speed; in some ways, sleep deprivation is like being drunk without any alcohol in your system. If you believe you can perform well in any endeavour without a good night's sleep, you're wrong!

HealthStyle Basket Case

Every now and again I encounter a patient who is in desperate need of a complete HealthStyle makeover. This patient typically has a poor diet, is highly stressed and is physically inactive. Here are my instructions: Go home and go to bed. You can't live healthily if you don't sleep, and chronic sleep debt makes other healthy activities difficult to achieve. You won't exercise if you're exhausted. You won't make good food choices if your appetite control system is out of whack – as it will be if you're sleep deprived. And you sure can't control stress when you're struggling to stay awake and function on a high level. I prescribe a full week of adequate sleep before you begin to think about setting other healthy goals. When you've achieved that, you're ready to take on all the HealthStyle challenges.

Close Your Eyes: Avoid Diabetes

Data from the Nurses' Health Study showed that healthy women who reported getting less than five hours or more than nine hours of sleep were more apt to develop diabetes in the next ten years than women who initially averaged seven to eight hours of sleep. A sleep deficit of three to four hours a night over a few days can result in metabolic changes that mimic a prediabetic state.

Close Your Eyes: Lose Weight

Perhaps one of the most interesting recent findings about sleep is the effect that it has on obesity. It's interesting to note that as Americans' nighttime sleep duration lessened by one to two hours over the second half of the twentieth century, the incidence of obesity *doubled over roughly the same time period*. While sleep deprivation alone doesn't explain the rise in obesity and diabetes, it surely plays a contributing role.

One study showed that the less you sleep the more likely you are to become obese. This study, conducted at Columbia University, demonstrated a clear link between the risk of being obese and the number of hours of sleep each night even after controlling for depression, physical activity, alcohol consumption, ethnicity, level of education, age and gender. The study subjects – ages thirty-two to fifty-nine – who slept four hours or less per night were 73 percent more likely to be obese than those who slept seven to nine hours per night. Those who got only five hours each night had a 50 percent higher risk than those who got a full night's sleep, and those who got six hours of sleep were still 23 percent more likely to be substantially overweight. In another study, adolescents with greater sleep disruption or generally poor quality of nighttime sleep also demonstrated lower daytime activity and for each hour of sleep lost, the odds of obesity increased by 80 percent.

> Trying to lose weight while suffering from sleep deprivation is like walking up a down escalator. You may find yourself trying very hard and getting nowhere.

One of the reasons that sleep seems to have such a dramatic effect on weight is the intimate relationship between sleep and hormones. When you experience sleep deprivation, your blood levels of leptin, a hormone that acts as an appetite suppressant, appear to decrease. Leptin is a hormone that's produced by fat cells. It helps to regulate your appetite and metabolism. High levels of leptin help you to eat less while low levels increase your appetite and cause you to eat more. In a study on sleep and leptin, it was found that subjects who slept less than five hours a night had a significant decrease in leptin and additionally a significant increase in gherlin, a hormone that triggers hunger.

Another factor when considering the relationship between sleep deprivation and obesity is perhaps more obvious: When we're tired we're less likely to make good choices about health-related activities. It's difficult to keep up with exercise routines or to cook a healthy dinner if you're just totally exhausted. So getting sufficient sleep not only contributes to your long-term health and your overall performance, it also helps reduce your chances of becoming obese.

How Much Do You Need?

While we know that adequate sleep is crucial to optimum health, we don't know the precise amount of sleep to recommend for everyone. We do know that as we age over a lifespan, our need for sleep seems to change and diminish. In the first days of life, our total sleep time is roughly sixteen hours, falling to about fourteen hours by the end of the first month. At six months of age, we're sleeping about twelve hours, and this amount declines about thirty minutes per year to the age of five. By adolescence we're sleeping from nine to ten hours, and as adults, seven to eight hours. There are, of course, individual differences in needs for sleep and abilities to sleep. We know that women have a greater need for sleep than men, and on average, though they retire earlier than men and fall asleep faster, they report more time spent awake during the night and generally poorer sleep quality.

Fifty percent of drivers report driving while sleepy and nearly 25 percent report falling asleep at the wheel, though not crashing. Approximately 5 percent of people have crashed while being drowsy. If you drive while sleep deprived, you're facing a risk comparable to that of someone who drives with an illegal blood alcohol level.

While not getting enough sleep is clearly associated with increased health risks, so is getting too much sleep. In the Nurses' Health Study, 82,969 women responding to the questionnaire revealed that those who slept five hours or less a night had a 15 percent greater mortality risk compared with those sleeping seven hours. But those who slept nine hours had a 42 percent increase in risk. Other studies have reported similar patterns.

I recommend seven to eight hours of sleep each night. While some people may claim that they do well on less, even six hours of sleep a night does not prevent cumulative performance deficits.

Health care professionals should ask patients in detail about their sleep habits and should stress the importance of adequate sleep for all.

Sleep-disordered Breathing

Sleep-disordered breathing, or sleep apnea, is a condition that is estimated to affect 2 to 4 percent of middle-aged adults and an even higher percentage of older people. Approximately 30 percent of those who snore regularly may have sleep-disordered breathing. This condition is most often diagnosed in overweight men with a large neck circumference. Even mild sleep-disordered breathing is related to an increased risk for hypertension, cardiovascular disease, diabetes and mortality. Obesity is a worldwide problem and is probably a cause of sleep-disordered breathing, thus weight loss and prevention of weight gain offer the best hope of reducing the incidence of this disorder. If snoring is an issue for you, an evaluation to rule out sleep-disordered breathing at a sleep clinic near you is a good step to take.

Insomnia

Insomnia is a special problem in the dark world of sleep deprivation. It's a condition affecting 9 to 19 percent of adults in the United States and Europe. The incidence of insomnia seems to increase with age and to be more common in women than men. A 1991 Gallup survey found that insomnia had a direct impact on the daily lives of one-third of American adults. Insomnia is generally described as the perception or complaint of inadequate or poor quality of sleep due to: difficulty falling asleep, waking up frequently during the night with difficulty going back to sleep, waking up early in the morning, or, finally and generally, unrefreshing sleep. Insomnia takes a toll similar to that of sleep debt: Sufferers feel tired, lack energy, have trouble concentrating, and are irritable. Insomnia, among thirty-seven other variables, is the most predictive factor for absenteeism at work.

As with sleep debt, the long-term toll that insomnia takes on health can be serious. Chronic insomnia is associated with an increased risk for alcohol and drug abuse, anxiety, neurosis, personality disorders, as well as dependence on sedatives, depression, diminished quality of life, and, in the case of older adults with cognitive disorders, placement in long-term-care facilities.

If you suffer from chronic or even occasional insomnia, read 'How to Get a Good Night's Sleep' (see page 307) and follow the recommendations. In addition, consult your doctor to be sure that medical problems such as angina, chronic pain, congestive heart failure, chronic lung disorders, endocrine disorders or prescription or over-the-counter medications are not contributing to your difficulty in sleeping.

Only one in twenty patients sees a physician specifically about chronic insomnia, even though chronic sleep disturbance is associated with substantial health consequences, including hypertension, chronic lung disease, arthritis, chronic pain or headaches, and diabetes. Untreated insomnia is a major risk factor for the development of psychiatric disorders, especially major depression but also anxiety and substance abuse disorders. Many people think that insomnia is a function of ageing. While it's true that some need less sleep as they age, it's also true that insomnia in the aged is often a function of increased rates of illness, medication usage, other sleep disorders and the isolation and inactivity that is often seen in older people.

A Note to Parents

Many of our kids are desperately in need of some sleep. Too often they're stressed both at school and at home with lots of demands on their time and little downtime. Help your kids get a good night's sleep. Learning good sleep habits early on will pay off. One US study found that just one hour of additional sleep restriction or extension on boys and girls in the fourth or sixth grade had a considerable effect on neurobehavioural functioning. Extension of sleep leads to improved memory function and alertness. The study concluded that most children can extend their sleep with demonstrable benefits. This has obvious implications for learning and school success. In another study on children and sleep habits, boys who had trouble sleeping as toddlers were more likely to become early users of alcohol and marijuana. Don't let this strike fear into your heart if your child is a poor sleeper; other factors could well have been at work in this study. It's worth knowing that healthy sleep hygiene can promote a host of beneficial effects in children, and that children suffer health consequences just as adults do when they suffer regular sleep deprivation. It's also significant to know that REM (rapid eye movement) sleep is important for learning; children who are lacking sufficient REM sleep will be at a disadvantage in the classroom.

Tips for Sleepy Kids and Parents

- Look at the tips for adults given below. Many of them are good for babies and children as well.

Even our babies are not getting enough sleep. According to a poll of more than 1,400 parents and others who care for children by the National Sleep Foundation, infants average almost ninety minutes less sleep a day than the fourteen-hour minimum that doctors recommend. The poll also reported that toddlers get on average at least two hours a week less and preschoolers more than four hours less than the minimum sleep they need to function at their best.

- It's particularly important to establish a bedtime routine for your child. Many parents find that a postdinner bath, followed by reading and quiet time, is a good prelude to a restful night's sleep.
- Many soft drinks contain caffeine, which can have a disastrous effect on children's ability to sleep. Eliminate caffeinated beverages from your child's diet, at least in the afternoon hours.
- Sleepless babies are the bane of parents. We now know that good sleep habits are learned and you may have to 'teach' your baby to sleep. There are a number of books that give good guidelines on this. *Solve Your Child's Sleep Problems* by Richard Ferber, M.D., is especially useful.

Schools should consider later starting times – about one hour later than usual – to accommodate teenagers' biological clocks. Some US universities such as Duke have already done this by eliminating 8 a.m. classes. Experts are beginning to recognize the close connection that stress, substance abuse and lack of sleep have with the increasing prevalence of depression in college students.

For Older People

The amount of sleep we need does not decrease with age, but the ability to sleep well does. Many older people face particular sleep challenges. For one thing, many seniors don't realize that their body rhythms shift as they age: As

306

we get older we feel an urge to retire sooner and wake earlier. Unfortunately, many people fight this urge: They stay up late as they always did, but they wake earlier. This creates a state of chronic sleep deprivation that takes its toll on health. In addition, many older people don't sleep as deeply as they once did, waking more often during the night. This, too, can make seniors feel less rested and refreshed. In addition to the tips listed in 'How to Get a Good Night's Sleep', the following conditions can affect sleep: hot flushes during menopause, frequent urination from an enlarged prostate, carpal tunnel syndrome or restless leg syndrome and chronic pain. Keep in mind that untreated depression as well as high blood pressure and heart disease can all encourage insomnia. Consult your doctor if you think you could be suffering from any of these conditions.

> Putting aside time in the early afternoon to nap appears to help older adults compensate for the sleeping problems that tend to occur with age, new research shows. US investigators found that people between the ages of fifty-five and eighty-five who had the opportunity to nap between 2:00 p.m. and 4:00 p.m. performed better on tests of mental ability, and had little trouble falling asleep at night. Older adults who took naps got an average of one hour more sleep each day they napped, giving them more than seven hours – close to the average for young adults.

How to Get a Good Night's Sleep

- Try to go to bed and arise at the same time each day.
- Sleep in a dark, cool room. You sleep more soundly when your body temperature is cool. Indeed, lowering your body temperature is a signal to your body to sleep. If you and your partner cannot agree on a room

temperature, use separate blankets or sew a thin twin-size blanket to a thicker one to create a full-size two-zone blanket.

- Take a warm bath an hour before bedtime. The resulting boost in body temperature will trigger a corresponding drop in body temperature a short while later, which helps induce sleep. If the bath is too hot, it may cause more difficulty in falling asleep.

- If you exercise in the late afternoon, it should not be less than four hours prior to your regular bedtime. Like a bath, exercise will raise your body temperature and trigger a rise in temperature, but could keep it elevated near bedtime, making sleep elusive.

- Minimize alcohol consumption. Alcohol may help you fall asleep, but it will not be a deep, restorative sleep. You'll also be more likely to wake in the middle of the night. The more alcohol you drink, and the closer it is to bedtime, the greater this effect. You may also find yourself going to the bathroom more often during the night due to alcohol's diuretic effect.

- Avoid caffeine eight to twelve hours before bedtime. Caffeine can stay in your system about twelve hours. Even decaffeinated coffee can cause sleeplessness in some people. So, if you have difficulty sleeping, avoid any caffeinated beverages, including soft drinks, after lunchtime.

- Don't eat dinner too close to bedtime. A late-evening meal can affect your ability to sleep.

- Complex carbohydrates can boost serotonin levels in your brain, which in turn relax you and help induce sleepiness. If you do have an evening snack, make it a complex carb like a slice of toasted whole-wheat bread with some peanut butter.

- Be careful about the supplements you use to promote sleep. While the herbal supplement valerian is touted to make you sleepy, studies have been inconclusive. Also avoid the herb kava kava, as there have been several reports of liver damage with this herb.

Studies of Okinawa and other elderly Japanese highlight the synergy between lifestyle and sleep health. These studies suggest that exercise, walking, short naps and a healthy diet were important factors in good sleep habits. A twenty-minute nap during the day can be beneficial.

- Check any medications you may be taking to be sure that they don't interfere with sleep. Calcium channel blockers like Cardizem and Procardia as well as steroids, decongestants and some pain relievers can interfere with a restful sleep.
- Some people find that an open window and/or a fan in the room helps them sleep. Circulating air and the steady drone of a fan can be sleep inducing.
- Do you love your pillow? A great pillow is a great encouragement to a good night's sleep. Invest in a new one if you're spending your nights punching and rearranging the one you have now.
- Drink some warm milk before bedtime. Milk and dairy products contain tryptophan, a natural sleep enhancer.
- Throw out the cigarettes. When smokers go to bed they may experience nicotine withdrawal, which has been linked to difficulty falling asleep.
- Let the sun shine in. As sunlight is an essential element in helping us to synchronize our body clocks, leave your sunglasses off until after 8:00 a.m.

For more information on sleep and sleep-related disorders, here are some resources:
American Insomnia Association, www.americaninsomnia
association.org

A New Autumn SuperFood
Apples

A source of:

- Polyphenols
- Fibre
- Vitamin C
- Potassium

SIDEKICKS: pears
TRY TO EAT: an apple a day

Autumn and apples go together. Apples are a SuperFood as well as the inspiration for a superactivity, apple picking, something the whole family can enjoy. Autumn is the time to indulge in all the glories of apples. Perhaps you've noticed that foods wax and wane in popularity. While the beloved apple has not been in the headlines lately, it has never lost favour with the public. The traditional gifts to teachers, the standard lunchbox treats, perhaps because of their ready availability, portability and overall deliciousness, apples are one of the most popular fruits. Apples well deserve their popularity, and research demonstrates that it's time to recognize them as a SuperFood. A number of studies have shown that apple consumption is associated with the reduced risk for a number of diseases, including cancer, particularly lung cancer, as well as cardiovascular disease, asthma and type II diabetes. If you take a look at the power of apples to prevent disease, you'll never take them for granted again.

Apple Power

An apple a day is perhaps one of the most delicious and efficient prescriptions ever made. Apples have proven themselves to be potent weapons against cancer, heart disease, asthma and type II diabetes compared with other fruits and vegetables, according to a recent major review study. The reasons for apples' potent health benefits are varied and synergistic. For one thing, apples are a rich and important source of phytochemicals, including flavonoids and phenols. In the United States, 22 percent of the phenolics (a class of polyphenols) consumed from fruits are from apples, making them the largest source of phenols in the American diet. Apples also contain two polyphenols – phloridzin and phloretin xyloglucoside – which to date have not been detected in any other fruits. Not only are apples particularly rich in phenols, they also have the highest concentration of 'free phenols'. These are phenols that seem to be more available for absorption into the bloodstream.

Eat a wide variety of apples. Different apple varieties have different skin colours, meaning the phytonutrient content of the skins varies in concentration and type of polyphenols.

Apples are also filled with superantioxidants. The antioxidant activity of approximately one apple is equivalent to about 1,500 mg of vitamin C, even though the amount of vitamin C in one apple is only about 5.7 mg.

And, by the way, apples with peel have a *far* greater antioxidant capacity than those with the peel removed. In cell culture in the laboratory, apple peel alone inhibits cancer cell proliferation better than whole apples. The apple peel contains more antioxidant compounds, especially polyphenols and vitamin C, than the flesh. A peel provides anywhere from two to six times (depending on the variety) more phenolic compounds than the flesh, and two to three times more flavonoids. The antioxidant activity of apple peel is about two to six times the activity of the apple flesh. So, eat the peel if you want to get the full protective benefits of apples.

Red Delicious apples have a high phenolic and flavonoid content. But don't limit yourself: Variety is the key.

One of the flavonoids found in apples, quercetin, seems to play a protective role against chronic conditions like heart disease and cancer. Quercetin is a plant pigment that has anti-inflammatory and antioxidant properties. It may be helpful in preventing the oxidation of bad cholesterol and in inhibiting cancerous changes to cells. Studies have suggested that people with the highest intakes of quercetin may have a reduced risk of heart disease and lung cancer.

Apples and Your Heart

Regular apple consumption seems to be a delightful way to protect yourself from heart disease. The fibre in apples – both soluble and insoluble – helps to reduce cholesterol levels, thus promoting heart and circulatory health. One large apple supplies almost 30 percent of the minimum amount of the US government's DV (daily value) for fibre (5.7 grams), and about 81 percent of the fibre in apples is soluble, the type that helps to reduce cholesterol levels.

Apples, along with pears, are loaded with soluble fibre, which plays an important role in normalizing blood lipids. In fact, adding just one large apple to your daily diet can reduce serum cholesterol levels 8 to 11 percent and eating two large apples daily has lowered cholesterol levels by up to 16 percent in some people. In one study, ten thousand Americans were studied for nineteen years. In this group, those eating the most fibre – 21 grams daily – had 12 percent less coronary heart disease and 12 percent less cardiovascular disease compared with those eating the least fibre – 5 grams daily. The people who ate the most water-soluble dietary fibre did better yet with a 15 percent reduction in their risk of coronary heart disease and a 10 percent reduced risk of cardiovascular disease.

Apples are also useful in preventing cardiovascular problems. A study of forty thousand women from the Women's Health Study found a 35 percent reduction in the risk of cardiovascular disease in the women with the highest flavonoid consumption, and in this study both apple and broccoli intake were associated with reductions in the risk of cardiovascular disease and events. Women ingesting apples had a 13 to 22 percent decrease in cardiovascular disease risk. Some of the apples' protective effect against cardiovascular disease may come from their potential cholesterol-lowering ability. In a 2003 study, it was found that combined apple pectin and apple phenolics (a class of polyphenols) lowered plasma and liver cholesterol, triglycerides and apparent cholesterol absorption to a much greater extent than either apple pectin or apple phenolics alone, once again demonstrating that it is the synergy of the whole food that makes the best insurance against disease.

Moreover, in a Finnish study, those who had the highest consumption of apples had a lower risk of thrombotic stroke compared with those who had the lowest consumption. In addition, apple and wine consumption was inversely associated with death from coronary heart disease in postmenopausal women in a study of nearly 35,000 women in Iowa. This would argue for the healthful effects of a wine and apple party.

Apples can help you lose weight. Soluble fruit fibre has been shown to be inversely associated with long-term weight gain, and in one study the daily consumption of either three apples or three pears was associated with weight loss in overweight women.

Apples and Cancer

Apples have proven themselves to be potent cancer fighters. In the Nurses' Health Study and the Health Professionals Follow-up Study, fruit and vegetable intake was associated with a 21 percent reduced risk of lung cancer in women. Subjects who consumed at least one serving per day of apples and pears had a reduced risk of lung cancer (apples were one of the individual fruits associated with a decreased risk).

A study in Hawaii found that apple and onion intake was associated with a reduced risk of lung cancer in men and women. There was a 40 to 50 percent decreased risk of lung cancer in participants with the highest intake of apples and onions compared with those who consumed the lowest amount of these foods.

Apples and Lung Health

In addition to all the ways that apples boost heart health, they're beneficial to lung function. Apple consumption has been inversely linked with asthma and has also been positively associated with general pulmonary health. For example, an Australian study found apple and pear intake to be associated with a decreased risk of asthma, and a United Kingdom study found that apple intake, as well as selenium intake, was associated with less asthma in adults. In the latter study, the clearest effect was in those consuming at least two apples per week. And, in a study of more than thirteen thousand adults in the Netherlands, it was found that apple and pear intake was positively associated with pulmonary function and negatively associated with chronic obstructive pulmonary disease. Another study showed that those who consumed five or more apples a week had a significantly greater forced expiratory volume (a measure of pulmonary function) compared with those who did not consume apples.

Apples and Diabetes

Not only may apples help decrease the risk of heart disease, cancer and asthma, but apple consumption may also be associated with a lower risk of diabetes. In a study of ten thousand Finnish people, a reduced risk of type II diabetes was associated with apple consumption and higher inake of quercetin (a polyphenol), a major component of apple peel, was also associated with a decreased risk of type II diabetes.

Apples in the Kitchen

While they are at their freshest obtained from local sources in the autumn, apples are readily available all year long. When shopping for apples, look for ones that are firm and unblemished. Choose different types of apples depending on how you plan to use them. Sweet apples like Red or Golden Delicious are great, so are slightly tarter Braeburn apples. Granny Smith and Bramleys are good choices for cooking, as they are tart and retain their texture. Apples should be kept cold after purchase.

The key to getting the best from apples is to eat the whole fruit, peel and all, and to eat a variety of apples, as each type offers different health-promoting benefits.

Here are some ideas for getting more apples into your life:

- A great snack is a sliced apple smeared with peanut or soy butter.
- For a healthy dessert, wash and core an apple. Put it in an oven-proof dish with a dash of honey, a sprinkle of walnuts, and a dusting of cinnamon (all SuperFoods). Bake in a preheated 350°F oven for about 30 minutes. Serve warm or cold.
- Dice an unpeeled, washed, cored apple and mix it with raisins, cranberries (dried or fresh), and any chopped dried fruit. Bake until soft and use to top yogurt or oatmeal.
- Add thinly sliced apples or pears to a spinach salad and top with walnuts and thinly sliced red onions. Dress with raspberry vinaigrette.
- Homemade apple sauce, made with cored, unpeeled apples, is always a favourite, served either as a dessert or as a side dish. Don't forget the cinnamon.

HOW TO PACK A 'GRADE A' LUNCHBOX

Now here's a challenge worthy of any survivor-type show: Pack five healthy, nutritious lunches that an eight-year-old will actually eat. Children can be so finicky in their food tastes and so sensitive to dining-room food fashions that getting them to eat what you pack is a daunting task. Don't give up: If you're willing to experiment and are open to hearing the truth from your child ('Did you really eat those baby carrots?'), then you can come up with some lunch ideas that are not only nutritious but also popular with your child. Here are some suggestions and tips for packing a lunch that's both healthy and delicious.

Parents sometimes lose touch with what their child's daily nutrition needs are. According to the American Medical Association, children between six and ten years old need about 1,800 to 2,400 calories a day. This translates roughly to two cups of low-fat milk; two servings of meat or a protein alternative; six servings of whole grains, such as pastas, cereals and breads; and at least five servings of fruits and vegetables. Of course, these calorie needs will vary widely with your child's activity level. A very active child who plays sports daily will need more calories than one who is more sedentary.

The first thing parents often forget when packing a lunchbox is the preferences of their child. Many of us pack a lunch for a fantasy child who will eat the foods we believe are nourishing. Many of us don't know that this lunch lands in the rubbish bin in the school cafeteria. So, the first rule in successful lunch packing is to keep your child's tastes in mind. If she never eats a turkey sandwich at home, there's not much chance she's going to eat one at school. This may mean bending the rules a bit. If you know he'll happily eat cereal for lunch, give it to him! If she'd rather have some fresh carrot sticks and onion dip, with perhaps a slice of whole-wheat bread smeared with honey, that's fine, too.

Two important food categories to keep in mind when preparing school lunches are protein and complex carbohydrates. Children's growing bodies need high-protein foods during periods of growth and complex carbs to break down slowly for sustained energy. Make up a list of foods in both these categories that your child likes. You can even create a 'lunchbox menu' so your child can pick which foods he'd like on which day. Often, the more involved a child feels in the process of selecting and preparing foods, the better the chances that she'll actually eat them.

Here are some ideas:

- Use whole-wheat flour tortillas to make healthy wraps. Fill them with tuna, turkey or lean ham, and add lettuce, some grated low-fat cheese, some grated carrot and a light smear of mayo.
- Most kids love rice cakes. Pack peanut butter or another nut butter separately for the child to spread onto the cracker.
- There's nothing wrong with cold pizza if your child likes it. Go light on the cheese and add sliced vegetables if your child will eat them.
- Kids love mini-muffins. Find a recipe for healthy ones without much sugar – a carrot muffin or a raisin bran muffin – and bake them in the small tins.
- Yogurt is a great lunch choice. Send along a separate container of fresh (or no-sugar-added tinned) fruit to be mixed in.
- Mix up a personalized trail mix of your child's favourite cereal, adding raisins, unsalted nuts, other chopped dried fruits and mini-pretzels.
- Send along crackers spread with cream cheese and dotted with raisins.
- Baked tortilla chips with a small container of bean dip or salsa make a great accompaniment to fresh fruit and perhaps diced cheese.
- Use a whole-wheat pitta pocket instead of bread for favourite sandwich fillings. Stuff with tuna and vegetables, hummus and shredded lettuce, or any other preferred filling.
- Peanut butter and banana bread or even plain old peanut butter and jelly on whole wheat makes a fine lunch.
- Air-popped popcorn is always a welcome treat. Salt it lightly.
- Fruit, of course, makes a great dessert. Just don't send fruit that's too messy or difficult to peel or eat easily.

Cut-up fruit is an alternative to whole. Be sure that it's not a fruit that will discolour once exposed to air.

■ Look for healthy chips for snacks. Two good choices are salsa with mesquite kettle chips and flaxseed tortilla chips.

Autumn SuperFood Update
Pumpkin

A source of:

■ Alpha-carotene
■ Beta-carotene
■ High fibre
■ Low calories
■ Vitamins C and E
■ Potassium
■ Magnesium
■ Pantothenic acid

SIDEKICKS: carrots, butternut squash, sweet potatoes, orange peppers
TRY TO EAT: ½ cup 5 to 7 days per week

It's time to unleash the power of pumpkin! If you think of pumpkin only at Halloween, it's time to update your appreciation of this extraordinary SuperFood. Pumpkins offer a host of health benefits, including their bountiful supply of fibre and various vitamins and minerals, but pumpkin deserves SuperFood status because of its rich and powerful supply of carotenoids. Indeed, think of pumpkin as the queen of the carotenoids. Carotenoids are the deep orange or yellow or red fat-soluble compounds that are present in a variety of plants. About six hundred carotenoids have been identified by scientists and every day we're learning more about the contributions these substances make to better health. Carotenoids have a wide range of biologic functions with an essential role in human health. Two of the carotenoids that are in rich supply in pumpkin – beta-carotene and alpha-carotene – are particularly powerful phytonutrients. Their presence in the body has been associated with a reduction in risk of the following diseases:

- Cancer, including lung, breast, prostate, skin, bladder and colon cancers
- Cardiovascular disease
- Inflammatory conditions, including asthma, osteo-arthritis and rheumatoid arthritis
- Diabetes mellitus

The most common carotenoids found in human tissue include beta-carotene, lycopene, lutein, zeaxanthin, alpha-carotene and beta-cryptoxanthin. These carotenoids help to protect us from free radicals, enhance cell-to-cell communication, modulate our immune response, and possibly stimulate the production of naturally occurring detoxification enzymes. Interestingly, carotenoids protect plants from sun damage and also provide the same protection to us: The primary purpose of carotenoids in the skin is to neutralize the free radicals produced by normal metabolism and exposure to sunlight, and they play a major role in protecting our skin and our eyes from the damaging effects of ultraviolet light.

Daily Carotenoid Recommendation

The US Food and Nutrition Board of the Institute of Medicine of the National Academy of Sciences is charged with setting the recommended daily allowances for various nutrients. While they have recognized that 'higher blood concentrations of beta-carotene and other carotenoids obtained from foods are associated with lower risk of several chronic diseases', as yet they have been unable to arrive at a recommended daily intake of carotenoids. In the meantime, my recommendations, based on all the available peer-reviewed literature, ensure that you are consuming the optimum daily protective amounts of these nutrients.

Alpha-carotene: 2.4 mg or more from food sources

Beta-carotene: 6 mg or more from food sources

Lycopene: 22 mg or more from food sources

Lutein and zeaxanthin: 12 mg or more from food sources

Beta-cryptoxanthin: 1 mg or more from food sources

It's not only the carotenoids in pumpkin that are working to keep us functioning at our best. It's the fibre, vitamin C, potassium as well as folate, omega-3 fatty acids (in pumpkin seeds), vitamin B1, niacin and pantothenic acid.

Here are some of the major benefits of including pumpkin and its sidekicks in your diet:

Cancer Protection. There's ample evidence that consuming carotenoid-rich foods reduces the risk of various types of cancer. In one recent study, dietary and lifestyle data collected over eight years from 63,257 adults in Shanghai, China, was reviewed and it revealed that those who ate the most beta-cryptoxanthin – an orange-red carotenoid – enjoyed a 27 percent lower risk of developing lung cancer. Even the smokers in the analysed group were found to have a 37 percent lower risk of developing lung cancer when they ate a diet rich in carotenoids compared with those eating the least amount of carotenoids. Another study, combining data from the Nurses' Health Study and the Health Professionals Study, found a significant risk reduction for lung cancer in subjects with a high intake of lycopene and alpha-carotene.

Carotenoids also seem to lessen the risk of breast cancer.

At least one study of premenopausal women reported a significant reduction in breast cancer risk in females with an increased dietary intake of alpha- and beta-carotene, lutein and zeaxanthin, and in another study, high lycopene intake was associated with a reduced risk of breast cancer. Yet another study found an inverse association between increasing levels of carotenoid intake and bladder cancer risk. This same study also suggests that a high carotenoid intake can have special chemopreventive benefits for those people susceptible to DNA damage.

Pumpkin seems to have a dual ability to fight colon cancer. The rich supply of fibre along with the beta-carotene has an ability to prevent cancer-causing chemicals from attacking colon cells. This is one reason why diets that are high in fibre-rich foods as well as beta-carotene have been found to reduce colon cancer risk.

Cardiovascular Disease. The carotenoids so richly present in pumpkin play a significant role in preventing cardiovascular disease. The beta-carotene in pumpkin and its sidekicks has powerful antioxidant and anti-inflammatory abilities. Beta-carotene is able to prevent the oxidation of cholesterol and, since oxidized cholesterol is the kind that coats the walls of blood vessels and contributes to the risk of heart disease and stroke, a diet rich in beta-carotene would be expected to promote heart health. Indeed, studies have demonstrated this to be true. A recent study examined the reasons for the declining life expectancy in central and eastern Europe. The decline seems to be largely the result of rising rates of cardiovascular disease. Traditional risk factors like smoking, hypertension, obesity, high dietary saturated fat and cholesterol intake do not appear to explain this decrease in longevity. The researchers ultimately concluded that a diet low in foods containing folate and carotenoids – particularly beta-carotene and lutein/zeaxanthin – appears to be a contributing factor to the increased coronary risk observed in this part of the world.

Inflammation. Inflammation has been associated with the development of various diseases. A recent laboratory study demonstrates that beta-carotene can downregulate the pro-inflammatory COX-2 pathway – in other words, suppress the activation of inflammation. This pathway is a major cause of inflammation and the same one that is disabled with nonsteroidal anti-inflammatories like aspirin. Although further work is needed to verify the relevance of these cellular studies, this is the first promising report showing beta-carotene as a natural COX-2 inhibitor or natural anti-inflammatory.

Want to boost your carotenoid intake? Here are some top sources:

Alpha-carotene

Pumpkin (cooked, 1 cup)	13 mg
Carrots (cooked, 1 cup)	6.4 mg
Butternut squash (cooked, 1 cup)	2.3 mg
Orange pepper (1 cup)	0.3 mg
Spring greens (cooked, 1 cup)	0.2 mg

Beta-carotene

Sweet potato (cooked, 1 cup)	19 mg
Pumpkin (cooked, 1 cup)	18.8 mg
Carrots (cooked, 1 cup)	12.5 mg
Butternut squash (cooked, 1 cup)	9.4 mg
Spinach (cooked, 1 cup)	9.4 mg

Pumpkin in the Kitchen

Winter squash, which count pumpkin as a family member, are usually available fresh only in the autumn. They're a treat when you can find them, and I advise you to search them out at farmers' markets where you can find unique varieties. Buy pumpkins or butternut squash that are rock hard. Winter squash do spoil and the first sign is a softened rind. Try to find squash with the stem still on, which protects them from bacteria. Varieties of winter squash that are particularly flavourful include butternut, buttercup, delicata and Hubbard squash. If they're not too large, prepare them by cutting them in half, drizzling on a bit of honey and a sprinkling of black pepper, and baking in a 350°F oven until the flesh is soft.

Pumpkin Seeds

Pumpkin seeds – often called pepitas, 'little seeds' in Spanish – are a nutritional bargain. They're rich in vitamin E, iron, magnesium, potassium and zinc, and are a good plant-based source of omega-6 and omega-3 fatty acids. You can buy them roasted or do it yourself. If you're removing seeds from a fresh pumpkin, remove any pulp or strings from them and rinse them in fresh water. Air-dry them on a baking sheet overnight. Drizzle with a bit of olive oil and some sea salt and roast at 350°F for 15 to 20 minutes. Sprinkle them with curry or chilli powder if you like. Cool completely and store in an airtight container.

When winter squash are not in season, you can take advantage of a more modern version of this vegetable by stocking up on tinned pumpkin, which should be a staple in every pantry. It's inexpensive, widely available, and can be called upon at a moment's notice to provide a nourishing soup, casserole or dessert, or even a delicious instant snack when mixed with some yogurt and perhaps nuts and honey.

Many people are surprised to learn that tinned pumpkin is rich in fibre; it's so creamy that you might not expect this to be the case. Low in calories, it has a truly impressive nutrient profile. I use tinned pumpkin frequently. It's always been popular in our house especially as the main ingredient in my wife Patty's Pumpkin Pudding, a recipe that appeared in *SuperFoods*, but I'm including it again here.

Let's not forget the pumpkin sidekicks. Carrots, butternut squash, sweet potatoes and orange peppers are a powerful group of foods that give us opportunities to consume a beneficial amount of the carotenoids often. Most people tend to eat pumpkin, butternut squash and sweet potatoes in the cooler weather and carrots and orange peppers when it's warm.

Baby carrots are great little bites, rich in beta-carotene and alpha-carotene. They're not really 'babies'; they are the clever marketing idea of a farmer in California who searched for a way to use up his broken or misshapen regular carrots. They're easy to use and worth the higher price if they help you serve carrots frequently. Put them out with a healthy dip for an after-school snack. Stick some in lunch-boxes. Keep a bowl in the fridge to satisfy snackers looking for something crunchy.

Sliced orange peppers are a good addition to any salad or platter of crudités. I find that kids really love these crunchy treats, and a plate set out in the evening will disappear. Serve them with your favourite healthy yogurt dip.

Don't forget sweet potatoes. With a little creativity, they can jazz up a simple meal. Peel and dice them, then toss the cubes in some extra virgin olive oil, dust with cumin, freshly ground pepper, and some ground chillies if you like. Roast them on a baking sheet in a 425°F oven for about 20 minutes until they're tender. Drizzle with fresh lime juice before serving.

Patty's Pumpkin Pudding

Here's an encore appearance of a favourite dessert at our house.

¼ to ½ cup sugar
2 to 4 teaspoons cinnamon
¼ teaspoon ground ginger, optional
¼ teaspoon ground cloves, optional
2 large eggs (use eggs with omega-3 content, as noted on label)
One 15-ounce tin Libby's 100% pure pumpkin
One 12-ounce tin Carnation evaporated nonfat milk (or evaporated 2% milk)

Mix all the ingredients together and pour into an 8- by 8-inch casserole and bake in a preheated 350°F oven for about 30 minutes. Don't overbake; the centre should be slightly wiggly. Cool and enjoy or refrigerate for later use.

Carrot-Chickpea Soup

Here's a great way to get some carrots as well as those fibre-rich chickpeas into your diet. For another layer of flavour, add some baby spinach during the last few minutes of cooking.

2 pounds carrots, peeled and cut into small chunks
1 large onion, diced
1 vegetable stock cube
1 tin chickpeas, rinsed and drained
¼ teaspoon cinnamon
Dash of mild curry powder

Dash of ground coriander
Salt and pepper

In a large pan, boil the carrots, onion and stock cube in 10 cups water until the carrots are soft. Turn off the heat and blend the soup until smooth. Add the chickpeas and blend into the soup. Add the remaining ingredients and stir well. Add more spices if needed.

If you prefer a chunkier, soup, remove a cup or two of the soup and purée it in a blender or food processor, and return the puréed soup to the original pan.

A TIP FROM CHEF MARK
How to Tame a Winter Squash
Winter squash are very hard, requiring brute force to penetrate them, even with the sharpest knives. Here's how to tame a winter squash: Wash it well and place the whole squash on a parchment-lined baking tray. Bake in a 325°F preheated oven 15 to 30 minutes, depending upon the size and variety, just until the skin is soft to the touch and the back of a spoon makes a slight indentation. Remove from the oven, and when cool enough to handle, cut in half, scoop out the seeds, then the pulp, and proceed with the recipe.

Autumn HealthStyle Focus
How to Avoid Hypertension

People are often surprised that I pay attention to the sodium content of foods. Why, they wonder, does a healthy guy bother to look for, say, low-sodium tinned tuna or no-salt-added salsa? Excess sodium intake is contributing to a looming crisis in national and international health. I'm talking about hypertension and the disastrous consequences of this syndrome.

Of course, sodium and excess salt intake aren't the sole causes of hypertension. For some people, salt intake seems to have no effect on their health whatsoever. Paying attention to sodium intake is a simple signal and reminder that you should work every day to ensure that your blood pressure is in the optimal HealthStyle zone.

Under Pressure

Blood pressure refers to the resistance created each time the heart beats in an effort to send blood rushing through the arteries. Between beats, when the heart relaxes, blood pressure drops. Blood pressure is routinely expressed in two figures: the systolic (SBP), or peak pressure created when the heart contracts. This figure is normally written over the diastolic (DBP), or reduced pressure present between beats. A typical adult blood pressure reading is 120 (systolic) over 80 (diastolic).

Recently, the acceptable levels of blood pressure were reduced. The guidelines recognize that the risk of death from heart disease and stroke begins to increase even at blood pressures as low as 115/75 mmHG, and that it doubles for each 20/10 mmHg increase beyond that mark. Previously, the normal or optimal mark was 120/80 mmHg. While this was considered optimal, it is now considered borderline. High blood pressure is now divided into the following different levels:

- Prehypertension SBP 120–139 or DBP 80–89
- Stage I hypertension SBP 140–159 or DBP 90–99
- Stage II hypertension SBP 160 or higher or DBP 100 or higher
- Residual hypertension is an SBP of 140 mmHg or more even after treatment
- HealthStyle goal is an SBP less than 120 and a DBP less than 80

> Have your blood pressure checked every time you see a health care professional for whatever reason. If you're over age sixty, have your pressure checked at least once a year.

Hypertension is the term that describes a state of chronic elevated blood pressure. Approximately one billion people worldwide suffer from hypertension. More than half of all Americans aged sixty-five to seventy-four and almost three quarters of African Americans in the same age group also suffer from elevated blood pressure. (The hypertension epidemic is especially dangerous for African Americans, whose rate of stroke deaths is 40 percent higher than that of the general population.) Data from the Framingham Heart Study suggests that about 90 percent of Americans will eventually develop hypertension. Ironically, and really tragically, many of these people don't even know they're suffering because hypertension generally is painless and has no symptoms.

Here's the truly frightening aspect of hypertension: It isn't an isolated ailment. Hypertension affects many bodily systems. If you have hypertension, you are also subject to:

- Increased risk of dying from a heart attack
- Increased risk of congestive heart failure
- Increased risk of dying from a stroke
- Increased risk of developing dementia and Alzheimer's disease
- Increased risk of kidney damage
- Increased risk of atherosclerosis and arteriosclerosis
- Increased risk of developing macular degeneration

If you have hypertension, you are pushing your heart and circulatory system to their limit every single day.

The good news about hypertension is that most people are in the borderline-to-moderate range, and most of them can bring their pressure down by making lifestyle and diet changes – in other words, by adopting the general recommendations of HealthStyle.

Don't expect to notice any symptoms from hypertension. It's typically picked up at a routine medical screening. A crisis resulting from hypertension could include the following symptoms:
- Headache, drowsiness or confusion
- Numb or tingling hands and feet
- Nosebleeds
- Severe shortness of breath
- A vague but intense feeling of discomfort

The Scourge of Salt

There are many reasons why hypertension rates around the world are soaring. For one thing, obesity is on the rise and obesity contributes to hypertension. We also know that the population is ageing, and as we age the likelihood of developing hypertension also increases. Indeed, since most adults develop blood pressure readings that put them at risk for negative health consequences, paying attention to your blood pressure and taking steps to control it, whatever your age, is a wise move.

Myth: Sea salt is a healthier product than table salt. In fact, there are no documented health advantages to sea salt and the sodium content of the two is similar. Sea salt, however, tastes better because it has no additives to make it free flowing.

Salt is a major hidden health menace to us and to our children. If you eat out, eat prepared foods, and/or eat fast foods, you're probably eating too much salt. We do need sodium to live. It helps us maintain fluid balance, regulates blood pressure, and transmits nerve impulses as well as helping in maintaining the body's acid-alkaline balance and playing a role in muscle movement. The average adult body contains about 250 grams of salt – enough to fill three small saltshakers. This salt is constantly lost through sweat and urine and replaced through the diet. The problem is that most of us are consuming far more salt than is required for healthy functioning. While the amount of salt the body needs daily, depending on circumstances like exercise and climate, is usually less than 500 mg a day, the typical American diet consists of 4,000 to 7,000 mg a day. We know that a diet containing more than 2,400 mg of salt a day is associated with higher blood pressure readings, and in fact there's some evidence that difficulties begin at consumption of more than 1,500 mg of sodium daily. It's generally agreed by researchers that much of the rise in blood pressure that seems inevitable as we age is actually a result of a lifetime of overconsumption of salt.

Attention parents: A low-sodium diet during the first six months of life not only lowers infant blood pressure, but these 'low-sodium babies' become adolescents whose SBP (systolic blood pressure) is lower than that of 'normal sodium babies'.

There is some disagreement among experts about an acceptable level of salt intake. For example, the Institute of Medicine in 2004 said that for people under fifty years of age, 1,500 mg of sodium daily was acceptable, while the 2005 Dietary Guidelines Advisory Committee said that for 'young adults' no more than 2,300 mg daily was acceptable. If even these two important US groups studying sodium can't agree on an appropriate intake, it's no wonder that the public might be somewhat confused. I think that we can take our cue from the past: Since our Stone Age ancestors ingested about 813 mg sodium daily and our genetic makeup hasn't changed much since then, it seems obvious that when it comes to sodium, the less the better. Unless you are training for or running a marathon or are physically active in hot humid environments, the need for sodium above that which you would consume in a whole-foods, low-sodium SuperFoods HealthStyle diet will rarely occur.

Does salt affect us all equally? No. It's true that some people who overuse salt will not elevate their blood pressure. On the other hand, it's difficult to determine who is and is not salt sensitive. We know for sure that where salt has not been added to the diet, there is virtually no hypertension. We also know that only in industrialized countries does blood pressure rise with age.

> The terms 'salt' and 'sodium' are used interchangeably, but they're not the same thing. Sodium is an element that joins with chlorine to form sodium chloride, or table salt. Sodium occurs naturally in most foods, and salt is the more common source of sodium in the diet.

You say you don't use that much salt and you guess your blood pressure is OK. That's the delusion too many of us labour under until it's too late and we're either on medication or suffering serious health consequences. The truth is that most of us are eating far more salt than necessary and that, combined with obesity and lack of physical activity, is putting our health at risk.

The best way to reduce salt in your diet is to read labels for salt content and avoid fast foods. Many fast foods are loaded with salt and for that reason, as well as the fat in those foods, they should be avoided. People are often surprised to discover how much salt there actually is in prepared foods. Here's an exercise: Take that bottle of salad dressing in the fridge and a box of any processed food in the cupboard – macaroni and cheese or taco seasoning or even salad croutons. Check the sodium content on the labels of these foods. Remember that you're aiming for less than 1,500 mg of sodium daily from all sources. Chances are that the labels will reveal that one serving of both the salad dressing and the prepared food will put you over the limit.

In the US about 10 to 20 percent of the population is 'salt sensitive'. The percentages are greater among African Americans, and also in the elderly and those who have diabetes.

Here are some tips on getting the salt out of your diet:

- Reeducate your taste buds. If you crave salt, it's because your taste buds have become used to very salty foods. By gradually cutting back on salt, after a few weeks you'll find that heavily salted foods will lose their appeal.
- Avoid bottled salad dressings or look for ones that are low in sodium. Make your own dressing with extra virgin olive oil and balsamic vinegar and fresh herbs. If you use dressing in a restaurant, request that it be served on the side and use it sparingly.
- Remove the saltshaker from the table and try salt substitutes.
- Avoid salt when cooking or reduce the amount called for. You can use less salt in most recipes without anyone noticing.
- Avoid processed meats and deli foods, as they are high in sodium.

- Check all tinned foods and processed foods as well as frozen dinners for salt content.
- Look for low-sodium tinned tuna and salmon.
- Home water softeners can add considerable amounts of sodium to your drinking water. Consider using bottled water for drinking and cooking if your household water is high in sodium.

Other reasons to shake the salt habit:
- Sodium increases urinary calcium loss, and although the literature is mixed, there is data to suggest that high salt intake may be related to loss of bone mass and to osteoporosis.
- High salt intake may have an adverse effect on lung function and asthma symptoms.
- Salt may promote the formation of kidney stones.
- High dietary salt may lead to a higher infection rate of *Helicobacter pylori*, the bacterium that causes stomach ulcers.
- High salt intake seems to increase your risk for stomach cancer.
- High salt intake has been associated with insomnia and preeclampsia of pregnancy.

Other Causes of Hypertension

While critically important, salt is not the only cause of hypertension. There are a number of steps you can take to ensure that your blood pressure remains at healthy levels throughout your lifetime.

- Stop smoking.
- Maintain an optimum weight. Obesity is a significant contributor to hypertension. Sometimes losing just a few pounds can make a significant difference to your blood

334

pressure. If you're overweight, your systolic blood pressure drops about one point for every two pounds you lose.

- Exercise. It's important to be physically active. See 'Exercise' (page 32) for some suggestions on how to work physical activity into your daily life. Exercise can not only lower your blood pressure, it can also help you lose weight and make major overall positive contributions to your health.

- Reduce your saturated fat intake. A high intake of saturated fat has been conclusively linked to high cholesterol levels and atherosclerosis, which in turn contributes to hypertension.

Only two out of three people who have hypertension know they do and only one in three has the condition under control.

- Increase your potassium, magnesium and calcium intakes by eating a diet that is rich in foods containing these nutrients. Most Americans have a sodium-to-potassium ratio greater than 2:1, which means that they eat twice the amount of sodium as potassium. Researchers suggest that a sodium-to-potassium ratio of 1:5 is optimum (see 'Potassium', page 267). Many of us also do not consume enough magnesium and calcium, the lack of which contributes to hypertension. A diet rich in fruits and vegetables can help you restore the optimal balance of these nutrients.

Foods rich in magnesium: Swiss chard, spinach, whole grains, pumpkin/sunflower seeds, soybeans, beans, halibut, nuts, avocado
Foods rich in calcium: low-fat/nonfat dairy, sardines, tinned wild salmon with bones, almonds, kale, spring greens, tofu, calcium-fortified orange juice or soymilk

- Investigate the DASH diet. This diet, which is rich in fruits, vegetables, and low-fat dairy products, has been shown to lower blood pressure. Check the DASH homepage at www.nhlbi.nih.gov/health/public/heart/hbp.dash for more details on this diet.
- Limit alcohol to a maximum of three to seven drinks per week for women and six to fourteen drinks per week for men. My own HealthStyle recommendations on alcohol are one to three drinks per week for women and two to eight drinks per week for men.
- Control stress. A number of studies suggest that relaxation techniques like meditation can play a role in lowering blood pressure (see 'Whole Mind/ Whole Body Health', page 219).

> A recent study reported that drinking alcohol outside of meals increased the risk of hypertension no matter what type of alcohol was consumed. The lesson: It's probably best to drink with your meals or immediately following them.

- Increase your fibre intake. Some studies show an inverse association between the consumption of dietary fibre and both high blood pressure and risk of hypertension (see 'Fibre', page 195).

A New Autumn SuperFood
Pomegranates

A source of:

- Vitamin B6
- Vitamin C
- Polyphenols
- Potassium

SIDEKICKS: plums
TRY TO DRINK: 4 to 8 ounces of 100 percent pomegranate juice multiple times a week or any amount of seeds

Did you know that it may have been a pomegranate – not an apple – that tempted Eve in the Garden of Eden? Ancient and beloved, the pomegranate figures prominently in history and mythology. The art, literature and culinary traditions of Europe, the Middle East, Africa and India all revere the mighty garnet-coloured jewel. For the ancient Chinese, pomegranates symbolized longevity, immortality and abundance, perhaps because of the roughly eight hundred seeds that each pomegranate contains.

One of the joys of autumn, pomegranates have been around since ancient times and their health benefits have long been recognized. Pomegranates can range in colour from yellow orange to red to deep purple. Rich in potassium, vitamin C, polyphenols and vitamin B6, pomegranates are real phytochemical powerhouses. Pomegranate juice may have two to three times the antioxidant power of equal amounts of green tea or red wine. In one study pomegranate juice was a potent fighter in the battle against atherosclerosis. As little as ¼ cup of pomegranate juice daily may improve cardiovascular health by reducing oxidation of LDL cholesterol. In addition, animal studies suggest that pomegranates may cause regression of atherosclerotic lesions. So don't avoid pomegranates just because it takes some work to get to the seeds.

Pomegranates possess potent anti-inflammatory phytochemicals, and consumption of pomegranate juice has been shown to lower blood pressure in hypertensive volunteers. Studies of several fruit juices and wines have reported the highest polyphenol concentration in pomegranate juice followed by red wine and cranberry juice.

If you've never tried a pomegranate, autumn is the ideal time. Select a pomegranate by weight: The seeds represent about half the weight of the fruit and so the heavier the fruit the better. The skin should be shiny without any cracks. You can store your pomegranate in a cool place for about a month, but it will keep in the fridge for up to two months.

Pomegranate juice, mixed with soda water and a slice of lemon or lime, can be enjoyed year-round. This cocktail will give you a powerful antioxidant boost as you enjoy the bright flavour and colour.

What do you do with pomegranates? The best way is to use the juice for sauces, vinaigrettes and marinades. The whole seeds can be added to salads and desserts, or as a garnish for meat or fish dishes. To get to the seeds, cut the top off the fruit and slice the rind vertically (from top to bottom) in about four places. Then put the fruit in a bowl of water. Peel away the sections of the fruit, releasing the seeds from the bitter white membrane. The seeds will sink to the bottom of the water and the remaining part of the fruit will float. Skim off and discard the floating bits and pour the seeds into a colander to rinse. You can then use the seeds in a recipe or put them in a blender or food processor to make juice. If you freeze the seeds first, they'll yield more juice. Each medium fruit yields about a half cup of pomegranate juice.

If you want the benefits of pomegranate without the fuss of preparation, you can buy pomegranate juice such as Pomegreat. Avoid brands that contain added sugar. Liven up your autumn recipes with pomegranate molasses, a highly concentrated form of pomegranate juice. It's a traditional ingredient in Middle Eastern dishes and can be found in speciality food markets.

Turkey (skinless turkey breast)

A source of:

- Low-fat protein
- Riboflavin
- Niacin
- Vitamin B6
- Vitamin B12
- Iron
- Selenium
- Zinc

SIDEKICKS: skinless chicken breast
TRY TO EAT: 3 to 4 servings per week of 3 to 4 ounces

It's lean, it's delicious, it's versatile, it's readily available and it's inexpensive. These attributes are enough to make turkey an excellent choice for dinner, but there's more: Turkey has health benefits that elevate it to SuperFood status. The leanest source of meat protein on the planet, skinless turkey breast is rich in heart-healthy nutrients that also cut your risk of cancer. The niacin, selenium, vitamins B6 and B12 and zinc in turkey breast make valuable contributions to your health and your diet. It's time to think about eating turkey more than once or twice a year.

Turkey is a standout in the SuperFood pantheon because perhaps one of its most valuable qualities is what it *doesn't* have: lots of saturated fat. It's a real challenge today to find sources of animal protein that aren't overloaded with disease-promoting saturated fat. Much of the poultry and red meat in markets today has too much bad fat and little or no good fat. Did you know, for example, that 3 ounces of fresh ham has 5.5 grams of saturated fat? And 3 ounces of sirloin steak has 4.5 grams of saturated fat? On the other hand, 3 ounces of skinless turkey breast meat has less than 0.2 gram of saturated fat. We are well aware these days that saturated fat is linked to a host of health problems, including everything from cardiovascular disease to cancer. Many studies indicate a relationship between increased dietary saturated fat and colon cancer, coronary heart disease and Alzheimer's disease. Remember that your dietary intake of saturated fat has a much stronger influence on increasing serum cholesterol than does your dietary intake of cholesterol. Saturated fat raises LDL cholesterol, which in turn promotes cardiovascular disease. This means that turkey can make a valuable contribution to your diet. This is especially welcome news to those who are eager to improve the quality of their everyday diets but are not willing to rely exclusively on vegetarian sources of protein.

Turkey is rich in various vitamins and minerals that are powerful health promoters. While lacking the disease-promoting fat contained in many other meats, turkey is high in the beneficial nutrients common to meats, including protein, of course, but also riboflavin, niacin, vitamin B6, vitamin B12, selenium, iron and zinc.

Selenium is perhaps the first nutrient that comes to mind when I think of turkey. One of my SuperNutrients, the trace mineral selenium is of critical importance to human health. It plays a role in thyroid hormone metabolism, antioxidant defence systems and immune functions. Studies have shown a strong inverse relationship between selenium intake and cancer incidence. While research is ongoing, there are a variety of explanations for selenium's role in preventing cancer. Proposed anticancer mechanisms associated with selenium include improved immune system function, inhibition of cancer cell growth, enhanced detoxification of carcinogens, and improved antioxidant status. Other good sources of selenium include Brazil nuts, crabmeat, wild salmon, halibut and whole grains.

Selenium is not the only nutrient in turkey that helps to prevent cancer and promote health. The B vitamins niacin, B 6 and B 12 all play important roles. The B vitamin niacin is essential for healthy DNA, and deficiencies of niacin, along with other B vitamins, have been linked to DNA damage. Niacin plus B 6 and B 12 are also crucial players in energy production in the body.

Zinc is another mineral in turkey that plays a role in many fundamental bodily processes. Perhaps most important for its contribution to a healthy immune system, zinc also promotes wound healing and healthy cell division. A 4-ounce serving of turkey supplies almost 20 percent of the daily value for zinc.

Turkey in the Kitchen

We're extremely fortunate these days, as turkey, which used to appear in the markets only around the holidays and most commonly as whole frozen birds, are now available all year round in a wide variety of forms. You can choose from whole turkey breast halves, cutlets or minced turkey meat.

When buying sliced turkey at a deli, ask for fresh roasted turkey meat, if available. Avoid 'turkey breast', which contains fillers as well as high amounts of fat and sodium. Buy fresh, roasted white meat to get all the SuperFood benefits.

Substitute ground (minced) turkey for ground beef in a variety of favourites, including pasta sauces, casseroles and even grilled burgers. When buying fresh-ground turkey, however, be sure to read the label carefully. Look for ground turkey that is 99 percent fat free, which usually means it consists only of ground white meat turkey. Higher-fat ground turkey can contain skin as well as other turkey parts and can be high in fat as well as cholesterol.

Here are a few ways to get turkey into your diet more often:

- The favourite all-round turkey preparation is roast turkey, the Christmas and Thanksgiving standard. At my house, we use a whole fresh turkey breast and remove the skin before eating it. Cooking the turkey with the skin on doesn't add any fat to the meat, but remove the skin after cooking.
- For turkey burritos, stir-fry ground turkey or diced left-over turkey breast in a bit of extra virgin olive oil with onions, garlic and sweet peppers. Fold the cooked meat in a whole-wheat wrap.
- Make a quick turkey chilli by lightly browning chopped onions and garlic, then adding ground turkey and cooking it until the meat is browned. Add 2 tins rinsed and drained red or white beans, a tin of chopped tomatoes and a chopped jalapeño pepper, if you like, and your favourite chilli spices, including cumin, oregano, fresh-ground black pepper, paprika and cayenne.
- Make turkey soup with the leftover meat.
- For sandwiches, put leftover sliced turkey on whole-wheat bread with avocado slices, sliced red onion and shredded spinach leaves.
- Make turkey Bolognese by sautéing onion, garlic, green pepper and fresh-ground turkey in a bit of olive oil. Add a tin of chopped tomatoes, a drizzle of honey and 2 tablespoons tomato purée, and simmer until the flavours blend. Serve on toasted whole-wheat buns.

SUPERSPICES

Most of us think of spices as incidental to our diets, but perhaps it's time to update our appreciation of these flavourful, and powerfully health-promoting, seasonings.

Spices are defined as any 'aromatic vegetable substance'. The key word is 'vegetable'. Derived from vegetables in the form of tree bark (cinnamon), seed (nutmeg) or fruit (peppercorns), spices have potent anti-cancer, anti-inflammatory and other health-promoting effects that are daily being confirmed by researchers. The following spices have been identified by the National Cancer Institute as having cancer-preventive properties: sage, oregano, thyme, rosemary, fennel, turmeric, caraway, anise, coriander, cumin and tarragon. Indeed, in one comparison of anti-oxidant power from the Agricultural Research Center, the compounds in oregano rank higher than vitamin E.

We've chosen cinnamon as a Superspice because of its general popularity and usefulness, but here are a few other spices that make major contributions to a healthy diet.

Cumin, a nutty, peppery seed, is popular in Indian, Middle Eastern and Mexican cuisines. In addition to being rich in iron, cumin seed has been found in animal studies to have anti-cancer properties.

Turmeric, sometimes known as the 'Indian saffron' because of its rich yellow-orange colour, has been used throughout history as a spice, healing food and textile dye. Numerous studies have shown that the yellow or orange pigment in turmeric – known as curcumin – has anti-inflammatory effects comparable to the potent drug hydrocortisone as well as other anti-inflammatory drugs. Turmeric has also been associated in preliminary research with providing relief for rheumatoid arthritis and cystic fibrosis and promoting liver function and cardiovascular health as well as possibly providing protection against Alzheimer's disease.

Oregano, the spice commonly associated with Mediterranean and Mexican cuisines, is a warm, aromatic herb with a variety of health-promoting abilities. The volatile oils in oregano have potent antibacterial properties. In addition, the various phytonutrients in oregano have powerful antioxidant properties. In fact, research has indicated that oregano has demonstrated forty-two times more antioxidant activity than apples and thirty times more than potatoes.

Thyme is a delicate herb with a delightful fragrance. The primary volatile oil in thyme – thymol – has been found to significantly increase the healthy fats found in the brains of ageing rats. Thyme has long been associated with healing abilities in connection with chest and respiratory problems. A rich source of flavonoids, thyme is now recognized as a powerful antioxidant food.

The bottom line on spices is that they can make significant contributions to your health, and you should make efforts to include them in your diet frequently. Don't forget that in addition to the health-promoting benefits described above, spices also make major contributions to our health by allowing us to reduce the amounts of salt, sugar and fat in our foods.

Rancho La Puerta Hibiscus Tea

The hibiscus plant is an annual herb whose flowers have been used to make hot and cold beverages in many of the world's tropical and subtropical countries. Hibiscus flowers contain large amounts of polyphenols with antioxidant, anti-inflammatory and antitumour activity. One study has shown that hibiscus tea can lower blood pressure in patients with hypertension.

Here's a recipe for Hibiscus Tea from the famous Rancho La Puerta spa in Mexico. Hibiscus (Jamaica) flowers can be found in the ethnic sections of many large supermarkets or even in health food shops.

Agua de Jamaica
2 pints water
½ cup dried Jamaica flowers (hibiscus)
1 cinnamon stick
½ cup honey, or agave nectar

Simmer the jamaica and cinnamon stick in the water for 20 minutes. Cool slightly before adding honey. Taste and add honey or more water to suit your preference.

Store in the refrigerator for up to a week. This can also be made as a concentrate and diluted when ready to serve.

Autumn SuperFood Update
Walnuts

A source of:

- Plant-derived omega-3 fatty acids
- Vitamin E
- Magnesium
- Polyphenols
- Protein
- Fibre
- Potassium
- Plant sterols
- Vitamin B6
- Arginine
- Resveratrol
- Melatonin

SIDEKICKS: almonds, pistachios, sesame seeds, peanuts, pumpkin and sunflower seeds, macadamia nuts, pecans, hazelnuts, cashews
TRY TO EAT: 1 ounce, 5 times a week

What's the single easiest, most delicious and health-promoting snack on the planet? My vote goes to walnuts and their sidekicks. The power of nuts to improve your health is extraordinary. Rich in vitamins, antioxidants, fibre, trace minerals, and a bounty of healthy fat, just a handful of walnuts a day can reduce your risk of heart disease and may help ward off Alzheimer's disease, type II diabetes and cancer. There's also evidence that nuts could play a role in reducing inflammatory diseases like asthma and rheumatoid arthritis as well as eczema and psoriasis. Indeed, the evidence supporting walnuts' important contributions to health is so convincing that the US Food and Drug Administration in March 2004 allowed walnuts to be the first whole food that can be labelled with a qualified health claim: 'Eating 1.5 ounces per day of walnuts as part of a diet low in saturated fat and cholesterol may reduce the risk of heart disease.' Shortly after that date, the FDA allowed two walnut sidekicks, peanuts and almonds, to be so labelled as well.

Nuts and Your Heart

There's no question about it: Nut consumption correlates with a reduced risk for coronary artery disease. For one thing, the fat in nuts is the healthy monounsaturated fat that is known to have a favourable effect on high cholesterol levels and other cardiovascular risk factors. Walnuts contain alpha-linolenic acid (ALA), a precursor to the omega-3 fatty acids found in fish oils. The ALA that is abundant in walnuts makes a major contribution to heart health. The omega-3s 'thin' the blood much like aspirin, reducing the risk of clots and heart attacks. Omega-3s also help prevent erratic heart rhythms and reduce inflammation – an important step in the process that transforms cholesterol into artery-clogging plaques. In one study of sixty-seven patients with borderline high total cholesterol, it was found that adding 64 grams (a little over 2 ounces) a day of walnuts to a low-fat, low-cholesterol diet caused a significant reduction of total cholesterol and low-density lipoprotein cholesterol (LDL) and a slight increase in high-density lipoprotein cholesterol (HDL).

Another study followed twenty-one men and women with high cholesterol who ate either a typical low-calorie Mediterranean Diet or one in which walnuts were substituted for about one-third of the calories supplied by other sources of monounsaturated fats like olive oil. After four weeks, the subjects switched diets for an additional four weeks. Walnuts made an impressive contribution to the heart health of those consuming them: The walnut diet reduced total cholesterol and LDL 'bad' cholesterol and, in addition and most impressively, walnuts increased the elasticity of the arteries by 64 percent.

The extraordinary antioxidant ability of walnuts is also responsible, in ways not yet completely understood, for reducing the risk of heart disease as well as a host of other ailments. In one recent study, researchers identified various polyphenols in walnuts that, along with the polyphenols ellagic and gallic acid, demonstrate 'remarkable' antioxidant abilities. These polyphenols seem to play an important role in reducing free-radical damage to cholesterol, thus promoting cardiovascular health. The hormone melatonin has recently been identified in walnuts, and in animal studies the blood levels of this substance after eating walnuts increased to values that could be protective against cardiovascular damage and cancer.

Omega-3s are essential for the optimal development and function of every cell in our bodies. Unfortunately, evidence of mercury in certain types of fish – a rich source of omega-3s – has led to warnings about safe levels of fish consumption for pregnant and postpartum women. If you are trying

Nuts and Diabetes

Given the impending epidemic of type II diabetes, it's encouraging to learn that just a handful of nuts can prove beneficial to those diagnosed with this disease. In one study, men and women with diabetes were assigned to follow one of three diets in which 30 percent of calories were from fat: a low-fat diet, a modified low-fat diet, and a modified low-fat diet that included an ounce of walnuts daily. After six months, the subjects who had been on the walnut diet enjoyed a significantly greater improvement in their HDL-to-total-cholesterol ratio than the other groups. Moreover, the walnut people had a 10 percent reduction in their LDL cholesterol. Another study that included more than 83,000 nurses found that women who ate nuts at least five times a week had a 30 percent lower risk of diabetes than women who almost never ate nuts. Even women who ate nuts one to four times a week or ate peanut butter at least five times a week enjoyed a 20 percent lower risk. As people with type II diabetes are at increased risk of heart disease, it's encouraging to know that a simple handful of nuts can help them to reduce that risk.

Institute of Medicine that women consume 1.1 grams per day of alpha-linolenic acid (an omega-3 fatty acid) and that men consume 1.6 grams per day.

Think Nuts

Walnuts have had a reputation as brain food, probably because their wrinkled shape actually resembles a human brain. However, there's more than appearance to link walnuts and the brain: As our brains are more than 60 percent fat, they rely on a steady supply of good fats – like the type found in walnuts – to promote the varied activities of the brain. Interestingly, there have been studies that have proposed a connection between increased rates of depression and our decreased consumption of omega-3 fats. Some of the research has suggested that there may be a connection between low omega-3 fat intake and ADHD (attention-deficit/hyperactivity disorder) in children. One recent study from Purdue University in the US showed that children with a low consumption of omega-3 fats are significantly more likely to be hyperactive, have learning disorders and exhibit behavioural problems.

There also may be a link between dietary intake of certain antioxidants – particularly vitamins C and E – and the development of Alzheimer's disease. Various studies have pointed to this connection. In one study more than five thousand participants were followed for six years, beginning at age fifty-five. Of that group, 146 developed Alzheimer's. When adjustments were made for age, sex, cognitive ability, alcohol intake, education, smoking habits and other variables, a high dietary intake of vitamin C and vitamin E was definitely associated with a lower risk of Alzheimer's disease. Since nuts are one of the richest dietary sources of vitamin E, this is yet another argument for making them a part of your diet.

Interesting recent research shows that a rich supply of dietary vitamin E may help to protect against Parkinson's disease, the chronic neurological condition that impairs motor function. Almonds, as well as other nuts, are good sources of vitamin E.

Nuts for Your Eyes

A 2003 study reported that a high intake of nuts reduced the risk for the progression of age-related macular degeneration. Elevated C-reactive protein has been shown to be an independent risk factor for both cardiovascular disease and age-related macular degeneration, and results from a study published in 2004 showed that eating walnuts and walnut oil can significantly reduce C-reactive protein and other markers of inflammation.

Nuts in Perspective

Few foods offer the health benefits of nuts, benefits that result from eating just a small amount weekly. An important issue is to remember that nuts must be eaten in limited amounts. Ideally, you should introduce them into your diet as a substitute for some other food, not as an addition to, or more than, what you're currently eating. Why? Nuts are high in calories and some people make the mistake of simply grabbing a handful a few times a day only to find that after a few weeks they've gained some unwanted pounds. Remember that a serving of nuts is generally a 'handful', or 1 ounce. In general, a single serving of nuts provides between 150 and 200 calories. Here's a list of the serving sizes of some common nuts:

Nut Calories
(All, except where noted, are for 1 ounce)

Almonds, 24 nuts, raw	164 calories
Almonds, 22 nuts, dry roasted	169 calories
Walnuts, 14 halves	185 calories
Hazelnuts, 20 nuts, raw	178 calories
Peanuts, 48, dry roasted, no added salt	166 calories
Peanut butter, 2 tablespoons	190 calories
Pecans, 20 halves, raw	195 calories
Pistachios, 47 kernels, dry roasted, no added salt	162 calories
Pistachios, 47 kernels, raw, no added salt	158 calories

Powerful Peanuts

Many of my patients are thrilled to learn that peanut butter, eaten in moderation, can be considered a 'health food'. Peanuts are not really nuts; they're legumes and are closely related to beans. However, most people consider them nuts and they share a similar nutritional profile with nuts. Peanuts are rich in vitamin E – 1 ounce (about forty-eight peanuts) provides about 15 percent of your daily requirement, as well as fibre, calcium, copper, iron, magnesium, niacin, folate and zinc. And don't forget that peanuts provide about 7 grams of healthy protein. The caveat with peanuts, as with all nuts, is to eat them in moderation. The serving size for peanut butter is 2 tablespoons, just enough to cover a slice of whole-wheat bread. When shopping, look for peanut butter with no trans fats, which you can identify by checking the label. Avoid products with partially hydrogenated oil. I prefer peanut butter with no added sugar and salt. If you store it upside down for a few days before opening, it will be easier to incorporate the oil on the surface. Other healthy nut butters include almond, cashew and soy.

Nuts in the Kitchen

It couldn't be easier to work nuts into your diet. Of all the SuperFoods, they could win the prize for giving you the most nutritional bang for your money. All it takes is a few plastic containers in your fridge of a few different types of nuts and a jar of good-quality peanut butter and you're good to go.

The key to tasty nuts is freshness. Because they are high in fats, they have a tendency to go rancid. Make sure before you buy nuts that they smell fresh and 'nutty'. If they taste sharp or bitter, it's a sign that they're rancid. They must be stored in a cool, dry spot. They'll keep in a cool place in an airtight container for about four months, in the fridge for about six months, and in the freezer for about a year. I keep a variety of nuts in the freezer in heavy plastic bags. I move small amounts at a time into the fridge, where I keep them in plastic containers so they're handy. If I haven't had any nuts in a meal, I make sure to eat a handful before the end of the day.

Always look for dry-roasted or raw nuts. Avoid nuts with added salt or oil or sweeteners. If you buy raw nuts, you can toast them yourself in the oven at a low temperature on a baking tray. Monitor the nuts carefully, as they can burn quickly.

Here are some great ways to get nuts into your diet:

■ Sprinkle chopped, toasted nuts on a salad. Walnuts are delicious on a spinach salad with a raspberry vinegar dressing and red onion rings. Pine nuts, toasted briefly in a nonstick pan, add flavour and crunch to any mixed green salad.

- Whole-wheat toast with 2 tablespoons peanut butter is a healthy snack.
- Top steamed spinach or kale with toasted pine nuts, walnuts or any chopped nuts instead of cheese.
- Sprinkle nuts on top of oatmeal (porridge) or yogurt in the morning to add fibre and protein to your breakfast.
- Nut oils also have health benefits and make good choices for salad dressings. Try almond, walnut and hazelnut oils.
- Nuts make a tasty 'instant' snack. Take some with you in a small container when you travel or to keep at your desk. Add raisins or other dried fruit and a handful of oatmeal to nuts for a supernutritious snack.
- Toasting nuts brings out their flavour. Preheat the oven to 325°F and toast nuts in a single layer on a baking tray, checking every 5 to 6 minutes until they turn a deep colour. Watch them carefully, as nuts can burn in seconds.

FAMILY MEALS

Twenty-first-century living is all about time. Most of us have far too little of it. With work and family obligations sometimes overwhelming, we trim our free time to the minimum, multitask, and always focus on the future to bring us our reward. Is that any way to live? We now know that not only does constant stress play havoc with our health, we also realize that taking steps to reduce this stress and enhance family and social ties can actually make us healthier. That fast-food meal, grabbed on the run, not only takes a nutritional toll, it's keeping you and your children from the proven benefits of family mealtime. Food eaten at leisure in a peaceful setting with loved ones is not a luxury; it is actually an activity crucial to your health and the health of your family.

The simple fact is that families who eat together are more healthy in many ways. A survey conducted by the University of Minnesota, found that frequent family meals are related to better nutritional intake and a decreased risk for unhealthy weight control practices and substance abuse. Another study conducted at Harvard found that families that ate together every day or almost every day generally consumed higher amounts of important nutrients, such as calcium; fibre; iron; vitamins B6, B12, C and E; and consumed less overall fat compared with families who 'never' or 'only sometimes' ate meals together.

Here are some tips on how to achieve satisfying family meals:

- Make family meals a priority. Mark them on the calendar. Arrange other activities around family meals whenever possible.
- It's most common to enjoy your family meal right in your own home, but sometimes a family meal can take place in a restaurant, at a sporting event or in the park – anywhere you can be together as a family, eat healthy foods and enjoy conversation and connecting with one another.
- Enjoy a wide variety of SuperFoods at meals. Dishes don't have to be fancy or take hours of preparation to be healthy and tasty. Develop a repertoire of quick, wholesome meals that you can get on the table fast, so you can spend more time enjoying your family.
- Enlist help from the family. You don't have to go it alone: Part of the pleasure of family meals can be the prep time that is spent together, engaged in conversation. If your children are small, assign them manageable tasks so they can be part of the process. Learning to set the table is a valuable lesson for a small child and makes him or her feel competent.

- Eliminate distractions. Don't answer the phone or the door while eating if at all possible. The time your family spends together is precious and shouldn't be interrupted.
- Make mealtimes a pleasure for all. Avoid arguments and emotionally draining conversations. Save lectures for another time. Share news of the day, discuss current events and plan future activities.

Autumn SuperFood Update
Broccoli

A source of:

- Sulphoraphane
- Indoles
- Folate
- Fibre
- Calcium
- Vitamin C
- Beta-carotene
- Lutein/zeaxanthin
- Vitamin K

SIDEKICKS: Brussels sprouts, red and green cabbage, kale, turnips, cauliflower, spring greens, bok choy, mustard greens, Swiss chard, swede, kohlrabi, rocket, watercress, daikon root, wasabi
TRY TO EAT: ½ to 1 cup most days

Delicious, versatile, almost ubiquitous – that's broccoli. Best of all, broccoli is one of the most nutrient-dense foods known to man, with more polyphenols than any other commonly eaten vegetable. Broccoli well deserves its SuperFood rating, as it's one of the best-studied, most nutritious foods in the world. There are several groups of compounds in broccoli and its sidekicks that show powerful abilities to prevent or alleviate disease and promote health. These include glucosinolates, vitamins, sulphur compounds, and carotenoids. These substances make major contributions to keeping us healthy.

Broccoli promotes health by:

- Fighting cancer
- Boosting the immune system
- Lowering the incidence of cataracts
- Supporting cardiovascular health
- Building bones
- Fighting birth defects
- Promoting the production of the primary intracellular antioxidant: glutathione
- Decreasing inflammation

There's some evidence that the best way to cook broccoli in order to preserve nutrients is to steam it lightly. Using the least amount of water possible preserves the most nutrients.

Cruciferous vegetables, such as broccoli and cauliflower, have become known for their cancer-fighting abilities in particular, which makes them a produce standout. Most cancers take years to develop, and broccoli acts as a natural chemopreventive, mitigating the progress of cancer at many stages. It's the chemicals called glucosinolates in broccoli that are the potent cancer fighters. Interestingly, these chemicals were first written about in the beginning of the seventeenth century. Glucosinolates are fairly unique to crucifers. When broccoli is cut or chewed, the glucosinolates are released and are converted into phytonutrients called isothiocyanates and indoles. Isothiocyanates have been shown to inhibit or block tumours from forming. Indoles seem to work as chemoprotective agents against hormone-related cancers like breast and prostate cancer through their effect on oestrogen.

A recent study confirms the power of these vegetables to fight cancer. A seven-year study in Australia followed 609 women who had been diagnosed with ovarian cancer – an aggressive form of cancer. It seems that by including five servings a day of vegetables, particularly cruciferous vegetables, in their diet, the women experienced a beneficial effect on their survival rates. The women who survived the longest after diagnosis ate the most vegetables, especially cruciferous ones.

Another interesting recent study found that the sulphoraphane in broccoli stopped the proliferation of breast cancer cells, even in the later stages of their growth. This is excellent news and also a reminder that it's never too late to improve your health by adopting a healthy diet and trying to include a wide variety of SuperFoods routinely in your meals.

Men, too, can benefit from a diet rich in broccoli as well as other fibre-rich vegetables. In one recent study, it was reported that men whose diets were highest in fibre had an 18 percent lower risk of prostate cancer compared with men in the study who ate the least fibre. It was mainly fibre from vegetables like broccoli, cabbage and peas that made the difference.

It's important to eat cruciferous vegetables both cooked and raw to gain optimum health benefits. For example, the bioavailability of isothiocyanates from raw broccoli is approximately three times greater than from cooked broccoli. Best solution: Eat cooked broccoli and Brussels sprouts and raw shredded cabbage – red and green – in salads. Eat raw broccoli sprouts on sandwiches and in salads; eat kale, spring greens and mustard greens cooked.

While broccoli's effectiveness against cancer has perhaps received the most attention, let's not forget the important role that cruciferous vegetables play in other aspects of health promotion:

- Broccoli is rich in folate – the B vitamin that's essential to prevent birth defects. As folic-acid deficiency may be the most common vitamin deficiency in the world, this is a significant benefit. Folate prevents neural tube defects for newborns, is itself a potent anticancer nutrient, and is also effective in helping to remove homocysteine – linked to cardiovascular disease and dementia – from the circulatory system.
- Broccoli is a good source of lutein, the carotenoid that promotes eye health and helps prevent cataracts.
- Broccoli and its sidekicks are also helpful in promoting healthy bones with their rich mix of calcium and vitamins C and K.
- Interesting research is indicating that a compound in broccoli and broccoli sprouts may be effective against *Helicobacter pylori*, the bacterium that is responsible for most peptic ulcers and may also be implicated in gastric cancer. An animal study found that a phytochemical found in broccoli sprouts was able to completely eradicate *H. pylori* in eight of eleven infected mice.
- The Women's Health Study found both apples and broccoli intake to be associated with reductions in the risk of both cardiovascular disease and cardiovascular events.

Vitamin K is a fat-soluble vitamin known as the clotting vitamin because of its role in promoting blood clotting. If you take a prescribed anticoagulant or blood thinner, you should be careful about your K intake. Don't increase your consumption of K-rich foods like broccoli, cauliflower or cabbage, leafy greens or Brussels sprouts without checking with your health care professional.

Broccoli in the Kitchen

Broccoli is available all year round and easy to find in every supermarket. Don't forget frozen broccoli. It's handy to use in stir-fries, soups and side dishes. When buying fresh broccoli, look for deep green heads with tight, dense florets. Avoid yellowing florets, as they're a sign of age. Keep broccoli in the fridge for up to a week. Wash just before using to prevent mould.

Recent studies have shown that lightly steaming broccoli preserves most of the nutrients. While boiled broccoli lost as much as 66 percent of its folate content, no significant loss of folate occurred when the broccoli was steamed.

- Add chopped broccoli to pasta sauces, lasagnes and casseroles.
- Top whole-wheat pasta with sautéed garlic, olive oil and broccoli (all SuperFoods). Add a dash of red chilli pepper flakes if you like.
- Add some shredded green or red cabbage to salads. I always keep a small head of red cabbage in the fridge to be shredded into salads.

Does your child hate broccoli? It could be all in the genes. A study done in Philadelphia found that a gene called TAS2R38 could be responsible for your child's aversion to certain vegetables. Each of us carries two of these genes, and one version of the gene is more sensitive to bitter tastes than the other. In the study of 143 children, almost 80 percent had two copies of the 'bitter gene'. The presence of this gene had a big impact on a child's food choices; the same gene in the mother didn't seem to play as big a role in diet. The solution? Serve vegetables like broccoli with a slightly sweet or salty sauce. And don't give up. It sometimes takes half a dozen tries before a child will develop a taste for new foods.

Here are two kid-friendly broccoli toppers:

- Mix 1/4 cup peanut butter with 2 tablespoons brewed hot black or green tea. Mix until smooth and stir in 1 tablespoon reduced-sodium soy sauce, 1 tablespoon lemon juice, 1 teaspoon brown sugar.
- Mix 2 tablespoons reduced-sodium soy sauce with 2 tablespoons orange juice, 1 tablespoon rice vinegar, 1 tablespoon toasted sesame oil, 2 teaspoons honey and 2 teaspoons minced fresh ginger.

- Lay cut-up cauliflower or broccoli in a roasting tin with a sprinkle of olive oil and a dash of sea salt. Roast at 425°F for 30 minutes or until the cauliflower or broccoli becomes sweet and browned at the edges.
- Purée cooked broccoli or cauliflower with some cooked rice and a dash of nutmeg and olive oil for a side dish.

A New Autumn SuperFood
Onions

A source of:

- Selenium
- Fructans (including inulin)
- Vitamin E
- Vitamin C
- Potassium

- Diallyl sulphide
- Saponins
- Fibre
- Polyphenols

SIDEKICKS: garlic, spring onions, shallots, leeks, chives
TRY TO EAT: multiple times a week

It's hard to imagine a culinary life without onions. A staple of so many cuisines, onions lend a unique savoury and pungent flavour to an endless variety of dishes. Eaten cooked and raw, available all year round, onions are hard to avoid, and once you know about their considerable health benefits, it's difficult to imagine why anyone would want to. While onions' health-promoting abilities have long been recognized, it's only recently that their considerable curative abilities have been conclusively demonstrated and thus their elevation to SuperFood status.

Cultivated for more than five thousand years, onions are native to Asia and the Middle East. The name 'onion' comes from the Latin *unis*, meaning 'one' or 'single', and it refers to the fact that onions, unlike their close relative garlic, have only one bulb.

Onions are a major source of two phytonutrients that play a significant role in health promotion: flavonoids and the mixture of more than fifty sulphur-containing compounds. The two flavonoid subgroups found in onions are the anthocyanins that impart a red-purple colour to some varieties, and the flavonoids, such as quercetin and its derivatives, that are responsible for the yellow flesh and brown skins of many other varieties. In general, the phytonutrients in onions, and in other fruits and vegetables, are concentrated in the skin and outermost portions of the flesh.

We now know that the health-promoting compounds in onions, like those in garlic, are separated by cell walls.

Slicing an onion ruptures these walls and releases the compounds, which then combine to form a powerful new compound: thiopropanal sulphoxide. In addition to mitigating various diseases, this substance also gives cut onions their pungent aroma and their ability to make us cry.

> To get the most health benefits from onions, let them sit for 5 to 10 minutes after cutting and before cooking. Heat will deactivate the thiopropanal sulphoxide and you want to give it time to develop fully and to become concentrated before heating.

Onions and Your Heart

While chopping onions may make you cry, their considerable cardiovascular benefits should bring a smile through your tears. As with garlic, onion consumption has been shown to lower high cholesterol levels and high blood pressure. Onions, along with tea, apples and broccoli – the richest dietary sources of flavonoids – have been shown to reduce the risk of heart disease by 20 percent in one recent meta-analysis that reviewed the dietary patterns and health of more than 100,000 individuals.

Onions and Cancer

Regular consumption of onions has also been associated with a reduced risk of colon cancer. It is believed that quercetin in onions is the protective factor, since it's been shown to stop the growth of tumours in animals and to protect colon cells from the negative effects of some cancer-promoting substances. There's also evidence that onions may lower the risk of cancers of the brain, oesophagus, lung and stomach.

From a health promotion standpoint, the most pungent onions and their sidekicks pack the biggest wallop. In one test of the flavonoid content of onions, shallots had six times the amount found in Vidalia onions, the variety with the lowest phenolic content. Shallots also had the most antioxidant activity. Western yellow onions had the most flavonoids – eleven times the amount found in Western white onions, the type with the lowest flavonoid content. Many of us have been opting for the sweeter onions of late. All types of onions are good additions to your diet, but choose the stronger-tasting ones when appropriate to your recipe.

Onions as Anti-Inflammatories

Onions contain several anti-inflammatory compounds that contribute to reducing the symptoms associated with a host of inflammatory conditions like osteoarthritis and rheumatoid arthritis, the allergic inflammatory response of asthma, and the respiratory congestion that is a symptom of the common cold. Onions and garlic both contain compounds that inhibit the enzymes that generate inflammatory prostaglandins and thromboxanes. Both vitamin C and quercetin contribute to this beneficial effect. They work synergistically to spell relief from inflammation, making both onions and garlic good choices as ingredients in many dishes during the cold and flu season. Onions also exhibit antimicrobial activity against a range of bacteria and fungi.

Onions in the Kitchen

Onions and their cousins, shallots, green onions or spring onions, are widely available all year round. Choose onions that are clean and firm with no soft or mouldy spots. Avoid sprouting onions or ones with any dampness. When choosing spring onions, look for those having green, fresh-looking tops with a whitish base. Avoid any that look wilted, brown or yellow at the tips.

Onions and potatoes, while delicious combined in foods, are not storage friends. The moisture and ethylene gas from the spuds will cause onions to spoil more quickly. Keep them separate. Onions should be kept in a well-ventilated dark place. Spring onions should be stored in a perforated plastic bag in the fridge.

If cutting an onion makes you weep, chill the onion for an hour or so before chopping to slow the enzyme activity. Allow the chopped onion to come to room temperature and rest after cutting to promote the beneficial enzyme activity before cooking.

- Onions are welcome additions to almost any cooked dish, including soups, stews and casseroles.
- Onions are a pungent addition to salads. Use red onions for colour and a polyphenol boost.
- Grilled or roasted onions are flavourful and sweet. Brush lightly with olive oil before cooking.

AUTUMN HEALTHSTYLE RECIPES
Balsamic Roasted Onions

8 medium onions, cut into 6 wedges each
¼ cup aged balsamic vinegar
1 tablespoon honey
Freshly ground black pepper
1 tablespoon extra virgin olive oil

Put the onion wedges in a bowl of ice water and soak for about 2 hours. Drain in a colander for 10 minutes.

Preheat the oven to 400°F. Arrange the onions on an oiled baking dish.

Whisk the vinegar and honey together, and season with

pepper. Pour over the onions, tossing gently to coat. Drizzle the onions with the olive oil.

Cover with foil and bake for 25 minutes. Uncover and bake an additional 45 minutes, or until tender.

Pumpkin Seed Dip

Serves 7

This is a healthy dip for parties or for snacking. Use a quality, light mayonnaise made with heart-healthy fats like grapeseed, extra virgin olive oil or soy oil in this recipe. Serve with a platter of cut-up vegetables.

1 small shallot
1 garlic clove
1 small jalapeño pepper
⅓ cup flaxseeds
1 cup roasted and salted pumpkin seeds
½ bunch coriander
¼ cup light mayonnaise
1 teaspoon ground cumin
½ teaspoon ground coriander
Freshly ground black pepper
2 medium oranges, juice and zest
1 small lemon, juice and zest
Paprika
Extra virgin olive oil

Process the shallot, garlic, and jalapeño pepper to a fine mince in a food processor. Add the flaxseeds and pumpkin seeds and process again. Cut the coriander with scissors into the food processor. Add the mayonnaise, spices, orange and lemon juices and zests, and process to a fine spreading consistency. Add more orange juice if necessary to create a creamier texture. Place in a bowl, and garnish with paprika and a drizzle of olive oil.

Pine Nut-Stuffed Basil Tomatoes

Serves 10

When you can find organic heirloom tomatoes, this recipe is a showstopper!

1 cup pine nuts, toasted
1¾ cups chopped fresh basil
¼ cup extra virgin olive oil
3 cups cooked brown rice
10 medium tomatoes
Salt and pepper

Toast the pine nuts on a baking tray or in a cast-iron pan in a preheated 325°F oven until just golden. Toss the pine nuts, basil and olive oil with the cooked brown rice. Cut off and discard the tops of the tomatoes. Remove the pulp and seeds. Fill each tomato with the rice mixture. Serve warm or chilled.

Roasted Turkey Breast

Serves 8

This makes a fine dinner and you can serve the leftovers in sandwiches, tacos, salads and many other dishes. A 4-pound turkey breast with bone should yield 2½ to 3 pounds of meat when the bone is removed. Always purchase organic turkey.

4 pounds turkey breast, bone in
1 tablespoon extra virgin olive oil
Salt and pepper
2 medium onions, coarsely diced
4 medium carrots, coarsely diced
3 celery stalks, coarsely diced

Preheat the oven to 325°F. Wash the turkey breast and pat dry. Place the turkey in a roasting tin and rub it with oil all over. Sprinkle with salt and pepper. Roast until the internal temperature is 165°F on an instant-read thermometer. Tent with foil if the breast browns too quickly. Add the diced vegetables to the roasting tin about 45 to 60 minutes before the bird is ready.

Calories: 169
Protein: 29 g
Carbohydrates: 6 g
Cholesterol: 6 g
Total fat: 2.6 g
  Saturated fat: 0.5 g
  Monounsaturated fat: 1.5 g

Polyunsaturated fat: 0.4 g
  Omega-6 linoleic acid: 0.2 g
  Omega-3 linoleic acid: <0.1 g
  EPA/DHA: <0.1 g
Sodium: 80 mg
Potassium: 517 mg
Fibre: 1.7 g

Lime Pecan–Crusted Turkey Breast

Serves 5

Roasting a turkey breast means you'll always have this SuperFood on hand for sandwiches. Buy organic turkey; it does make a difference.

1¾ pounds turkey breast
2 medium limes, zest and juice
1 tablespoon Dijon mustard
⅔ cup coarsely chopped pecans
Freshly ground black pepper

Preheat the oven to 375°F. Place the turkey breast in a roasting tin. Whisk together the lime juice and zest, mustard, pecans and black pepper. Pack the mixture on the top of the breast to create a crust, and roast until the turkey is heated through and the pecans are lightly browned. Check after 20 minutes. If the nuts don't brown well, put the breast under a low grill for a few minutes more.

Calories: 262
Protein: 35 g
Carbohydrates: 5.1 g
Cholesterol: 84 mg
Total fat: 11.5 g
  Saturated fat: 1.2 g
  Monounsaturated fat: 6.2 g

Polyunsaturated fat: 3.4 g
  Omega-6 linoleic acid: 3.1 g
  Omega-3 linoleic acid: 0.2 g
  EPA/DHA: <0.1 g
Sodium: 84 mg
Potassium: 490 mg
Fibre: 2.2 g

Curried Squash Corn Soup

Serves 8

Make this soup with unpeeled organic red or white potatoes, whichever you prefer.

    1 medium butternut squash
    1 medium acorn squash
    1 medium potato
    1 large red onion, diced
    1 tablespoon crushed garlic
    2 tablespoons extra virgin olive oil
    Black pepper
    1 small leek, diced
    2 teaspoons curry powder, or more to taste
    2 bay leaves
    4 pints soymilk or vegetable stock
    ¼ cup dark sherry
    1½ cups corn kernels
    ¼ cup pumpkin seeds, roasted

Preheat the oven to 300°F. Wash and roast the squash and the potato for 30 to 45 minutes, or until tender when pierced with a knife. Cool, then cut in half and scoop out

368

the squash seeds (reserving them for garnish if desired). Use a spoon to scoop out the pulp. Sauté the onion and garlic in the oil. Add a few grinds of black pepper, the leek, curry powder and bay leaves. When fragrant and soft, add the milk and sherry. Add the squash and potato. When the vegetables are tender, add the corn. Divide among warmed bowls and garnish with pumpkin seeds.

Calories: 264
Protein: 11.3 g
Carbohydrates: 32.3 g
Cholesterol: 0.0 mg
Total fat: 12 g
  Saturated fat: 1.6 g
  Monounsaturated fat: 4.5 g

Polyunsaturated fat: 3.6 g
  Omega-6 linoleic acid: 1.8 g
  Omega-3 linoleic acid: 0.3 g
  EPA/DHA: 0.0 g
Sodium: 157 mg
Potassium: 983 mg
Fibre: 6.5 g

Tarragon Turkey-Walnut Salad

Serves 4

A good way to use up those turkey leftovers.

¼ cup nonfat yogurt
2 tablespoons light mayonnaise
Salt and pepper
2 cups cooked turkey, cubed
1 large shallot, chopped
2 celery stalks, sliced
¼ cup dried cranberries
2 tablespoons chopped walnuts
1 tablespoon chopped tarragon or dill
Lettuce
Whole-wheat bread
Sweet pickles, low sodium

In a medium bowl, whisk the yogurt and mayonnaise together with the salt and pepper. Add the turkey, shallot, celery, cranberries, walnuts and tarragon. Serve as a salad on lettuce leaves or on whole-wheat bread with sweet pickle slices.

Calories: 295
Protein: 22 g
Carbohydrates: 36 g
Cholesterol: 51 g
Total fat: 8.8 g
  Saturated fat: 1.1 g
  Monounsaturated: 2.2 g

Polyunsaturated: 4.5 g
  Omega-6 linoleic acid: 4.0 g
  Omega-3 linoleic acid: 0.8 g
  EPA/DHA: <0.1 g
Sodium: 186 mg
Potassium: 370 mg
Fibre: 6.5 g

Acorn Squash with Pineapple

Serves 4

Pineapple and allspice bring out the inherent sweetness in squash.

2 medium acorn, butternut or delicata squash
⅓ cup pineapple juice
1 tablespoon extra virgin olive oil
¼ teaspoon allspice
Salt and pepper

Preheat the oven to 350°F. Place the whole squash on a baking sheet lined with parchment or foil and roast for 40 to 45 minutes, or until tender. Remove from the oven, allow to cool for 10 minutes, then cut in half horizontally. Scoop out the seeds; reserve them to roast if you'd like. Divide the juice, oil, allspice, salt and pepper among the four halves and use a fork to fluff and incorporate. Serve in their shells with a spoon.

Calories: 128
Protein: 1.8 g
Carbohydrates: 25 g
Cholesterol: 0.0 mg
Total fat: 3.7 g
  Saturated fat: 0.6 g
  Monounsaturated fat: 2.8 g

Polyunsaturated fat: 0.4 g
  Omega-6 linoleic acid: <0.1 g
  Omega-3 linoleic acid: 0.1 g
Sodium: 7 mg
Potassium: 777 mg
Fibre: 3.9 g

Penne with Broccoli and Nuts

Serves 6

This is a superfast one-dish meal that everyone will enjoy. You can use red or yellow peppers as you wish.

2 heads broccoli
2 medium orange peppers, diced
1 pound whole-wheat pasta
2 tablespoons grapeseed or extra virgin olive oil
1 garlic clove or more, crushed or sliced
Black pepper
¼ cup orange juice
2 tablespoons soy sauce
5 medium spring onions
⅔ cup roasted mixed nuts

Bring a large pan of salted water to a boil. Cut the broccoli into florets. Peel the stems and dice them. Dice the peppers. While the pasta is cooking, heat the oil over medium heat in a large frying pan. Add the garlic and the black pepper, and toss until just fragrant. Add the broccoli, peppers, orange juice and soy sauce, and cook until the broccoli begins to brighten in colour and is almost tender. If it gets too dry or sticks, add some of the pasta cooking water. Add the spring onions and nuts and heat through. Drain the pasta and toss with the broccoli.

Calories: 219
Protein: 6 g
Carbohydrates: 21.4 g
Cholesterol: 0.0 g
Total fat: 13.6 g
  Saturated fat: 2.0 g
  Monounsaturated fat: 7.3 g

Polyunsaturated fat: 3.7 g
  Omega-6 linoleic acid: 3.2 g
  Omega-3 linoleic acid: 0.1 g
  EPA/DHA: 0.0 g
Sodium: 15 mg
Potassium: 415 mg
Fibre: 3.3 g

Notes and Bibliography

Winter • Season of Resolution

Abraham, C., and P. Sheeran, Deciding to exercise: The role of anticipated regret. *British Journal of Health Psychology*, May 2004; 9(2):269–78.

Anderson, L.B., et al. All-Cause Mortality Associated with Physical Activity During Leisure Time, Work, Sports, and Cycling to Work. *Arch Intern Med* 2000; 160:1621–28.

Anderson, R.A., et al. Isolation and Characterization of Polyphenol Type-A Polymers from Cinnamon with Insulin-like Biological Activity. *J Agric Food Chem* 2004; 52:65–70.

Bacon, C., et al. Sexual Function in Men Older Than 50 Years of Age: Results from the Health Professional Follow-up Study. *Ann Intern Med*, 2003; 139:161–68.

Baghurst, K., The Health Benefits of Citrus Fruits. Report to Horticulture Australia Ltd.: CSIRO Health Sciences and Nutrition; June 2003.

Bazzano, L.A., et al. Dietary fiber intake and reduced risk of coronary heart disease in U.S. men and women: The

National Health and Nutrition Examination Survey I Epidemiologic Follow-up Study. *Arch Intern Med* 2003, Sep 8; 163(16):1897– 1904.

Berlin, J.A., et al. A meta-analysis of physical activity in the prevention of coronary heart disease. *Am J Epidemiol* 1990; 132:612–28.

Biomechanics 2003; 10, no. 7, 67–76.

Boileau, T.W., et al. Prostate carcinogenesis in N-methyl-N-nitrosourea (NMU)-testosterone-treated rats fed tomato powder, lycopene, or energy-restricted diets. *J Natl Cancer Inst* 2003, Nov 5; 95(21):1578–86.

Calucci, L., et al. Effects of gamma-irradiation on the free radical and antioxidant contents in nine aromatic herbs and spices. *J Agric Food Chem* 2003, Feb 12; 51(4):927–34.

Cartee, G.D. Aging skeletal muscle response to exercise. *Exerc Sport Sci Rev* 1994; 22:91–120.

Chevaux, K., et al. Proximate, Mineral and Procyanidin Content of Certain Foods and Beverages Consumed by the Kuna Amerinds of Panama. *J Food Cmpstn & Anal* 2001; 14:553–63.

Choung, M.G., et al. Anthocyanin profile of Korean cultivated kidney bean *(Phaseolus vulgaris L.)*. *J Agric Food Chem* 2003, Nov 19; 51(24):7040–43.

Cleveland, L.E., et al. Dietary intake of whole grains. *J Am Coll Nutr* 2000; 19:331S–38S.

Clyman, B. Exercise in the Treatment of Osteoarthritis. *Current Rheumatology Reports* 2001; 3:520–23.

Colcombe, S., and A.F. Kramer. Fitness Effects on the Cognitive Function of Older Adults: A Meta-Analytic Study. *Psychological Science* (March 2003); 14, no. 2, 125–29.

Costacou, T., et al. Nutrition and the prevention of type 2 diabetes. *Ann Rev Nutr* 2003; 23:147–70.

Darmadi-Blackberry, I., et al. Legumes: The most important dietary predictor of survival in older people of different ethnicities. *Asia Pacific Journal of Clinical Nutrition* 2004, June 13(2):217–20.

The Diabetes Prevention Program Research Group. Reduction of the Incidence of Type 2 Diabetes with Lifestyle Intervention or Metformin. *N Eng J Med* 2002; 346:393–403.

Dunn, A.L., et al. Comparison of lifestyle and structured interventions to increase physical activity and cardio-respiratory fitness: A randomized trial. *JAMA* 1999; 281 (4):327–34 (from *KM Active Living Every Day*).

Estabrooks, P.A., et al. Physical activity promotion through primary care. *JAMA* 289, no. 22, 2913–16.

Etminan, M., et al. The role of tomato products and lycopene in the prevention of prostate cancer: A meta-analysis of observational studies. *Cancer Epidemiol Biomarkers Prev* 2004, Mar; 13(3):340–45.

Exercise and Women. *National Health Interview Survey*, 2000.

Finson, J.A., et al. Phenol antioxidant quantity and quality in foods: Fruits. *J Agric Food Chem* 2001; 49:5315–21.

Frontera, W.R., et al. Strength conditioning in older men: skeletal muscle hypertrophy and improved function. *J Appl Physiol* 1988; 64:1038–44.

Frontera, W.R., et al. Strength training and determinants of VO2 max in older men. *J Appl Physiol* 1990; 68:329–33.

Gertner, J. Eat Chocolate, Live Longer? *New York Times Sunday Magazine*, October 10, 2004; 33–37.

Get your daughters off the sofa and into the gym. *WSJ*, Dec 23, 2003, D1.

Girard, B., et al. Functional Grape and Citrus Products. In *Functional Foods*, ed. G. Mazza. Lancaster, PA: Technomic Publishing Co., Inc., 1998; 139–92.

Gorton, H.C., and K. Jarvis. The effectiveness of vitamin C in preventing and relieving the symptoms of virus-induced respiratory infections. *Manipulative and Physiological Therapeutics* 1999; 22(8):530–33.

Gregg, Edward W., et al., for the Study of Osteoporotic Fractures Research Group. Relationship of Changes in Physical Activity and Mortality Among Older Women. *JAMA* 2003; 289:2379–86.

Gulati, M., et al. Exercise Capacity and the Risk of Death in Women. The St. James Women Take Heart Project. *Circulation*, American Heart Association. Abstract available online at http://circ.ahajournals.org/cgi/content/abstract/01.CIR .0000091080.57509.E9v1.

Guraloik, J., et al. Maintaining mobility to late life. *Am J Epidemiol* 1993; 137:845–57.

Hannum, S.H., et al. Chocolate: A Heart Healthy Food? Show Me the Science. *Nutrition Today* 2002; 37:103–109.

Harnack, L., et al. Dietary intake and food sources of whole grains among US children and adolescents: Data from the 1994–1996 continuing survey of food intakes by individuals. *Journal of the American Dietetic Association* 2003; 103:1015–19.

Harvard Men's Health Watch, May 2004.

Hawkins, S., et al. Rate and mechanism of maximal oxygen consumption decline with aging: Implications for exercise training. *Sports Medicine* 2003; 33:877–888.

Hodge, A.M., et al. Glycemic index and dietary fiber and the risk of type 2 diabetes. *Diabetes Care* 2004, Nov; 27(11):2701–706.

Hodge, A.M., et al. Glycemic index and dietary fiber and the risk of type 2 diabetes. *Diabetes Care* 2004, Feb; 27:538–46.

Holick, M.F. McCollum Award Lecture, 1994: Vitamin D: New horizons for the 21st century. *Am J Clin Nutr* 1994; 60:619–30.

Hu, F., et al. Diet, Lifestyle and the Risk of Type 2 Diabetes

Mellitus in Women. *N Eng J Med* 2001; 790–97.

Institute of Medicine, Food and Nutrition Board. Dietary Reference Intakes: Calcium, Phosphorus, Magnesium, Vitamin D and Fluoride. Washington, DC: National Academy Press, 1999.

Ishida, B.K., and M.H. Chapman. A comparison of carotenoid content and total antioxidant activity in catsup from several commercial sources in the United States. *J Agric Food Chem* 2004, Dec 29; 52(26):8017–8020.

Ivarsson, T., et al. Physical exercise and vasomotor symptoms in postmenopausal women. *Maturitas* 1998, June 3; 29(2):139–46. (Original material from *Harvard Health Letter.*)

Jacobs, D.R., Jr., et al. Whole-grain intake and cancer: An expanded review and meta-analysis. *Nutr Cancer* 1998; 30(2):85–96.

Jensen, M., et al. Intakes of whole grains, bran, and germ and the risk of coronary heart disease in men. *Am J Clin Nutr* 2004, Dec; 80:1492–99.

Jiang, R., et al. Nut and Peanut Butter Consumption and Risk of Type 2 Diabetes in Women. *JAMA* 2002; 288:2554–60.

Johnston, C. Vitamin C. In B.A. Bowman and R.M. Russell, eds., *Present Knowledge in Nutrition*, 8 ed. Washington, DC; ILSI Press, 2001; 175–83.

Joshipura, K., et al. Fruit and vegetable intake in relation to risk of ischemic stroke. *JAMA* 1999; 282:1233–39.

The Joys and Benefits of Getting into Shape. *Harvard Health Letter*, July 2002.

Jung, U.J., et al. The Hypoglycemic Effects of Hesperidin and Naringin Are Partly Mediated by Hepatic Glucose-Regulating Enzymes in C57BL/KsJ-db/db Mice. *J Nutr* 2004; 134:2499–2503.

Kamel, H.K., et al. Sarcopenia and aging. *Nutrition Reviews* 2003; 61:157–67.

Kelemen, L.E., et al. Associations of dietary protein with disease and mortality in a prospective study of post-menopausal women. *Am J Epidemiol* 2005, Feb 1; 161(3):239–49.

Kemmler, W., et al. Benefits of 2 Years of Intense Exercise on Bone Density, Physical Fitness, and Blood Lipids in Early Postmenopausal Osteopenic Women: Results of the Erlangen Fitness Osteoporosis Prevention Study (EFOPS).

Khan, A., et al. Cinnamon improves glucose and lipids of people with type 2 diabetes. *Diabetes Care* 2003; 26:3215–218.

Khfgaard, H., et al. Function, morphology and protein expression of aging, skeletal muscle: a cross-sectional study of elderly men with different training backgrounds. *Acta Physiol Scand* 1990; 140:41–54.

Kris-Etherton, P.M., et al. Effects of a milk chocolate bar per day substituted for a high-carbohydrate snack in young men on an NCEP/AHA Step I Diet. *Am J Clin Nutr* 1994; 60:1037S–42S.

Kris-Etherton, P.M., et al. The role of fatty acid saturation on plasma lipids, lipoproteins, and apolipoproteins: 1. Effects of whole food diets high in cocoa butter, olive oil, soybean oil, dairy butter, and milk chocolate on the plasma lipids of young men. *Metabolism* 1993; 42:121–29.

Kurowska, E.M., and J.A. Manthey. Hypolipidemic effects and absorption of citrus polymethozylated flavones in hamsters with diet-induced hypercholesterolemia. *J Agric Food Chem* 2004, May 19; 52(10):2879–86.

Lam, T.H., et al. Leisure Time Physical Activity and Mortality in Hong Kong: Case-control Study of All Adult Deaths in 1998. *Ann Epidemiol* 2004; 14:391–98.

Lazarus, S.A., et al. Tomato juice and platelet aggregation in type 2 diabetes. *JAMA* 2004, Aug 18; 292(7):805–806.

Lazarus, S.A., and M.L. Garg. Inhibition of platelet aggregation from people with type 2 diabetes mellitus following consumption of tomato juice. *Asia Pacific Journal of Clinical Nutrition* 2004; 13 (Suppl):S65.

Lee, C., et al. Cocoa Has More Phenolic Phytochemicals and a Higher Antioxidant Capacity Than Teas and Red Wine. *J Agric Food Chem* 2003; 51(25):7292–95.

Lemura, L.M., et al. The effects of physical training on functional capacity in adults. Ages 46 to 90: A meta-analysis. *Journal of Sports Medicine and Physical Fitness* 2000; 40:1–10.

Liebeerman, L.S. Dietary, Evolutionary, and Modernizing Influences on the Prevalence of Type 2 Diabetes. *Annu Rev Nutr* 2003; 23:345–77.

Liu, S., et al. Relation between changes in intakes of dietary fiber and grain products and changes in weight and development of obesity among middle-aged women. *Am J Clin Nutr* 2003, Nov; 78(5):920–27.

Liu, S., et al. Whole grain consumption and risk of ischemic stroke in women: A prospective study. *JAMA* 2000, Sep 27; 284(12):1534–40.

McGuire, D.K., et al. A 30-year Follow-up of the Dallas Bed Rest and Training Study I. Effect of Age on the Cardiovascular Response to Exercise II. Effect of Age on Cardiovascular Adaptation to Exercise Training. *Circulation* 2001; 104:1358–1366.

McGuire, D.K., et al. A 30-year Follow-up of the Dallas Bed Rest and Training Study I. Effect of Age on the Cardiovascular Response to Exercise I. *Circulation* 2001; 104:1350–57.

Meyer, K.A., et al. Carbohydrates, dietary fiber, and incident type 2 diabetes in older women. *Am J Clin Nutr* 2000, Apr; 71(4):921–30.

Milgram, N.W., et al. Learning ability in aged beagle dogs is preserved by behavioral enrichment and dietary fortification: A two-year longitudinal study. *Neurobiol Aging* 2005; 26:77–90.

Mokdad, A.H., et al. The Coming Epidemic of Obesity and Diabetes in the United States. *JAMA* 2001; 286:1195–1200.

Mora, S., et al. Ability of Exercise Testing to Predict Cardiovascular and All-Cause Death in Asymptomatic Women. *JAMA* 290:1600–1607.

Mursu, J., et al. Dark Chocolate Consumption Increases HDL Cholesterol Concentration and Chocolate Fatty Acids May Inhibit Lipid Peroxidation in Healthy Humans. *Free Radical Biology & Medicine* 2004; 37:1351–59.

Nkondjock, A., et al. Dietary Intake of Lycopene Is Associated with Reduced Pancreatic Cancer Risk. *J Nutr* 2005, Mar; 135(3):592–97.

Ockene, I.S., et al. Seasonal variation in serum cholesterol levels. *Arch Intern Med* 2004; 164:868–70.

Otsuka, H., et al. Studies on anti-inflammatory agents. VI. Anti-inflammatory constituents of Cinnamomum sieboldii Meissn [author's transl]. *Yakugaku Zasshi* 1982, Jan; 102(2):162–72.

Ouattara, B., et al. Antibacterial activity of selected fatty acids and essential oils against six meat spoilage organisms. *Int J Food Microbiol* 1997, Jul 22; 37(2–3):155–62.

Pattison, D.J., et al. Vitamin C and the risk of developing inflammatory polyarthritis: Prospective nested case-control study, *Annals of Rheumatic Diseases* 2004, Jul; 63(7):843–47.

Pereira, M.A., et al. Dairy consumption, obesity, and the insulin resistance syndrome in young adults: The CARDIA Study. *JAMA* 2002; 287:2081–89.

Pereira, M.A., et al. Dietary fiber and risk of coronary heart disease: A pooled analysis of cohort studies. *Arch Intern Med* 2004, Feb 23; 164(4):370–76.

Quale, J.M., et al. In vitro activity of Cinnamomum zeylanicum against azole resistant and sensitive Candida species and a pilot study of cinnamon for oral candidiasis. *Am J Chin Med* 1996; 24(2):103–109.

Rein, D., et al. Cocoa inhibits platelet activation and function. *Am J Clin Nutr* 2000; 72:30–35.

Rockhill, B., et al. Physical Activity and Mortality: A Prospective Study Among Women. *Am J Public Health* 91(4), April 2001, 578–83.

Salmeron, L., et al. Dietary Fiber, Glycemic Load and Risk of Non-Insulin Dependent Diabetes in Men. *Diabetes Care* 1997; 20:545–50.

Sanchez-Moreno, C., et al. Effect of orange juice intake on vitamin C concentrations and biomarkers of antioxidant status in humans. *Am J Clin Nutr* 2003; 78:454–60.

Saris, W.H.M., et al. How much physical activity is enough to prevent unhealthy weight gain? Outcome of the IASO 1st Stock Conference and consensus statement. *Obesity Reviews* 2003; 4:101–14.

Schramm, D.D., et al. Chocolate procyanidins decrease the leukotriene-prostacyclin ratio in humans and human aortic endothelial cells. *Am J Clin Nutr* 2001; 73:36–40.

Serafini, M., et al. Plasma antioxidants from chocolate. *Nature* 2003; 424:1012.

Sesso, H.D., et al. Dietary lycopene, tomato-based food products and cardiovascular disease in women. *J Nutr* Jul; 133(7):2336–41.

Simonsick, E.M., et al. Risk due to inactivity in physically capable older adults. *Am J Public Health* 1993; 83:1443–50.

Slattery, M., et al. Plant Foods, Fiber and Rectal Cancer. *Am J Clin Nutr* 2004, Feb; 79(2):274–81.

Slattery, M., et al. Physical Activity and Colon Cancer: A Public Health Perspective. *Ann Epidemiol* 1997; 7:137–45.

Slavin, J. Whole Grains and Human Health. *Nutrition Research Reviews* 2004; 17.

Smith, D.T., et al. Effects of ageing and regular aerobic exercise on endothelial fibrinolytic capacity in humans. *J Physiol* 2003; Jan 1; 546(pt.1):289–98.

Smith, K., et al. Two Years of Resistance Training in Older Men and Women: The Effects of Three Years of Detraining on the Retention of Dynamic Strength. *Can J Appl Phys* 2003; 28, no. 3, 462–74.

Stone, W.J., et al. Long-term exercisers: What can we learn from them? ACSM's *Health & Fitness Journal*, March/April 2004, 11–14.

Thornton, E.W., et al. Health benefits of tai chi exercise: improved balance and blood pressure in middle-aged women. *Health Promotion International*, 2004; 19, no. 1, 33–38.

Tsai, C.J., et al. Dietary protein and the risk of cholecystectomy in a cohort of US women: The Nurses' Health Study. *Am J Epidemiol* 2004, Jul 1; 160(1):11.

U.S. Department of Health and Human Services. Physical Activity and Health: A Report of the Surgeon General. Atlanta, GA: U.S. Department of Health and Human Services, Centers for Disease Control and Prevention, National Center for Chronic Disease Prevention and Health Promotion, 1996.

Valero, M., and M.C. Salmeron. Antibacterial activity of 11 essential oils against Bacillus cereus in tyndallized carrot broth. *Int J Food Microbiol* Aug 15; 85(1–2):73–81.

Van Dam, R.M., et al. Dietary patterns and risk for type 2 diabetes mellitus in US men. *Ann Int Med* 2002; 136:201–9.

van den Berg, H. Bioavailability of vitamin D. *Eur J Clin Nutr* 1997; 51 Suppl 1:S76–S79.

Waladktani, A.R., et al. Preventive and therapeutic effects of dietary phytochemicals on cancer development. In

Functional Foods and Nutraceuticals in Cancer Prevention, Iowa State Press, 2003, 179–211.

Webb, A.R., et al. Influence of season and latitude on the cutaneous synthesis of vitamin D3: Exposure to winter sunlight in Boston and Edmonton will not promote vitamin D3 synthesis in human skin. *J Clin Endocrinol Metab* 1988; 67:373–78.

Wu, S., et al. Plasma cholesterol predictive equations demonstrate that stearic acid is neutral and monounsaturated fatty acids are hypocholesterolemic. *Am J Clin Nutr* 1995; 61:1129–39.

Wu, X., et al. Lipophilic and hydrophilic antioxidant capacities of common foods in the United States. J *Agric Food Chem* 2004, Jun 16; 52(12):4026–37.

Young, D.R., et al. The effects of aerobic exercise and tai chi on blood pressure in older people: Results of a randomized trial. *J Am Geriatrics Soc* 1999; 47:277–84.

Yuan, J.M., et al. Dietary cryptoxanthin and reduced risk of lung cancer: the Singapore Chinese Health Study. *Cancer Epidemiol Biomarkers Prev* 2003, Sep; 12(9):890–98.

Zoladz, P., et al. Cinnamon perks performance. Paper presented at the annual meeting of the Association for Chemoreception Sciences, Sarasota, FL, April 21–25, 2004.

Spring • Season of Joy

Ajani, U.A., et al. Dietary Fiber and C-Reactive Protein: Findings from National Health and Nutrition Examination Survey Data. *J Nutr* 2004; 134:1181–85.

Allred, C.D., et al. Soy processing influences growth of estrogen-dependent breast cancer tumors in mice. *Carcinogenesis* 2004, June.

The American Institute for Cancer Research. Understanding the Obesity-Cancer Connection. Awareness and Action: *AICR Surveys on Portion Size,*

Nutrition and Cancer Risk, p. 7. Available at http://www.aicr.org/press/awarenessandaction_03conf.pdf. Accessed March 4, 2004.

Apovian, C.M. Sugar-Sweetened Soft Drinks, Obesity, and Type 2 Diabetes. *JAMA* 2004; 292 (8):978–79.

Braam, L.A.J.L.M., et al. Vitamin K1 supplementation retards bone loss in postmenopausal women between 50 and 60 years of age. *Calcif Tissue Int* 2003; 73:21–26.

Brown, M.J., et al. Carotenoid bioavailability is higher from salads ingested with full-fat than with fat-reduced salad dressings as measured with electrochemical detection. *Am J Clin Nutr* 2004, Aug 1; 80(2):396–403.

Burke, J.D., et al. Diet and Serum Carotenoid Concentrations Affect Macular Pigment Optical Density in Adults 45 Years and Older. *J Nutr* 2005; 135:1208–14.

Carson, L., et al. Carotenoids and eye health. *Nutrition and the MD* 2004; 30:1–4.

Chandalia, M., et al. Beneficial Effects of High Dietary Fiber Intake in Patients with Type 2 Diabetes Mellitus. *N Eng J Med* 2000; 342:1392–98.

Cifuentes, M., et al. Weight loss and calcium intake influence calcium absorption in overweight postmenopausal women. *Am J Clin Nutr* 2004, Jul; 80 (1):123–30.

Clark, A., et al. *Int J Cardiol* 2001, Aug; 80(1):87–88.

Conceicao de Oliveir, M., et al. Weight loss associated with a daily intake of three apples or three pears among overweight women. *Nutrition* 2003; 19:253–56.

Cornuz, J., et al. Smoking, Smoking Cessation, and Risk of Hip Fracture in Women. *Am J Med* 1999; 106:311–14.

Correa, P., et al. Chemoprevention of gastric dysplasia: Randomized trial of antioxidant supplements and anti-helicobacter pylori therapy. *J Natl Cancer Inst* 2000; 92:1868–69.

Desroches, S., et al. Soy protein favorably affects LDL size independently of isoflavones in hypercholesterolemic men and women. *J Nutr* 2004, Mar; 134(3):574–79.

Duttaroy, A., and A. Jørgensen. Effects of kiwi fruit consumption on platelet aggregation and plasma lipids in healthy human volunteers. *Platelets* 2004, Aug; 15(5):287–92.

Dwyer, J.H., et al. Oxygenated carotenoid lutein and progression of early atherosclerosis. The Los Angeles Atherosclerosis Study. *Circulation* 2001; 103:2922–27.

Earnest, C.R., et al. Effects of preexercise carbohydrate feedings on glucose and insulin responses during and following resistance exercise. *Strength and Conditioning Research* 2000; 14:361.

Fujiki, H. Two stages of cancer prevention with green tea. *J Cancer Res Clin Oncol* 1999, Nov; 125:589–97.

Gheldof, N., et al. Buckwheat honey increases serum antioxidant capacity in humans. *J Agric Food Chem* 2003, Feb 26; 51(5):1500–505.

Gross, H., et al. Effect of honey consumption on plasma antioxidant status in human subjects. Paper presented at the 227th American Chemical Society Meeting, Anaheim, CA, March 28, 2004.

Gupta, S.K., et al. Green tea protects against selemite-induced oxidative stress in experimental cataractogenesis. *Exp Eye Res* 2001; 73:393–401.

Guzman-Maldonado, S.H., et al. Functional Products of Plants Indigenous to Latin America: Amaranth, Quinoa, Common Beans, and Botanicals. In *Functional Foods*, ed. G. Mazza. Lancaster, PA: Technomic Publishing Co. Inc., 1998, pp. 293–328.

Hakim, A.A. Effects of walking on mortality among non-smoking retired men. *N Eng J Med* 1998, Jan 8; 338:94–99.

Hannum, S.M., et al. Use of portion-controlled entrees enhances weight loss in women. *Obes Res* 2004, Mar; 12(3):538–46.

Jensen, M.K., et al. Intakes of whole grains, bran, and germ and the risk of coronary heart disease in men. *Am J Clin Nutr* 2004; 80:1492–99.

Keller, M.C., et al. (in press). A warm heart and a clear head: The contingent effects of weather on human mood and cognition. *Psychological Science*.

LaChance, P.A. Fruits in Preventative Health and Disease Treatment: Nutritional Ranking and Patient Recommendations. Presented at the 38th annual meeting of the American College of Nutrition, Sept 27, 1997, New York.

Lambert, J.D., et al. Piperine enhances the bioavailability of the tea polyphenol (-)-epigallocatechin-3-gallate in mice. *J Nutr* 2004, Aug; 134(8):1948–52.

Liebman, B. Breaking Up: Strong Bones Need More Than Calcium. *Nutrition Action* 2005, April; 32 (3):2.

Logue, E.F., et al. Longitudinal relationship between elapsed time in the action stages of change and weight loss. *Obes Res* 2004, Sep; 12(9):1499–1508.

Ludwig, D.S., et al. Dietary fiber, weight gain and cardio-vascular disease risk factors in young adults. *JAMA* 1999; 282 (16):1539–46.

Manson, J.E., et al. A prospective study of walking as compared with vigorous exercise in the prevention of coronary heart disease in women. *N Eng J Med* 1999, Aug 26; 341:650–8.

Mei, Y., et al. Reversal of cancer multidrug resistance by green tea polyphenols. *J Pharm Pharmacol* 2004, Oct; 56(10):1307–14.

Nagao, T., et al. Ingestion of a tea rich in catechins leads to a reduction in body fat and malondialdehyde-modified LDL in men. *Am J Clin Nutr* 2005, Jan; 81(1):122–129.

National Osteoporosis Foundation. *America's Bone Health: The State of Osteoporosis and Low Bone Mass in Our Nation*. Washington, DC: National Osteoporosis Foundation, 2002.

Ni, W., et al. Anti-atherogenic effect of soya and rice-protein isolate, compared with casein, in apolipoprotein E-deficient mice. *Br J Nutr* Jul; 90(1):13–20.

Nutrition and the M.D 2004; 30:6–7.

Nutrition and the M.D., 2004; 30:7–8, and this article referenced Brown, J.K., et al. *Cancer J Clin* 2003; 53:268.

Olshansky, S.J., et al. A Potential Decline in Life Expectancy in the United States in the 21st Century. *N Eng J Med* 2005, March 17; 352(11):1138–45.

Orlet, Fisher J., et al. Children's bite size and intake of an entree are greater with large portions than with age-appropriate or self-selected portions. *Am J Clin Nutr* 2003, May; 77(5):1164–70.

Rock, C.L., et al. *J Clin Oncol* 2004; 22:2379 (from *Nutrition and the M.D.* 2004, Oct; 30:6–7).

Rolls, B.J., et al. Portion size of food affects energy intake in normal-weight and overweight men and women. *Am J Clin Nutr* 2002, Dec; 76(6):1207–13.

Rush, E.C., et al. Kiwifruit promotes laxation in the elderly. 2001 (unpublished).

Sagara, M., et al. Effects of dietary intake of soy protein and isoflavones on cardiovascular disease risk factors in high risk, middle-aged men in Scotland. *J Am Coll Nutr* 2004, Feb; 23(1):85–91.

Sagon, C. It's Growing on Us. *Washington Post*, March 30, 2005, F01.

Sloan, E.A. What, when, and where Americans eat. *Food Technol* 2003; 38:91–94.

Stephanou, A., Role of STAT-1 and STAT-3 in ischaemia/reperfusion injury. *J Cell Mol Med* 2004, Oct–Dec; 8(4):519–25.

Subrahmanyan M. A prospective randomized clinical and histological study of superficial burn wound healing with honey and silver sulfadiazine. *Burns* 1998; 24:157–61.

Teixeira, S.R., et al. Isolated Soy Protein Consumption Reduces Urinary Albumin Excretion and Improves the Serum Lipid Profile in Men with Type 2 Diabetes Mellitus and Nephropathy. *J Nutr* 2004; 134:1874–80.

Tillotson, J.E. Pandemic Obesity. *Nutrition Today* 2004, Jan/Feb; 39(1):6–9.

Tsuneki, H., et al. Effect of green tea on blood glucose levels and serum proteomic patterns in diabetic (db/db) mice and on glucose metabolism in healthy humans. *BMC Pharmacol* 2004, Aug 26; 4(1):18.

UC Berkeley. *Wellness Letter*, Feb 2005, p. 8.

Wansink, B., and J. Kim. Bad Popcorn in Big Buckets: Portion Size Can Influence Intake as Much as Taste. *J Nutr Edu and Behavior* (forthcoming 2005).

Wellness Foods A to Z

White, J.W. Composition of honey. In *Honey, A Comprehensive Survey*, ed. E. Crane. New York: Crane, Russak & Co., 1975, pp. 157–206.

Wolk, A., et al. Long-term Intake of Dietary Fiber and Decreased Risk of Coronary Heart Disease Among Women. *JAMA* 1999; 281:1998–2004.

Wood, C.E., et al. Breast and uterine effects of soy isoflavones and conjugated equine estrogens in post-menopausal female monkeys. *J Clin Endocrinol Metab* 2004, Jul; 89(7):3462–68.

Yang, Y.C., et al. The protective effect of habitual tea consumption on hypertension. *Arch Inter Med* 2004, July; 164:1534–40.

Young, L.R., and M. Nestle. Expanding Portion Sizes in the US Marketplace: Implications for Nutrition Counseling. *J Am Diet Assoc* 2003; 103:231–4.

Zhao, Y., et al. Calcium Bioavailability from Fortified Soymilk and Bovine Milk. Abstract 972.1, *Experimental Biology*, March 31–April 5, 2005, San Diego, CA.

Zhou, J.R., et al. Soy phytochemicals and tea bioactive components synergistically inhibit androgen-sensitive human prostate tumors in mice. *J Nutr* 2003; 133:516–21.

Summer • Season of Peace

Adolfsson, O., et al. Yogurt and Gut Function. *Am J Clin Nutr* 2004; 80:245–56.

Allen, J.B., et al. The effects of glucose on nonmemory cognitive functioning in the elderly. *Neuropsychologia* 1966; 34(5):459–65.

Barnes, V. Impact of transcendental meditation on ambulatory blood pressure in African-American adolescents. *Am J Hypert* 2004, April; 17:366–69.

Bazzano, L.A., et al. Dietary intake of folate and risk of stroke in US men and women; NHANES I Epidemiologic Follow-up Study. *Stroke* 2002, May; 33(5):1183–89.

Berke, J., et al. Mortality Pattern and Life Expectancy of Seventh-Day Adventists in the Netherlands. *Int J Epidemiol* 1983; 12:455–59.

Bonadonna, R. Meditation's Impact on Chronic Illness. *Holist Nurs Pract* 2003; 17(6):309–19.

Castillo-Richmond, A., et al. Effects of stress reduction on carotid atherosclerosis in hypertensive African-Americans. *Stroke* 2000; 31:568–73.

Colditz, G.A., et al. Diet and risk of clinical diabetes in women. *Am J Clin Nutr* 1992; 55:1018–23.

Comstock, G.W., et al. Church Attendance and Health. *J Chro Dis* 1972; 25:665–72.

Couillard, C. Canadian Cardiovascular Society Annual Congress Meeting, Calgary, Alberta, Oct 23–27, 2004.

da Costa, A.P., and K.M. Kendrick. Face pictures reduce behavioural, autonomic, endocrine and neural indices of stress and fear in sheep. *Proc Royal Soc London B* 2004, Oct 7; 271:2077–84.

Erlund, I., et al. Consumption of black currants, lingonberries and bilberries increases serum quercetin concentrations. *Eur J Clin Nutr* 2003; 57:37–42.

Everson, S.A., et al. Anger expression and incident hypertension. *Psychosom Med* 1998; 60:730–35.

Everson, S.A., et al. Hopelessness and 4-year Progression of Carotid Atherosclerosis: The Kuopio Ischemic Heart Disease Risk Factory Study. *Arterioscler Thromb Vasc Biol* 1997; 17:1490–95.

Ferrara, L.A., et al. Olive oil and reduced need for antihypertensive medications. *Arch Intern Med* 2000; 160:837–42.

Frasure-Smith, N., et al. Gender, depression, and one-year prognosis after myocardial infarction. *Psychosom Med* 1999; 61:26–37.

Furberg, A.S., et al. Serum high-density lipoprotein cholesterol, metabolic profile, and breast cancer risk. *National Cancer Inst* 2004, Aug; 96(15):1152–60.

Gardner, J.W., et al. Cancer in Utah Mormon Women by Church Activity Level. *Am J Epidemiol* 1982; 116:258–65.

Ginkgo biloba for Alzheimer's disease: "promising evidence." www.cochrane.org. October 21, 2002.

Gold, P.E. Role of glucose in regulating the brain and cognition. *Am J Clin Nutr* 1995; 61(4 suppl): 987S–995S.

Graham, T.W., et al. Frequency of Church Attendance and Blood Pressure Elevation. *Journal of Behavioral Medicine* 1978; 1:37–43.

Hargrove, R.L., et al. Low fat and high monounsaturated fat diets decrease human low density lipoprotein oxidative susceptibility in vitro. *J Nutr* 2001; 131:1758–63.

He, K., et al. Fish consumption and incidence of stroke: A meta-analysis of cohort studies. *Stroke* 2004, Jul; 35(7):1538–42.

Hebert, Le, et al. Annual Incidence of Alzheimer Disease in the US projected to the Year 2000 through 2050. *Alzheimer Dis Assoc Dissord* 2001; 15:169–73.

Hojo, K., et al., of Tsurumi University, Yokohama, Japan. Paper presented at the International Association for Dental Research, Baltimore, March 10, 2005.

House, J.S., et al. The Association of Social Relationships and Activities with Mortality: Prospective Evidence from the Tecumseh Community Health Study. *Am J Epidemiol* 1982; 116:123–40.

Iribarren, D., et al. Dietary intake of n-3, n-6 fatty acids and fish: Relationship with hostility in young adults – the CARDIA study. *Eur J Clin Nutr* 2004, Jan; 58(1):24–31.

Kalijn, S., et al. Dietary intake of fatty aids and fish in relation to cognitive performance at middle age. *Neurology* 2004 Jan 27; 62(2):275–80.

Koenig, H.G., et al. Religion, spirituality, and acute care hospitalization and long-term care use by older patients. *Arch Intern Med* 2004, Jul 26; 164(14):1579–85.

Krantz, D.S., et al. Effects of Mental Stress in Patients with Coronary Artery Disease. *JAMA* 2000; 283:1800–1802.

Lee, Y.L., et al. Antibacterial activity of vegetables and juices. *Nutrition* 2003, Nov–Dec; 19(11–12):994–96.

Lewis, N.M., et al. Blueberries in the American Diet. *Nutrition Today* 2005; 40:92–96.

Lopez, L., et al. Monounsaturated fatty acid (avocado) rich diet for mild hypercholesterolemia. *Arch Med Res* 1996, Winter; 27(4):519–23.

Luchsinger, J.A., et al. Dietary Factors and Alzheimer's Disease. *The Lancet Neurology* 2004; 3:579–87.

Lupien, S.J., et al. Stress hormones and human memory function across the lifespan. *Psychoneuroendocrinology* 2005, Apr; 30(3):225–42.

Lutz, A., et al. Long-term mediators self-induce high-amplitude gamma synchrony during mental practice. *Proc Natl Acad Sci USA* 2004, Nov 16; 101(46):16369–16373.

Marrugat, J., et al. Effects of differing phenolic content in dietary olive oils on lipids and LDL oxidation: A randomized controlled trial. *Eur J Clin Nutr* 2004, Jun; 43(3):140–47.

Masella, R., et al. Extra Virgin Olive Oil Biophenols Inhibit Cell-Mediated Oxidation of LDL by Increasing the mRNA Transcription of Glutathione-Related Enzymes. *J Nutr* 2004, Apr; 134(4):785–91.

Mattson, M.P. Emerging neuroprotective strategies for Alzheimer's disease: Dietary restriction, telomerasc activation, and stem cell therapy. *Exp Gerontology* 2000; 35:489–502.

McEwen, B.S. Protective and damaging effects of stress mediators. *New Eng J Med* 1998, Jan 15; 338:171–79.

Menendez, J.A., et al. Oleic acid, the main monounsaturated fatty acid of olive oil, suppresses Her-2/neu (erbB-2) expression and synergistically enhances the growth inhibitory effects of trastuzumab (HerceptinTM) in breast. *Ann Oncol* 2005, Jan. 10.

Mittleman, M. Harvard Medical School. American Heart Association Conference on Cardiovascular Disease and Epidemiology, 1996. *Fam Pract News* 1996; 26:8.

Morello, J.R., et al. Changes in commercial virgin olive oil (cv Arbequina) during storage, with special emphasis on the phenolic fraction. *J Agric Food Chem* 2004, May; 85(3):357–64.

Morris, M.C., et al. Consumption of fish and n-3 fatty acids and risk of incident Alzheimer disease. *Arch Neurol* 2003, Jul; 60(7):940–46.

Morris, M.C., et al. Dietary Fats and the Risk of Incident Alzheimer Disease. *Arch Neurology* 2003; 60:194–200.

Morris, M.C., et al. Dietary niacin and the risk of incident Alzheimer's disease and of cognitive decline. *J Neurol Neurosurg Psychiatry* 2004; 75:1093–99.

Mozaffarian, D., et al. Fish intake and risk of incident atrial fibrillation. *Circulation* 2004, Jul 27; 110(4):368–73.

Mukamal, K.J., et al. Prospective study of alcohol consumption and risk of dementia in older adults. *JAMA* 2003; 289:1405–13.

Music and Blood-Pressure Reduction. *Harvard Heart Letter* 1995; 5(adapted from JAMA, Sep 21, 1994).

Okello, Ed J., et al. In vitro anti-beta-secretase and dual anti-cholinesterase activities of Camellia sinensis L. (tea) relevant to treatment of dementia. *Phytotherapy Research* 2004; 18:624–27.

Oleckno, W.A., et al. Relationship of Religiosity to Wellness and Other Health-Related Behaviors and Outcomes. *Psychological Reports* 1991; 68:819–26.

Pearsall, P. *The Pleasure Prescription*. Salt Lake City, UT: Publishers Press, 1996.

Pilaczynska-Szczesniak, L., et al. The Influence of Chokeberry Juice Supplementation on the Reduction of Oxidative Stress Resulting from an Incremental Rowing Ergometer Exercise. *International Journal of Sport Nutrition and Exercise Metabolism* 2005; 14:48–58.

Polk, D.E., et al. State and trait affect as predictors of salivary cortisol in healthy adults. *Psychoneuroendocrinology* 2005, Apr; 30(3):261–72.

Psaltopoulou, T., et al. Olive oil, the Mediterranean diet, and arterial blood pressure: The Greek European Prospective Investigation into Cancer and Nutrition (EPIC) study. *Am J Clin Nutr* 2004, Oct; 80(4):1012–18.

Rimando, A. Pterostilbene as a new natural product agonist for the peroxisome proliferators-activated receptor alpha isoform. Paper presented at the 228th American Chemical Society National Meeting, Philadelphia, PA, August 23, 2004.

Rimando, A., et al. Resveratrol, pterostilbene, and piceatannol in vaccinium berries. *J Agric Food Chem* 2004, Jul 28; 52(15):4713–19.

Ruiz-Gutierrez, V., et al. Plasma lipids, erythrocyte membrane lipids and blood pressure of hypertensive women after ingestion of dietary oleic acid from two different sources. *J Hypertens* 1996; 14:1483–90.

Ruo, B., et al. Depressive symptoms and health-related quality of life: The Heart and Soul Study. *JAMA* 2003; 290:215–21.

Sanchez-Moreno, C., et al. Anthocyanin and proanthocyanidin content in selected white and red wines. Oxygen radical absorbance capacity comparison with nontraditional wines obtained from highbush blueberry. *J Agric Food Chem* 2003, Aug 13; 51(17):4889–96.

Schneider, R.H., et al. A randomized controlled trial of stress reduction for hypertension in older African-Americans. *Hypertension* 1996; 26:820–27.

Selye, H. *The Stress of Life*. NY: McGraw-Hill, 1956; 2nd ed., paperback, 1978.

Seshadri, S., et al. Plasma homocysteine as a risk factor for dementia and Alzheimer's disease. *N Eng J Med* 2002, Feb 14; 346:476–82.

Singletary, K.W., et al. Non-nutritive components in foods as modifiers of the cancer process. In *Preventive Nutrition*, ed. A. Bendich and R.J. Deckelbaum. Totowa, NJ: Human Press, 2005, pp. 55–58.

Stoneham, M., et al. Olive oil, diet, and colorectal cancer: An ecological study and hypothesis. *J Epidemiol Community Health* 2000; 54:756–60.

Strike, P.C., and A. Steptoe. Psychosocial factors in the development of coronary artery disease. *Prog Cardiovasc Dis* 2004, Jan–Feb; 46(4):337–47.

Sun, J., et al. Antioxidant and Antiproliferative Activities of Common Fruits. *J Agric Food Chem* 2002; 50(25):7449–54.

Suvarna, R., et al. Possible Interaction between warfarin and cranberry juice. *BMJ* 2003, Dec 20; 327(7429):1454.

Toews, J. *Soul Care: The Importance of Spirituality in Life and Practice. Exploring Health and Healing.* Calgary Health Region, Kananaskis, Canada, June 2005.

Trichopoulou, A., et al. Cancer and Mediterranean dietary traditions. *Cancer Epidemiol Biomarkers Prev* 2000; 9:869–73.

Tsao, S.M., et al. Garlic extract and two diallyl sulphides inhibit methicillin-resistant Staphylococcus aureus infection in BALB/cA mice. *J Antimicrob Chemother* 2003, Dec; 52(6):974–80.

Tufts Health and Nutr Letter 2003, Aug; 21(6):2.

Unlu, N.Z., et al. Carotenoid absorption from salad and salsa by humans is enhanced by the addition of avocado or avocado oil. *J Nutr* 2005, Mar; 135(3):431–36.

Vanit Veer, P., et al. Consumption of fermented milk products and breast cancer: A case-control study in the Netherlands. *Cancer Res* 1989; 49:4020–23.

Votruba, S.B., et al. Prior exercise increases subsequent utilization of dietary fat. *Med Sci Sport Exerc* 2002; 34:1757–65.

Votruba S.B., et al. Prior exercise increases dietary oleate, but not palmitate oxidation. *Obes Res* 2003; 11(12):1509–18.

Weinbrenner, T., et al. Olive Oils High in Phenolic Compounds Modulate Oxidative/Antioxidative Status in Men. *J Nutr* 2004; 134:2314–21.

Whitemore-Burns, B., et al. Effect of N-3 Fatty Acid Enriched Eggs vs Walnuts on Blood Lipids in Free-Living Lacto-Ovo Vegetarians. *Experimental Biology* 2005, Mar 31–April 5; San Diego, CA, Abstract 591.17.

Williams, J.E., et al. Anger proneness predicts coronary heart disease risk: Prospective analysis from the atherosclerosis risk in communities (ARIC study). *Circulation* 2000; 101:2034–39.

Williams, K.A., et al. Evaluation of a Wellness-Based Mindfulness Stress Reduction Intervention: A Controlled Trial. *Am J Health Promot* 2001, Jul–Aug; 15(6):422–432.

Zemel, M.B., et al. Dairy (yogurt) augments fat loss and reduces central adiposity during energy restriction in obese subjects. *FASEB* 2003; 17 (5):A1088.

Autumn • Season of Transition

Arts, I., et al. Dietary catechins in relation to coronary heart disease among postmenopausal women. *Epidemiology* 2001; 12:668–75.

Aviram, M., et al. Pomegranate juice consumption inhibits erum angiotension converting enzyme activity and reduces systolic blood pressure. *Atherosclerosis* 2001; 158:195–98.

Aviram, M., et al. Pomegranate juice flavonoids inhibit LDL oxidation and cardiovascular diseases: Studies in atherosclerotic mice and in humans. *Proc Int Conf Mech Action Nutraceuticals (ICMAN)* 2002; 28:49–62.

Awash, P.B., et al. The effects of bulb extracts of onions and garlic on soil bacteria. *Acta but Ind* 1984; 12:45–49.

Bazzano, L.A., et al. Dietary fiber intake and reduced risk of coronary heart disease in US men and women: The National Health and Nutrition Examination Survey I Epidemiologic Follow-up Study. *Arch Intern Med* 2003, Sep 8; 163(16):1897–1904.

Boyer, J., and R.H. Liu. Apple phytochemicals and their health benefits. *J Nutr* 2004, May 12; 3(1):5.

Campbell, S., et al. Effects of a Nap on Nighttime Sleep and Waking Function in Older Subjects. *Journal of the American Geriatrics Society* 2005, Jan; (53):48.

Carskadon, M.A. Sleep deprivation: Health consequences and societal impact. *Med Clin N Am* 2004; 88:767–76.

Chinnici, F., et al. Improved HPLC determination of phenolic compounds in cv. Golden Delicious apples using a monolithic column. *J Agric Food Chem* 2004, Jan 14; 52(1):3–7.

Conceicao de Oliveir, M., et al. Weight loss associated with a daily intake of three apples or three pears among overweight women. *Nutrition* 2003; 19:253–56.

Connor, S., et al. Diets low in folic acid and carotenoids are associated with the coronary disease epidemic in Central and Eastern Europe. *J Am Diet Assoc* 2004; 104:1793–99.

Crouch, E.R., et al. Retinal Vascular Changes in Obstructive Sleep Apnea Syndrome. *ARVA* 2005; poster 3278–B831.

Culebras, A. Cerebrovascular disease and sleep. *Curr Neurol Neurosci Rep* 2004; 4:164–69.

Dorant, E., et al. A prospective cohort study on the relationship between onion and leek consumption, garlic supplement use and the risk of colorectal carcinoma in the Netherlands. *Carcinogenesis* 1996, Mar; 17(3):477–84.

Eisenberg, M., et al. Correlations between family meals and psychosocial well-being among adolescents. *Arch Pediatrics and Adolescent Medicine* 2004; 158:792–96.

Engle-Friedman, M., et al. The effect of sleep loss on next day effort. *J Sleep Res* 2003: 12:113–24.

Etminan, M., et al. Intake of vitamin E, vitamin C, and carotenoids and the risk of Parkinson's disease: A meta-analysis. *Lancet Neurology* 2005, Jun; 4(6):362–65.

Fernandez, M.L. Soluble fiber and nondigestible carbohydrate effects on plasma lipids and cardiovascular risk. *Curr Opin Lipidol* 2001, Feb; 12(1):35–40.

Ferrara, M., et al. How much sleep do we need? *Sleep Medicine Reviews* 2001; 5 (2):155–79.

Feskanich, D., et al. Prospective study of fruit and vegetable consumption and risk of lung cancer among men and women. *J Natl Cancer Inst* 2000; 92:1812–23.

Franco, V., et al. Role of dietary vitamin K intake in

chronic oral anticoagulation: Prospective evidence from observational and randomized protocols. *Am J Med* 2004, May 15; 116(10):651–56.

Fukuda, T., et al. Antioxidative polyphenols from walnuts *(Juglans regia L.)*. *Phytochemistry* 2003, Aug; 63(7):795–801.

Fukushima, S., et al. Cancer prevention by organosulfur compounds from garlic and onion. *J Cell Biochem Suppl* 1997; 27:100–105.

Gad, C.M., et al. Protective effect of allium vegetables against both esophageal and stomach cancer: A simultaneous case-referent study of a high epidemic area in Jianjsu province, China. *Jpn J Cancer Res* 1999; 90:614.

Gil, M.I., et al. Antioxidant activity of pomegranate juice and its relationship with phenolic composition and processing. *J Agric Food Chem* 2000; 48:4581–89.

Gillman, M.W., et al. Family Dinner and Diet Quality Among Older Children and Adolescents. *Arch Fam Med* 2000; 9:235–40.

Gupta, N.K., et al. Is obesity associated with poor sleep quality in adolescents? *Am J Hum Biol* 2002; 14:762–68.

Haristoy, X., et al. Efficacy of sulforaphane in eradicating Helicobacter pylori in human gastric xenografts implanted in nude mice. *Antimicrob Agents Chemother* 2003, Dec; 47(12):3982–84.

Hu, J., et al. Diet and brain cancer in adults: A case control study in northeast China. *Int J Cancer* 1999; 81:20.

Huxley, R.R., and H.A.W. Neil. The relation between dietary flavonol intake and coronary heart disease mortality: A meta-analysis of prospective cohort studies. *Eur J Clin Nutr* 2003; 57:904–908.

Jackson, S.J.T., and K.W. Singletary. Sulforaphane inhibits human MCF-7 mammary cancer cell mitotic progression and tubulin polymerization. *Am J Clin Nutr* 2004, Sep; 134(9):2229–36.

Jiang, R., et al. Nut and peanut butter consumption and risk of type 2 diabetes in women. *JAMA* 2002, Nov 27; 288(20):2554–60.

Knekt, P., et al. Flavonoid intake and risk of chronic diseases. *Am J Clin Nutr* 2002; 76:560–68.

Lamberg, L. Promoting Adequate Sleep Finds a Place on the Public Health Agenda. *JAMA* 2004; 2415–17.

Laurin, D., et al. Vitamin E and C supplements and risk of dementia. *JAMA* 2002, Nov 13; 288(18):2266–68.

Ledger, D. Public Health and Insomnia: Economic Impact. *Sleep* 2000; 23:S69– S76.

Mennella, J., et al. Flavor Programming During Infancy. *Pediatrics* 2004, April; 113(4):840–45.

Michand, D.S., et al. Intake of specific carotenoids and risk of lung cancer in 2 prospective US cohorts. *Am J Clin Nutr* 2000; 72:990–97.

Morgan, J.M., et al. Effects of walnut consumption as part of a low-fat, low cholesterol diet on serum cardiovascular risk factors. *Int J Vitam Nutr Res* 2002, Oct; 72(5):341–47.

Nagle, C.M., et al. Dietary influences on survival after ovarian cancer. *Int J Cancer* 2003, Aug 20; 106(2):264–69.

North American Association for the Study of Obesity, Nov 14–18, 2004, Las Vegas.

Palozza, P., et al. Beta-carotene downregulates the steady-state and heregulin-alpha-induced cox-2 pathways in colon cancer cells. *J Nutr* 2005; 135:129–36.

Patel, S.R., et al. A Prospective Study of Sleep Duration and Mortality Risk in Women. *Sleep* 2004; 27(3):440–44.

Pelucchi, C., et al. Fibre intake and prostate cancer risk. *Int J Cancer* 2004, Mar 20; 109(2):278–80.

Peppard, P.F., et al. Longitudinal study of moderate weight change and sleep-disordered breathing. *JAMA* 2000; 284:3015–21.

Reiter, R.J., et al. Melatonin in Walnuts: Influence on

Levels of Melatonin and Total Antioxidant Capacity of Blood. *Nutrition: Intl J Applied and Basic Nutr Sciences* 2005; 21:920–24.

Ros, E., et al. A walnut diet improves endothelial function in hypercholesterolemic subjects: A randomized crossover trial. *Circulation* 2004, Apr 6; 109(13):1609–1614.

Sable-Amplis, R., et al. Further studies on the cholesterol-lowering effect of apple in humans: Biochemical mechanisms involved. *Nutr Res* 1983; 3:325–28.

Sadeh, A., et al. The Effects of Sleep Restriction and Extension on School-Age Children: What a Difference an Hour Makes. *Child Development* 2003; 74:444–55.

Schabath, M.D., et al. Dietary carotenoids and genetic instability modify bladder cancer risk. *J Nutr* 2004; 134:3362–69.

Seddon, J.M., et al. Progression of Age-Related Macular Degeneration. *Arch Ophthalmol* 2003; 121:1728–37.

Sesso, H., et al. Flavonoid intake and risk of cardiovascular disease in women. *Am J Clin Nutr* 2003; 77:1400–1408.

Shaheen, S., et al. Dietary antioxidants and asthma in adult-population based case-control study. *Am J Respir Crit Care Med* 2001; 16:1823–28.

Song, K., and J.A. Milner. The influence of heating on the anticancer properties of onions. *J Nutr* 2001, Mar; 131(3s):1054S–1057S.

Spiegel, K., et al. Leptin levels are dependent on sleep duration: Relationships with sympathovagal balance, carbohydrate regulation, cortisol, and thyrotropin. *J Clin Endrocrinol Metab* 2004, Nov; 89(11):5762–71.

Stevens, L.J., et al. Essential Fatty Acid Metabolism in Boys with Attention-Deficit Hyperactivity Disorder. *Am J Clin Nutr* 1995, Oct; 62(4):761–68.

Stranges, S., et al. Relationship of Alcohol Drinking Pattern to Risk of Hypertension: A Population-Based Study. *Hypertension* 2004; 44:813–19, doi:10.1161/01.HYP .0000146537.03103.f2.

Taira, K., et al. Sleep health and lifestyle of elderly people in Ogimi, a village of longevity. *Psychiatry Clin Neurosci* 2002; 56:243–44.

Tapsell, L.C., et al. Including Walnuts in a Low-Fat/ Modified-Fat Diet Improves HDL Cholesterol-to-Total Cholesterol Ratios in Patients with Type 2 Diabetes. *Diabetes Care* 2004, Dec; 27(12):2777–83.

Vallejo, F., et al. Phenolic compound contents in edible parts of broccoli inflorescences after domestic cooking. *J Sci Food and Agric* 2003, Oct; 83(14):1511–16.

Van Dongen, H.P., et al. The cumulative cost of additional wakefulness: Dose-response effects on neurobehavioral functions and sleep physiology from chronic sleep restriction and total sleep deprivation. *Sleep* 2003; 26:247–49.

Wagner, H., et al. Antiasthmatic effects of onions: Inhibition of 5-lipoxygenase and cyclooxygenase in vitro by thiosulfinates and "Cepaenes." *Prostaglandins Leukot Essent Fatty Acids* 1990, Jan; 39(1):59–62.

Webb, W.B., et al. Are we chronically sleep deprived? *Bull Psychon Soc* 1975; 6:47–48.

Wolfe, K., et al. Antioxidant activity of apple peels. *J Agric Food Chem* 2003; 5:609–14.

Wong, Maria M. Alcoholism: Clinical and Experimental Research, April 2004.

Yang, J., et al. Varietal Differences in Phenolic Content and Antioxidant and Antiproliferative Activities of Onions. *J Agric Food Chem* 2004; 52(22):6787–93.

Yuan, J.M., et al. Dietary cryptoxanthin and reduced risk of lung cancer: The Singapore Chinese Health Study. *Cancer Epidemiol Biomarkers Prev* 2003, Sep; 12(9): 890–98.

Zhang, S., et al. Dietary carotenoids and vitamins A, C, E

and risk of breast cancer. *J Natl Cancer Inst* 1999; 91:547.

Zhao, G., et al. Dietary and Linolenic Acid Reduces Inflammatory and Lipid Cardiovascular Risk Factors in Hypercholesteaclemic Men and Women. *J Nutr* 2004; 134:2991–97.

Steven Pratt, M.D., is a world-renowned authority on the role of nutrition and lifestyle in the prevention of disease and optimising health. He is a senior staff ophthalmologist at Scripps Memorial Hospital in La Jolla, California. He lives in Del Mar, California.

Kathy Matthews has co-authored several health and medical bestsellers, including *Medical Makeover* and *Natural Prescriptions*. She lives in Pelham, New York.

They are also the authors of *SuperFoods*, also published by Bantam Books.

Index

407

motor skills, sleep deprivation and, 296, 297, 298
music, as stress reducer, 231
mustard greens, 170, 357

napping, for older adults, 307, 309
naringenin, 80, 84
National Academy of Sciences, Institute of Medicine of, *see* Institute of Medicine
National Cancer Institute, 208, 343
National Institute on Aging, 49
National Sleep Foundation, 293, 305–6
National Strength and Conditioning Association, 51
natural killer cells, sleep deprivation and, 295, 297
Nedd, Kenford, 225
niacin, 340
    Alzheimer's and, 250
    sources of, 250, 339, 340, 341, 351
night sweats, exercise and, 43
nobiletin, 83
Nurses' Health Study, 111, 112, 246, 300, 302, 314, 321
nuts, 100, 101, 345–50, 351–3
    amounts and calories of, 350–1
    nutrients in, 345–50
    penne with broccoli and, 371–2
    top fibre choices in, 204

oats, oatmeal, 106–12, 113, 114–15
    cinnamon-apricot cookies, 132
    nutrients in, 106, 108, 109, 110
obesity:
    Alzheimer's and, 247
    childhood, 143, 158–60
    exercise and, 52–4
    food ad exposure and, 158–9
    hypertension and, 330, 332, 334–5
    leptin and, 85, 301
    metabolic syndrome and, 258
    prediabetes and, 97, 98–9, 100
    sleep deprivation and, 294, 295, 296, 297, 300–1, 303
    type II diabetes and, 52–3, 97, 98–100, 102–3, 149
    whole grains and, 112
oesophageal cancer, substances protective against, 82, 362
oestrogen, circulating, fibre and reduction of, 200, 357
oleic acid, 76, 235, 280
oligosaccharides, 191–2, 194
olive oil, extra virgin, 234, 275–82
omega-3 fatty acids, 102, 174, 260, 261–4, 265, 266, 267, 346

    animal sources of, 246–7, 260–7, 347–8
    deficiencies of, 261–2, 349
    plant sources of, 112, 113, 173, 175, 247, 324, 346
    replaced in diet by omega-6, 261–2
    supplements of, 266
omega-6 fatty acids, 261–2, 324
onions, 314, 360–4
    balsamic roasted, 364
    nutrients in, 360–2, 363
orange juice, 82, 88
oranges, 78–88
    French toast à l'orange, 88
    garlic glaze, cedar plank salmon with, 285–6
    -poppyseed dressing, 88–9
oregano, 343–4
oropharyngeal cancers, citrus and, 82
osteoarthritis, substances protective against, 84, 363
osteoporosis, 164–9
    exercise and, 37, 41, 42, 69, 136, 165, 166–7
    hip fractures and, 118, 165, 167
    prevention of, 166–9, 180, 206, 256
    stress and, 222–3
ovarian cancer, substances protective against, 172, 199–200, 357

pancreatic cancer, nutrients protective against, 121
Parkinson's disease, 350
pasta e fagioli, 129–30
Patty's pumpkin pudding, 325, 326
peanut butter, 100, 351, 352, 353
peanuts, 345, 351–2
pears, 313, 314–15, 316
pea shoots, 170
pecan-crusted lime turkey breast, 367–8
pedometers, 141
penne with broccoli and nuts, 371–2
peppers, orange, 174, 325
periodontal disease, 206, 243
personal change, process of, 26–31
Personal Peace, 26, 221–2, 223–34
    meditation in, *see* meditation
    relaxation response in, see relaxation response
    simple techniques for achieving of, 226–7, 230–4
    spirituality and, 229–30
    as stress antidote, 223
phenolics, 311, 312
phloretin xyloglucoside, 311
phloridzin, 311
phosphoros, 271

412

413

414

415